Endocrine Pathophysiology

■ **Catherine B. Niewoehner, M.D.** ■

Professor of Medicine
University of Minnesota School of Medicine
Staff Physician, Endocrinology and Metabolism
Veterans Affairs Medical Center
Minneapolis, Minnesota

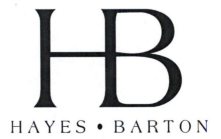

HAYES • BARTON

The authors and publishers have made every effort to ensure that the methods of treatment and drug recommendations are correct at the time of publication. However, new research and new therapies alter approaches constantly and usually there are several methods of diagnosis and treatment available for every condition. We have offered our best approach and advice. Nevertheless, we recommend consulting other sources (textbooks, Package inserts, *Physicians' Desk Reference*, and so on) before deciding on treatment.

Hayes Barton Press
a division of Vital Source Technologies, Inc.
Raleigh, North Carolina 27601-1300

08 07 06 05 04   2 3 4 5

Cover design by Linda de Jesus, Wing and Prayer Design, Springfield, Massachusetts, wingandprayerdesign@comcast.net

Composition by PerfecType, Nashville, Tennessee, and IC Corp., Portland, Oregon

Illustrations by Dave Carlson, Fort Collins, Colorado

Distributed by Ingram Book Group

ISBN (paper): 1-59377-174-6

Contents

Contributors

John P. Bantle, M.D., is a professor of medicine in the Division of Endocrinology and Diabetes of the University of Minnesota School of Medicine in Minneapolis.

Charles J. Billington M.D., is a professor of medicine at the University of Minnesota School of Medicine and director of the Special Diagnostic and Treatment Unit of the Veterans Affairs Medical Center in Minneapolis.

Nacide G. Ercan-Fang, M.D., is an assistant professor of medicine in the University of Minnesota School of Medicine and staff physician in Endocrinology and Metabolism at the Veterans Affairs Medical Center in Minneapolis.

Erica A. Eugster, M.D., is a clinical associate professor of pediatrics in the Department of Pediatrics of the Indiana University School of Medicine and at Riley Hospital for Children in Indianapolis.

Susan L. Freeman, M.D., is an assistant professor of medicine at the University of Minnesota School of Medicine in Minneapolis.

Angeliki Georgopoulos, M.D., is a professor of medicine at the University of Minnesota School of Medicine and medical director of the Women Veterans Program of the Veterans Affairs Medical Center in Minneapolis.

J. Michael Gonzales-Campoy, M.D., Ph.D., is a clinical assistant professor of medicine at the University of Minnesota School of Medicine in Minneapolis and medical director of the Minnesota Center for Obesity, Metabolism, and Endocrinology in St. Paul, Minnesota.

David M. Kendall, M.D., is a clinical assistant professor of medicine at the University of Minnesota School of Medicine and at Park Nicollet Clinic and International Diabetes Center in Minneapolis.

Virginia R. Lupo, M.D., is an assistant professor of obstetrics and gynecology at the University of Minnesota School of Medicine and director of Maternal-Fetal Medicine at Hennepin County Medical Center in Minneapolis.

Cary N. Mariash, M.D., is a professor of medicine, cell biology, and anatomy and director of the Division of Endocrinology and Diabetes at the University of Minnesota School of Medicine in Minneapolis.

Antoinette M. Moran, M.D., is an associate professor of pediatrics in the Department of Pediatrics at the University of Minnesota School of Medicine in Minneapolis.

Catherine B. Niewoehner, M.D., is a professor of medicine at the University of Minnesota School of Medicine and staff physician in the Department of Endocrinology and Metabolism at the Veterans Affairs Medical Center in Minneapolis.

Elizabeth R. Seaquist, M.D., is a professor of medicine in the Division of Endocrinology and Diabetes at the University of Minnesota School of Medicine in Minneapolis.

Joseph J. Sockalosky, M.D., is an assistant professor of pediatrics at the University of Minnesota School of Medicine in Minneapolis and director of Medical Education for Children's Health Care at St. Paul Children's Hospital in St. Paul, Minnesota.

Preface

While preparing the second edition of *Endocrine Pathophysiology*, we kept in mind three major principles of medical practice: (1) the human body and its disorders are complex and wonderful; (2) we must ask the right questions in order to get the right answers; and (3) if we do not understand the underlying pathophysiology, we will not know the right questions to ask.

Endocrinology is about the communication between tissues by chemical mediators called hormones. We begin with a brief review of general concepts of hormone and receptor interaction. Our discussion of specific areas of endocrinology begins with the pituitary gland, the "master gland," which, together with the hypothalamus, controls many target glands. This is followed by a discussion of other classic glands of the endocrine system: the thyroid and adrenal glands and their disorders; the parathyroid glands and regulation of calcium homeostasis; and normal and abnormal regulation of blood glucose by the endocrine pancreas. Chapters on lipid disorders and obesity emphasize control of fuel and energy metabolism. We conclude with the chapters on the complex hormone regulation of male and female reproduction, growth, sexual development, puberty, and pregnancy and lactation, which are affected by all the hormone systems described previously.

Since the first edition was written, we have gained new insight into the immensely complex reactions that allow hormone interactions with receptors to be translated into physiological responses. New fields of genomics and proteomics offer immense potential for exploring these interactions at a deeper level.

New studies have revealed the earlier onset, greater extent, and increased risk of metabolic disorders such as diabetes, the metabolic syndrome, obesity, hyperlipidemia, and vitamin D deficiency. New approaches to treatment based on increased understanding of the underlying physiology have major consequences for public health. New guidelines have been developed for management of blood glucose, cholesterol, and body weight.

Results of recent large, randomized, controlled trials have emphasized the need for evidence-based medicine and caused us to reexamine old assumptions. Changes in the use of estrogen and parathyroid hormone are particularly striking.

New synthetic hormones, hormone agonists, and hormone antagonists provide more approaches to treatment, but they also raise medical and ethical questions. Are the changes associated with aging "normal" or manifestations of "disease" in need of treatment? These questions are particularly relevant with regard to the reproductive system and bone health. Which short children should be treated with growth hormone? How should growth hormone be used in adults? New approaches for management of intersex disorders are being evaluated.

The field of endocrinology is expanding so rapidly that even endocrinologists become overwhelmed. We have concentrated on basic principles of endocrine pathophysiology and illustrated their significance with clinical problems. It seems more important to provide a framework that students can use to solve problems rather than to focus on details of treatment, because these change constantly.

We hope that you will find this material relevant and exciting.

Catherine B. Niewoehner
Spring 2004

Acknowledgments

The time and effort of the contributing authors is appreciated. We especially acknowledge the contribution of Frank Q. Nuttall, M.D., Ph.D. to the education of many of us. He is an outstanding scientist, clinician and mentor who has been a constant source of information during preparation of this manuscript. We are grateful to Nancy Gable Lucas for her assistance in preparing the manuscript for publication. They have done their best to protect us from errors; those that remain are our responsibility. Matt Harris at Fence Creek Publishing provided the original format for the book.

1

Endocrinology—General Concepts

Catherine B. Niewoehner, M.D.

■ CHAPTER OUTLINE ■

■ LEARNING OBJECTIVES ■

At the completion of this chapter, the student will:
1. recognize that endocrine glands produce hormones that exert effects in target tissues.
2. understand the role of cell membrane and nuclear receptors in determining the response to hormones.
3. be aware of the major hormone classes—peptide or glycoprotein hormones and steroid or steroid-type hormones—and how they differ.
4. recognize the interaction of the endocrine system and the nervous system.
5. understand that the endocrine system operates to maintain homeostasis, often by feedback loops.
6. recognize that gland and target tissue responses must be assessed together to determine whether hormone levels represent true excess or deficiency states.
7. understand the concept of hormone resistance.

Endocrinology Defined

The endocrine system and the nervous system are the two major systems by which cells and tissues communicate. Originally endocrinology was defined as the study of glands that produce chemical mediators called *hormones*. Hormones are secreted directly (not via ducts) into the circulation and exert their effects by binding to receptors in or on target cells. It is now clear that virtually every tissue can produce substances that act like hormones, and that hormones can act within the same cell (autocrine action) or on neighboring cells (paracrine action) or on distal cells (endocrine action). The boundaries of endocrinology are somewhat arbitrary, but include the following:

- Regulation of hormone synthesis and secretion
- Hormone-receptor interaction and how it results in specific biological effects
- Interaction between endocrine organs and target tissues, including normal feedback loops, perturbed feedback loops, and use of feedback loops to monitor endocrine therapy
- Symptoms and signs of hormone excess and deficiency
- Regulation of energy metabolism, reproduction, and growth

Hormone-Receptor Interactions

HORMONE-RECEPTOR COMPLEX

Hormone receptors are proteins that bind hormones with high affinity and specificity. Each receptor usually binds only one kind of hormone efficiently. Cells respond only to certain hormones because they have receptors only for certain hormones. Hormone binding alters receptor conformation. Each receptor has a domain that recognizes a specific hormone and a domain that generates a signal once the hormone is bound. Many hormone-receptor complexes (HR) must interact with another HR, forming homodimers (H_1R_1-H_1R_1) or heterodimers (H_1R_1-H_2R_2), to be active.

Response to hormones requires:
- normal receptor protein structure
- receptor availability
- intact receptor signaling
- normal post-receptor events

Receptors located in the cell membrane are usually present in excess of the amount needed for maximum biologic response. Since hormones are present in low concentrations in the circulation, the maximum biologic response of cell surface receptors is determined by the hormone concentration. Nuclear receptors are usually present only in low concentrations in the cell, and the number of receptors determines the extent of the biologic response.

Normal events at the postreceptor level are necessary for normal hormone action. Cells must also have a mechanism for release of bound hormone or destruction of the hormone-receptor complex to turn the action of a hormone off.

Major Classes of Hormones

Hormones are usually divided into two main classes: *the peptide* or *glycoprotein hormones* and the *steroid* and *steroid-type hormones* (Table 1-1). Steroid hormones are derived from cholesterol. The steroid-type hormones include thyroid hormones and 1,25-dihydroxyvitamin D. Although they are not true steroids in the structural sense, their mechanism of action places them in a class with steroid hormones.

PEPTIDE AND PROTEIN HORMONES

Peptide hormone synthesis follows the typical sequence for protein synthesis: gene activation, transcription of DNA, formation of messenger RNA, and translation of messenger RNA into protein. The initial large preprohormone enters the endoplasmic reticulum. A signal sequence is cleaved; the remaining prohormone or hormone undergoes

Table 1-1. Peptide vs. Steroid Hormones

PEPTIDE HORMONES		STEROID-TYPE HORMONES
Attach to receptors on cell surface	Luteinizing hormone (LH)	Enter cell cytoplasm and nucleus
Subsequent activation of second messengers	Growth hormone	Interact with receptors in cytoplasm and nucleus
Changes in cell phosphorylation state, calcium, etc.	Thyroid-stimulating hormone (TSH)	Hormone-receptor complex interacts with DNA
Changes in cell secretion and protein synthesis	Prolactin (somatomammotropin)	Changes in protein synthesis
Water soluble	**Posterior Pituitary Hormones**	Fat soluble
Catabolized in GI tract; poorly absorbed from skin	Antidiuretic hormone (ADH)	Absorbed from GI tract and skin
Short half-life	Oxytocin	Longer half-life if protein bound or stored in fat
Hypothalamic Hormones	**Pancreatic Islet Hormones**	**Adrenal and Gonadal Hormones**
Corticotropin-releasing hormone (CRH)	Glucagon	Aldosterone
	Insulin	Cortisol
Growth hormone–releasing hormone (GHRH)	Somatostatin	Dehydroepiandrosterone
	Calcium-Regulating Hormones	Dihydrotestosterone
Gonadotropic hormone–releasing hormone (GnRH)	Calcitonin	Estradiol
	Parathyroid hormone (PTH)	Progesterone
Thyrotropin-releasing hormone (TRH)	Parathyroid hormone–related protein (PTHrP)	Testosterone
Somatostatin	**Additional Peptide Hormones**	**Steroid-Type Hormones**
Anterior Pituitary Hormones	Epinephrine	Triiodothyronine (T_3)
Adrenocorticotropic hormone (ACTH)	Human chorionic gonadotropin (HCG)	Thyroxine (T_4)
Follicle-stimulating hormone (FSH)	Human chorionic somatomammotropin (HCS) (human placental lactogen[HPL])	1,25-Dihydroxyvitamin D (1,25[OH]$_2$ D)
	Inhibin	
	Insulin-like growth factor-1 (IGF-1)	

further modification, is packaged into vesicles, and is delivered to the Golgi apparatus. Peptide hormones can be stored *in* the gland in granules awaiting the appropriate stimulus for release. Sometimes peptide hormones are altered further while in the storage granules. For example, insulin is stored as a larger molecule, proinsulin, which is cleaved to insulin and another peptide at the time the insulin is released. Sugar molecules are added to some hormones to form glycoproteins. Hormones can also be modified by phosphorylation or acetylation. Major peptide hormones are listed in Table 1-1.

Once released into the circulation most peptide hormones travel unbound to other carrier proteins. The unbound proteins are subject to attack by proteases; therefore, they tend to have short half-lives. They cannot be given orally because they are hydrolyzed by acid in the stomach or peptidases in the intestine. Glycoprotein hormones are more stable, and usually last longer in the circulation.

Peptide hormones are water soluble and cannot cross cell membranes easily. They bind to receptors on the cell surface. Cell membrane receptors usually have an extracellular amino acid sequence that recognizes and binds the hormone, a transmembrane sequence that anchors the receptor in the membrane, and an intracellular sequence that initiates intracellular signaling. Coupling of peptide hormones (first messengers) to cell surface membrane receptors generates small, diffusible second messengers such as cyclic adenosine monophosphate (cAMP), diacylglycerol (DAG), or mobilized intracellular calcium, which activate protein kinases. The kinases produce a cascade of phosphorylated intermediates including regulatory proteins and DNA-binding proteins (transcription factors) that alter gene expression (Figs. 1-1 and 1-2).

For example, peptide hormone binding to one of the G-protein–coupled family of receptors activates a GTP-binding protein. This results in increased or decreased adenyl cyclase activity, which, in turn, increases or decreases cAMP formation. cAMP activates protein kinase A, initiating a series of phosphorylations mediated by other kinases. Alternatively, insulin binding to its receptor causes the receptor itself to become an active kinase, phosphorylating some of its own tyrosines. This initiates a very complex series of protein phosphorylations with many, many effects on the insulin target cell (see Fig. 1-2). Many changes that occur in response to peptide hormones can happen very quickly and can be very transient.

STEROID AND STEROID-TYPE HORMONES

Steroid and steroid-type hormones are lipid soluble and mostly are carried in the circulation attached to carrier proteins such as sex hormone-binding globulin, thyroid hormone-binding globulin, and cortisol-binding globulin. They can be given orally. Since they are fat soluble, they cross membranes and enter all cells. Only cells with receptors for the hormones can respond to them. Major steroid and steroid-type hormones are listed in Table 1-1.

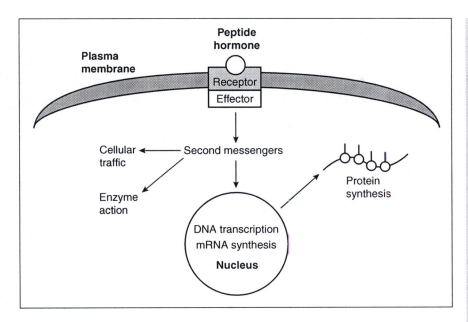

Fig. 1-1. Mechanism of Action of Peptide Hormones

Peptide hormones bind to receptors on the cell surface. Binding of hormones (first messengers) to their receptors changes the conformation of the receptors, which initiates reactions resulting in the formation of second messengers such as cyclic adenosine monophosphate (cAMP). Second messengers set off a reaction cascade, which results in changes in the phosphorylation state of cell components. This results in changes in cellular traffic, enzyme action, and protein synthesis.

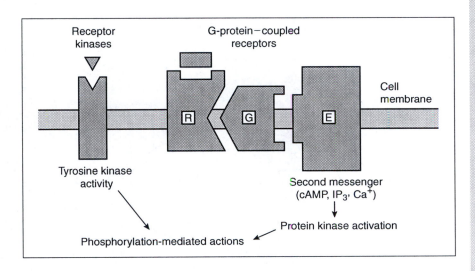

Fig. 1-2 Receptors for Peptide Hormones

Peptide hormone binding to its membrane receptor results in changes in receptor conformation, which are transmitted to the intracellular domain of the protein and initiate postreceptor events. The cell membrane receptors for hormones such as insulin and insulin-like growth factor-1 (represented by the triangle) have tyrosine kinase activity. Interaction of many peptide hormones (represented by the rectangle) with their membrane receptors (R) activates guanosine triphosphate-binding proteins (G). This results in increased concentrations of effectors (E), also called second messengers, such as cyclic adenosine monophosphate (cAMP), which activate protein kinases.

Steroid and steroid-type hormones bind to intracellular receptors, which can be in the cytoplasm or the nucleus. These intracellular receptors belong to the steroid hormone-receptor superfamily. They all have the same basic structure, which includes characteristic hormone-binding and DNA-binding domains. These domains allow the hormone-receptor complex to bind directly to DNA. Steroid and steroid-type hormone-receptor complexes bind as dimers. Binding alters interaction with transcription factors, which alters the rate of gene transcription. The binding site on the target gene is known as a hormone response element (Fig. 1-3).

Only a few hormone effects result from genes that bind hormone-receptor complexes directly (primary response genes). When this happens, changes in transcription can occur within 30 minutes. Most hormones act through secondary response genes. The hormone-receptor complex binds to primary response genes, initiating protein synthesis. The protein products then bind to the secondary response genes and initiate transcription. This process can take hours to days.

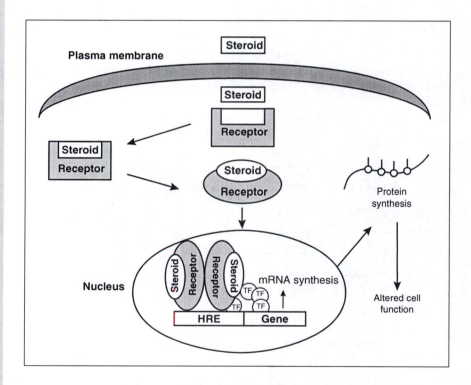

Fig. 1-3. Mechanism of Action of Steroid Hormones

Steroid hormones bind to intracellular receptors in the cytoplasm or nucleus. The receptor changes conformation once the hormone receptor complex has formed. The hormone-receptor complex (HR) enters the nucleus and binds directly to the DNA at the area of the gene known as the hormone response element (HRE). HRs bind to the HRE as either homodimers or heterodimers. Binding results in activation of transcription factors (TFs), altered gene transcription, protein synthesis, and altered cell function.

Hormone-receptor complexes can also exert their effects by increasing mRNA stability.

The steroid hormone-generated cascade of events can persist for days, even after the hormone-receptor complex releases from DNA. Steroid hormones are metabolized by the cytochrome P-450 system in the liver. The half-lives in plasma can be very long, especially for the synthetic preparations with added side chains, which slow hepatic metabolism.

The same hormone can affect different genes in different cells. Hormone action depends on the presence of other gene regulatory proteins (transcription factors), which can be specific to particular cells. Response to steroid and steroid-type hormones is abnormal if the receptor is defective or if there are mutations in the genes to which the hormone-receptor complexes bind.

Additional Considerations for Homeostasis

Hormones may have different actions at different times, depending on the presence of receptors and other modulators. The same hormone may produce some effects only in the fetus; different effects only during childhood, puberty, or pregnancy; and other effects in adults, which change with age.

The endocrine system interacts with the nervous system, the immune system, and other systems. This is particularly evident in the interaction between the hypothalamus and the pituitary gland. As a result of this interplay, peptide hormones are secreted in pulsatile fashion, and normal pulse amplitude and duration are important for normal hormone action. There are also diurnal rhythms of hormone secretion and rhythms that are tied to the sleep-awake cycle.

Major Moderators of Hormone Secretion/Action

- age
- pregnancy
- nervous system
- immune system
- sleep–wake cycle
- feedback loops

In general, the system operates to maintain homeostasis. Excess hormone down-regulates the number of receptors. Decreased receptor availability diminishes tissue response to the excess. Hormone depletion usually up-regulates receptors. Increased receptor availability increases the opportunity for tissue response.

Hormone secretion is also regulated by *feedback loops*. Hormones are secreted in response to a signal. The hormone acts on a target gland to produce a response. When this response has returned the initial signal to normal, hormone secretion decreases.

Hormone Excess, Hormone Deficiency, and Hormone Resistance

When control mechanisms fail, hormone excess and deficiency result in abnormal metabolism, growth, and reproduction. However, a high or low hormone level per se does not always represent the primary problem. A high hormone level can be an appropriate response to a persistent deficiency or represent an appropriate attempt by a gland to overcome hormone resistance (a problem at the receptor or postreceptor level in the target tissue). Some patients have polypeptide hormone receptors with abnormal GTP-binding proteins, which constantly initiate hormone action whether hormone is bound or not. Patients with these receptors appear as if they have hormone excess.

A low hormone level might indicate a true deficiency or be an appropriate response to an abnormally low stimulus from a higher center. Usually it is necessary to assess both gland and target organ response to find the true source of the problem.

Practical Clinical Considerations

Hormones are secreted in response to a specific signal (i.e., low calcium or low glucose), but some hormone is often secreted constitutively. New sensitive assays reveal that in deficiency states hormone levels may be low, but they are not zero.

Most hormones are synthesized as needed. However, since some peptide hormone is usually stored in secretory granules within a gland, the signal for secretion often elicits an initial burst of stored hormone into the circulation, followed by a decrease in secretion of the hormone until the peptide synthetic machinery can be geared up. Hormone stimulation or suppression tests are often needed to assess gland capacity for normal response.

Hormone replacement for deficiency states is becoming more and more sophisticated. Synthetic replacement hormones can be altered to prolong their half-lives in the circulation and increase their potency.

Genomics and Proteomics—Impact on Endocrinology

Hormones and hormone disorders were usually named at the time of discovery, often before the most important hormone action was known. This has become even more apparent with elucidation of the human genome (genomics) and sophisticated studies of the proteins expressed by gene translation (proteomics). New tools for analyzing large, complex databases (bioinformatics) and gene chips with probes that can identify tens of thousands of unique mRNAs in a sample are being used to examine changes in gene expression after hormone administration or deletion. Gene regulatory elements and transcription factors and receptor genes and proteins are undergoing the same level of scrutiny. The clinical impact of this research is just beginning to be felt.

REVIEW QUESTIONS

Directions: For each of the following questions choose the *one best* answer.

1 Several peptide hormone analogs are being considered for development. Based on hormone physiology, a hormone with prolonged action is most likely to be successful because

A it needs to be taken orally only once a day
B it is very tightly bound to its transport protein in plasma
C it inactivates its receptor guanosine triphosphate (GTP)-binding protein
D it is tightly bound to the hormone response element of DNA
E it elicits a prolonged second messenger response

2 A large family is remarkable because many members have reduced responses to all of their steroid hormones. The problem in this family is most likely to be

A increased binding of hormone-receptor complexes to DNA hormone response elements
B decreased steroid hormone catabolism by the hepatic cytochrome P-450 system
C more efficient production of transcription factors activating gene promoters
D inefficient production of steroid hormone plasma binding proteins

Directions: The group of questions below consists of lettered choices followed by several numbered items. For each numbered item, select the appropriate lettered option with which it is most closely associated. Each lettered option may be used once, more than once, or not at all.

Questions 3-5

Gland X produces hormone A, which stimulates target tissue Y to produce hormone B. For each clinical situation described below, select the expected hormone levels.

A High A, high B
B High A, low B
C Low A, high B
D Low A, low B

3 A patient has a congenital defect, causing gland X to function at a very low level.

4 A patient has a tumor, causing gland X to overproduce hormone A.

5 A patient is resistant to hormone A because of a receptor defect in target tissue Y.

References

Chandra PL, Hsu SY, Hsueh AJW: Hormonal genomics. *Endocr Rev* 23: 369–381, 2002.

Lazar MA: Mechanism of action of hormones that act on nuclear receptors. In *Williams Textbook of Endocrinology*, 10th ed. Edited by Larson PR, Kronenberg HM, Melmed S, Polonsky KS. Philadelphia, PA: W. B. Saunders 2003, pp 34–44.

Lefkowitz RJ. G proteins in medicine. *N Engl J Med* 332: 186–187, 1995.

Miller WL. Molecular biology of steroid hormone synthesis. *Endocr Rev* 9: 295–318, 1988.

Spiegel A, Carter-Su C, Taylor S: Mechanism of action of hormones that act at the cell surface. In: *Williams Textbook of Endocrinology*, 10th ed. Edited by Larson PR, Kronenberg HM, Melmed S, Polonsky KS. Philadelphia, PA: W. B. Saunders 2003, pp 45–64.

Stone DK: Receptors: structure and function. *Am J Med* 105: 244–250, 1998.

Thompson EB: Editorial: The impact of genomics and proteomics on endocrinology. *Endocr Rev* 23: 366–368, 2002.

2

The Anterior Pituitary

Susan L. Freeman, M.D.

■ CHAPTER OUTLINE ■

■ LEARNING OBJECTIVES ■

At the completion of this chapter, the student will be familiar with
1. basic pituitary anatomy.
2. the hormonal functions of the anterior pituitary gland.
3. the hypothalamic-pituitary-target organ axes and feedback mechanisms
   for their control.
4. the anatomic and hormonal effects of pituitary tumors.
5. disorders of pituitary failure.

CASE STUDY: *INTRODUCTION*

A 30-year-old man was referred to the endocrinology clinic for evaluation of impotence experienced over a period of 18 months. He also complained of fatigue, weakness, loss of libido, and intermittent headaches. There was no history of illness or trauma. His shoe size had increased two sizes over the last 3 years; he could no longer remove his wedding ring, which previously slipped off easily; and he was shaving every other day rather than daily, as he had in the past.

On physical examination, he was 6′2″ and weighed 260 lb. There was prominent frontal bossing (prominent supraorbital ridges) and a wide nose. There were no cranial nerve defects and extraocular eye motion was intact. Peripheral vision was diminished bilaterally to confrontation. His tongue appeared to be of normal size; however, there were spaces between the teeth and dental malocclusion consistent with mandibular enlargement. The hands were enlarged and of a spade-like configuration. The thyroid gland was of normal size and consistency. The lungs were clear bilaterally and the cardiovascular examination was unremarkable. The liver edge was palpable but the abdomen was otherwise unremarkable. The testes were small and soft.

Laboratory studies revealed an elevated serum prolactin level of 742 ng/mL (normal: 1–20). The growth hormone (GH) level was 7.5 ng/mL (normal in men: 0–5 ng/mL). The insulin-like growth factor-1 (IGF-1) level was elevated at 324 ng/mL (normal: 51–115 ng/mL). The serum testosterone level was low at 92 ng/dL (normal: 300–1200 ng/dL in men). Luteinizing hormone (LH) and follicle-stimulating hormone (FSH) levels were also low. The remaining laboratory tests, including serum cortisol, free thyroxine (FT$_4$), and thyroid-stimulating hormone (TSH) levels were all within normal limits. A fasting plasma glucose level was 110 mg/dL (normal: 70–110 mg/dL). An oral glucose tolerance test was ordered, but the patient failed to keep the appointment.

Introduction

The anterior pituitary gland is a central feature of the endocrine system. The word *pituitary* comes from the Greek *ptuo* (to spit) and the Latin *pituita* (mucus). It was thought that mucus produced by the brain was excreted through the nose by the pituitary gland. Today, of course, we know that the pituitary produces hormones, not mucus, and that its secretions are released into the bloodstream, not the nose. In fact, the pituitary is part of an elaborate hormonal system. It receives signals from the brain and hypothalamus and responds by sending pituitary hormones to target glands. The target glands produce hormones that provide negative feedback at the level of the hypothalamus and pituitary. It is the feedback mechanism that enables the pituitary to regulate the amount of hormone released into the bloodstream by the target glands. The pituitary's central role in this hormonal system and its ability to interpret and respond to a variety of signals has led to its designation as the "master gland."

ANATOMY

The pituitary gland is located at the base of the skull in a saddle-shaped cavity of the sphenoid bone called the sella turcica (Fig. 2-1).

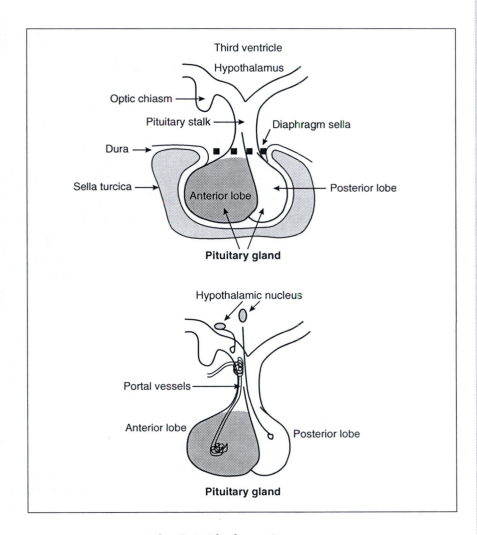

Fig. 2-1. Pituitary Anatomy

The pituitary gland, which is connected to the hypothalamus by the pituitary stalk, lies within the sella turcica below the diaphragm sella. Posterior pituitary hormones are synthesized in hypothalamic nuclei and transported through the pituitary stalk to nerve terminals in the posterior pituitary. Anterior pituitary hormones are made within the anterior pituitary in response to hypothalamic-releasing hormones. Hypothalamic-releasing hormones are made in hypothalamic neurons and secreted into the hypothalamic-hypophyseal portal vessels, which carry them to the anterior pituitary. Note the location of the optic chiasm above the anterior pituitary.

This bony structure protects and surrounds the pituitary bilaterally and inferiorly. The dura, a dense layer of connective tissue, forms the roof of the sella (the diaphragm sella). An external layer of the dura continues into the sella to form its lining. As a result, the pituitary is extradural and is not normally in contact with cerebral spinal fluid (CSF). The pituitary stalk (or infundibular stalk) passes through a foramen in the dura, resulting in the appearance of the pituitary as a cherry on a stem. The anterior pituitary gland is called the adenohypophysis; the posterior pituitary gland is also called the neurohypophysis. The anterior lobe of the pituitary comprises about 80% of the gland. It may double in size during pregnancy and shrinks in old age.

EMBRYOLOGY

The anterior pituitary is derived from Rathke's pouch, which is an ectodermal pouch of the primordial oral cavity. By 6 weeks, the connection between Rathke's pouch and the oropharynx is totally obliterated, and the pouch establishes a direct connection with the downward extension of the hypothalamus, which gives rise to the pituitary stalk. The lumen of Rathke's pouch in humans is eventually obliterated by the developing pituitary gland. (Remnants of Rathke's pouch can persist as small cysts, which can give rise to tumors called craniopharyngiomas.) Secretory granules are seen in the developing pituitary at the end of the first trimester of pregnancy, and hormones can be measured as early as the seventh week of gestation. However, functional maturation of the pituitary axes is not fully developed until well into postnatal life.

Two Tissues of the Pituitary Gland

Anterior pituitary (adenohypophysis) is derived from the primitive oral cavity.

Posterior pituitary (neurohypophysis) is an extension of the nervous system.

Several cell types in the pituitary gland depend on a nuclear transcription factor, pit-1, for normal development. A deletion or mutation of the gene for this protein is associated with failure of these cell types to develop.

VASCULAR SUPPLY

The arterial blood supply of the pituitary gland originates from the internal carotid arteries via the superior, middle, and inferior hypophyseal arteries (Figure 2-1). This network of vessels forms a unique portal circulation connecting the hypothalamus and the pituitary. The branches of the superior hypophyseal arteries penetrate the stalk and form a network of vessels. All of these vessels drain into a series of long portal vessels, which transverse the pituitary stalk and terminate in a network of capillaries within the anterior lobe. It is through this portal venous system that hypothalamic hormones are delivered to the anterior pituitary gland.

Anterior Pituitary Anatomy: Key Points

Well protected by bony sella

Highest blood flow of any tissue

Vascular (not physical) communication with hypothalamus

Hypothalamic hormones reach pituitary via portal venous system

---

CELL TYPES

The anterior pituitary is composed of a variety of cell types, which are responsible for synthesis, storage, and release of specific hormones. Most of these have been identified by immunohistochemical staining techniques using antisera for specific hormones and electron microscopy.

Anterior Pituitary Cell Types

Somatotrophs	50%
Lactotrophs	15%
Corticotrophs	15–20%
Gonadotrophs	10%
Thyrotrophs	5%

Somatotrophs produce growth hormone (GH). Lactotrophs produce prolactin (PRL). Corticotrophs produce adrenocorticotropic hormone (ACTH). Gonadotrophs produce luteinizing hormone (LH) and follicle-stimulating hormone (FSH), and thyrotrophs produce thyroid-stimulating hormone (TSH).

TSH, LH, and FSH are glycoprotein hormones comprised of an α-subunit noncovalently linked to a β-subunit. The α-subunit is the same for all three hormones. It is the β-subunit that confers specificity of action. GH and prolactin are composed of single chains of amino acids.

Anterior pituitary hormones are secreted in pulses. The pulsatile pattern of pituitary hormone release is essential for efficient and effective signaling of target tissues. Alterations in this pattern lead to target organ dysfunction.

Hypothalamic-Pituitary Regulation

Each pituitary hormone is regulated by one or more hormones synthesized and released by the hypothalamus. These hypothalamic hormones are transported into the pituitary via the hypothalamic-pituitary portal

Table 2-1. Hypothalamic-Pituitary-Target Organ Axes and Their Actions

HYPOTHALAMIC HORMONES	Growth hormone–releasing hormone and somatostatin (inhibitory)	Thyrotropin-releasing hormone	Corticotropin-releasing hormone	Gonadotropin releasing hormone	Dopamine (inhibitory)
PITUITARY CELL TYPE	Somatotroph	Thyrotroph	Corticotroph	Gonadotroph	Lactotroph
PITUITARY HORMONES	Growth hormone	Thyroid-stimulating hormone	Adrenocorticotropic hormone	Luteinizing hormone and follicle-stimulating hormone	Prolactin
TARGET ORGANS	Liver, cartilage, and other tissues	Thyroid gland	Adrenal cortex	Ovaries and testes	Breast
TARGET ORGAN HORMONES	Insulin-like growth factor-1	Thyroxine (T_4) and triiodo-thyronine (T_3)	Glucocorticoids (cortisol), miner-alocorticoids, and androgens	Estrogen, progesterone, and testosterone	
TARGET ORGAN HORMONES— MAJOR ACTIONS	Linear growth[a] and cell proliferation	Thermogenesis, growth[a], and CNS maturation[a]	Stress response and sodium retention	Sexual maturation, menstrual, cycle, gamete production, libido, and fertility	Milk produc-tion
PITUITARY HYPERFUNCTION	Acromegaly and gigantism[a]	Hyperthyroidism (rare)	Hypercortisolism (Cushing disease)		Galactorrhea, amenorrhea, infertility, and impotence
PITUITARY HYPOFUNCTION	Dwarfism[a]	Hypothyroidism	Adrenal insufficiency	Amenorrhea, infertility, decreased libido, and impotence	No lactation postpartum

Note. CNS = central nervous system.
[a] Seen only in children.

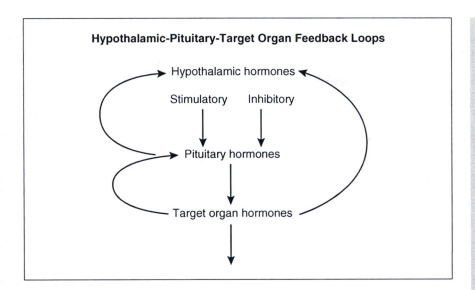

Hypothalamic-Pituitary-Target Organ Feedback Loops

Fig. 2-2. Feedback Loops

Hypothalamic hormones stimulate anterior pituitary hormone release. Anterior pituitary hormones in turn stimulate target gland hormone release. Target gland hormones provide feedback to both the hypothalamus and the anterior pituitary. Anterior pituitary hormones also provide some feedback to the hypothalamus.

circulation. The hormones produced by the different pituitary cell types and which hypothalamic hormones stimulate or inhibit their release are shown in Table 2-1.

The hypothalamic hormones bind to high-affinity cell membrane G-protein receptors on the appropriate pituitary cell types. The pituitary cells respond by secreting specific pituitary hormones that stimulate target glands. The target glands produce hormones that feed back to the hypothalamus and pituitary and regulate further release of pituitary hormones. This is called long-loop feedback (Fig. 2-2). Feedback can be positive or negative and involves both releasing factors and inhibitory factors. Short-loop feedback occurs when pituitary hormones feed back to the hypothalamus. If a target gland fails there is a reduction in negative feedback, which leads to increased secretion of the hypothalamic and pituitary hormones. The pituitary is truly the "master gland" because it integrates signals from the brain and target organs and modifies its own hormone secretion to maintain a normal endocrine state.

Hypothalamic-Pituitary Axes and Associated Anterior Pituitary Hormones

HYPOTHALAMIC-PITUITARY-THYROID AXIS AND TSH

TSH is stored in secretory granules and released into the circulation in response to thyrotropin-releasing hormone (TRH), which is produced by the hypothalamus (Fig. 2-3). When TRH is released, it interacts with a high-affinity membrane receptor on pituitary thyrotrophs and

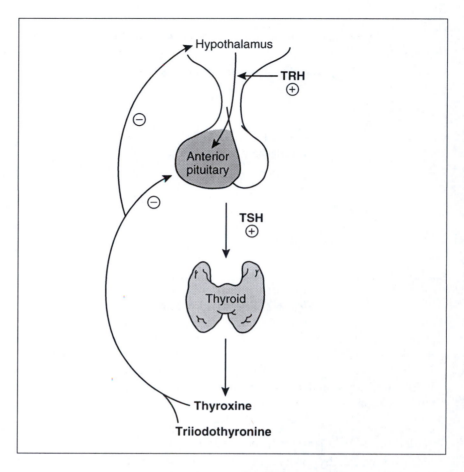

Fig. 2-3. Hypothalamic-Pituitary-Thyroid Axis

TRH = thyrotropin-releasing hormone; TSH = thyroid-stimulating hormone.

initiates a cascade of intracellular effects that leads to the synthesis and release of TSH. TRH has a direct effect on the transcription rates of both TSH α- and β-subunit genes. TRH also is necessary for glycosylation of the subunits. Glycosylation is necessary for appropriate folding to occur so that the tertiary structure of the peptides is stable.

After TSH is released into the bloodstream, it binds to specific thyroid cell membrane receptors. This activates adenylate cyclase, which increases intracellular cyclic adenosine monophosphate (cAMP) levels and activates protein kinase A. This results in phosphorylation of proteins that regulate the thyroid cells. These proteins increase the synthesis and release of thyroid hormones, thyroxine (T_4) and triiodothyronine (T_3). TSH also increases the size and vascularity of the thyroid gland.

Once T_4 and T_3 are released into the bloodstream they begin feedback inhibition of the production of TRH and TSH (see Fig. 2-3). Within the pituitary gland, T_3 binds to specific nuclear receptors to form an activated T_3-receptor complex. This complex binds to specific nucleotide sequences on the TSH subunit gene and inhibits transcription. T_3 suppresses TSH levels within hours. Thyroid hormones may also decrease TRH stimulation of TSH secretion.

If the thyroid gland fails, T_4 and T_3 levels decrease and TSH levels increase. If the thyroid is overactive, T_4 and T_3 levels increase and TSH levels fall. Although T_3 and T_4 are the main regulators of TSH, several other hormones interact with the hypothalamic-pituitary-thyroid axis. Dopamine and glucocorticoids inhibit TSH secretion. The hypothalamic hormone somatostatin inhibits both TRH and TSH secretion.

HYPOTHALAMIC-PITUITARY-ADRENAL AXIS AND ACTH

ACTH is a 39–amino acid peptide, which is synthesized in pituitary corticotrophs as part of a much larger precursor molecule called pro-opiomelanocortin (POMC). ACTH release is accompanied by release of other peptide components of POMC, including α-melanocyte–stimulating hormone (α-MSH) and corticotropin-like intermediate lobe peptide (CLIP), which are part of the ACTH molecule; and β-lipotropin, which contains the peptides β-melanocyte–stimulating hormone (β-MSH), γ-lipotropin (γ-LPH), and β-endorphin. The function of these other peptides is beyond the scope of this chapter. ACTH release is governed by the central nervous system (CNS) and hormonal mechanisms.

ACTH is secreted in a pulsatile manner, which is a reflection of its neural control. ACTH secretory bursts increase in frequency during sleep, resulting in a diurnal rhythm of hormone secretion. The highest levels of ACTH are present in the morning, about the time of normal awakening; levels gradually decrease through the day, reaching a trough around midnight. Reversal of the normal sleep-awake pattern results in a corresponding change in the diurnal pattern of ACTH secretion.

Corticotropin-releasing hormone (CRH) from the hypothalamus stimulates the production of ACTH. Psychological stress and physical stresses like trauma, surgery, hypoglycemia, and fever also increase ACTH production. Some of these responses are mediated through interleukin-1, -2, and -6. Stress also increases the production of ACTH through catecholamines, serotonin, acetylcholine (ACh), or angiotensin II, depending on the type of stress present. Even exercise increases ACTH and β-endorphin levels in proportion to the intensity of exercise and the level of training. The more intense the exercise, the higher the levels.

ACTH acts on the adrenal gland through specific cell membrane receptors located in the adrenal cortex. The actions of ACTH are mediated through an adenylate cyclase mechanism resulting in synthesis and secretion of glucocorticoids (cortisol), mineralocorticoids (aldosterone), and adrenal androgens. ACTH also stimulates protein synthesis, which can lead to adrenocortical hypertrophy and hyperplasia.

The cortisol that is produced by the adrenal cortex feeds back negatively to inhibit both CRH and ACTH secretion within seconds or minutes and ACTH production within days (Fig. 2-4). This is another example of a classic hypothalamic-pituitary-target gland feedback loop. If the adrenal glands fail, cortisol levels drop and ACTH levels rise.

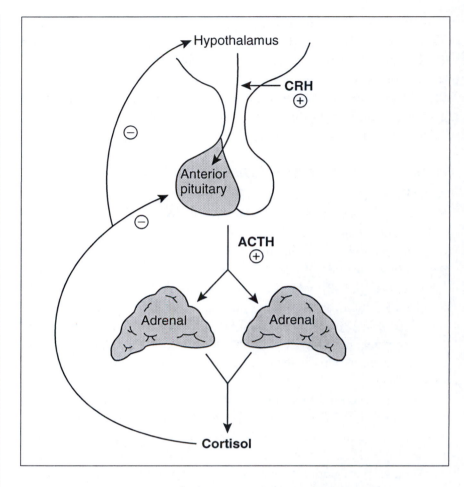

Fig. 2-4. Hypothalamic-Pituitary-Adrenal Axis

CRH = corticotropin-releasing hormone; ACTH = adrenocorticotropic hormone.

HYPOTHALAMIC-PITUITARY-GONADAL AXIS AND LH AND FSH

LH and FSH are the two anterior pituitary hormones that regulate gonadal function. Both hormones are released in response to the hypothalamic hormone gonadotropin-releasing hormone (GnRH). This hormone is also called luteinizing hormone–releasing hormone (LHRH).

There are several unique features of the hypothalamic-pituitary-gonadal axis. The first is that GnRH must be released in a pulsatile manner; the amplitude and frequency of the pulses determine the magnitude of the LH and FSH response. If GnRH is administered continuously, its receptors on pituitary cells are down-regulated, and LH and FSH release decrease.

Second, GnRH regulates the release of both LH and FSH, but the two hormones are secreted in different amounts at different times. There are variations in the sensitivity of LH and FSH to gonadal hormone feedback and also variations in sensitivity to the frequency and amplitude of GnRH pulses. If the GnRH pulse frequency increases, LH levels may rise more than FSH levels.

Third, LH and FSH have different functions in men and women. In men, LH binds to specific receptors on Leydig cells and stimulates production of testosterone, which is essential for spermatogenesis; development of secondary sexual characteristics and sexual function; and maintenance of bone, mineral, and protein metabolism. FSH is essential for the normal function of Sertoli cells and spermatogenesis. Testosterone exerts negative feedback at the level of the pituitary and the hypothalamus (Fig. 2-5). Gonadal failure results in increases in both LH and FSH.

In women, the hypothalamic-pituitary-gonadal axis regulates the complex events of the menstrual cycle. GnRH from the hypothalamus stimulates pituitary gonadotrophs to release LH and FSH (Fig. 2-6). FSH is critical for recruitment and maturation of a dominant ovarian follicle. As the follicle matures, the combined effects of LH and FSH stimulate the secretion of the ovarian hormone estradiol. This increase in estradiol actually inhibits FSH secretion and plasma FSH levels fall. On the other hand, LH pulse frequency increases. Positive feedback of estradiol on the production of LH is a unique feature of the female

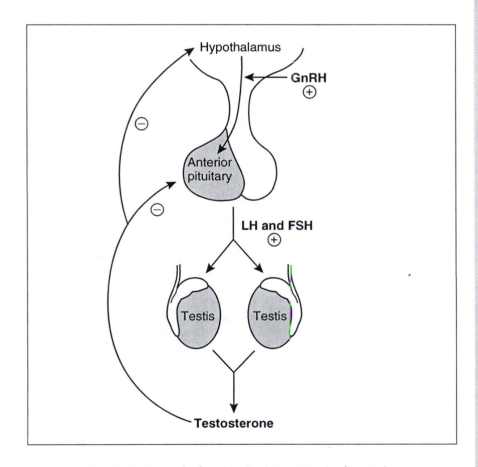

Fig. 2-5. Hypothalamic-Pituitary-Testicular Axis

In men, luteinizing hormone (LH) stimulates testosterone production from Leydig cells in the testes. Follicle-stimulating hormone (FSH) stimulates sperm formation in the seminiferous tubules. GnRH = gonadotropin-releasing hormone.

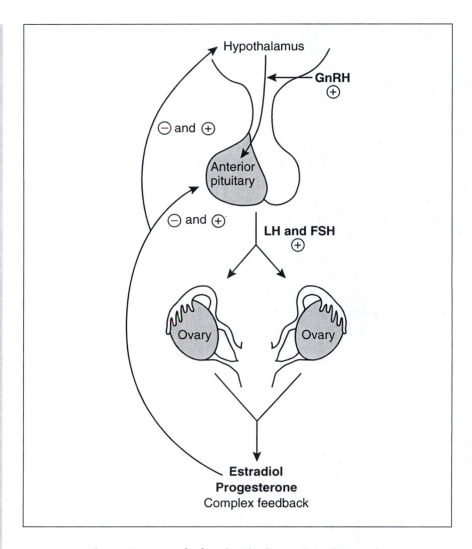

Fig. 2-6. Hypothalamic-Pituitary-Ovarian Axis

In women follicle-stimulating hormone (FSH) and luteinizing hormone (LH) regulate the events of the menstrual cycle. GnRH = gonadotropin-releasing hormone.

gonadotropin axis. The rise in LH triggers ovulation. After ovulation, LH stimulates production of progesterone and estrogen by the ovary. These hormones exert negative feedback, causing GnRH pulses and LH and FSH levels to fall. When LH and FSH levels fall, the GnRH pulse frequency rises again and the cycle repeats itself.

Menstrual cycles cease when there are no ovarian follicles left to produce estrogen and progesterone. This time is called menopause. FSH and LH levels are high after menopause because there is no negative feedback from the ovarian hormones.

Secretion and release of LH and FSH are also regulated by other peptides, including inhibin. Inhibin, synthesized by Sertoli cells in the testes and granulosa cells in the ovaries, exerts negative feedback on FSH secretion. Actions of inhibin are complex and are not well understood.

Unique Features of the Hypothalamic-Pituitary-Gonadal Axis

- Normal action requires pulsatile GnRH and LH and FSH secretion.
- GnRH regulates LH and FSH simultaneously but differently.
- The axis is different in men and women.
- In women ovarian hormones provide both negative and positive feedback.

Growth Hormone (GH)

Growth hormone is well named because its primary function is the promotion of normal linear growth. Growth hormone is a 191–amino acid single chain polypeptide, which is synthesized, stored, and secreted by the somatotroph cells in the pituitary. Growth hormone secretion is pulsatile and controlled by the action of two hypothalamic hormones, growth hormone–releasing hormone (GHRH), which stimulates GH release, and somatostatin, which inhibits GH release (Fig. 2-7). An increase of GH inhibits the action of GHRH and stimulates somatostatin. This is the short feedback loop.

The long feedback loop involves GH-induced production of insulin-like growth factor-1 (IGF-1). IGF-1 is produced and used locally by many tissues, but in the liver IGF-1 is regulated by action of GH on GH receptors. IGF-1 is secreted by the liver, exerts negative feedback on GH release, and stimulates somatostatin release. This creates the long feedback loop regulating GH production. Both GH and IGF-1 interact with different cell types to promote growth.

Physiologic factors also regulate GH secretion (Table 2-2). Sleep is associated with growth hormone peaks. Growth hormone is secreted in response to exercise and physical stress. Insulin-induced hypoglycemia stimulates GH release 30 to 45 minutes after the blood glucose level reaches its nadir. On the other hand, high blood sugar inhibits GH secretion. Low thyroid hormone levels are associated with low GH levels. Glucocorticoids (cortisol) inhibit somatic growth either by increasing somatostatin release or by causing damage to

Table 2-2. Major Regulators of Growth Hormone (GH)

INCREASE GH	DECREASE GH
GH-releasing hormone (GHRH)	Somatostatin
Sleep	Hyperglycemia
Exercise	Hypothyroidism
Trauma	Glucocorticoids (decrease GH action)
Acute illness	
Hypoglycemia	
Gonadal hormones (increase GH action)	

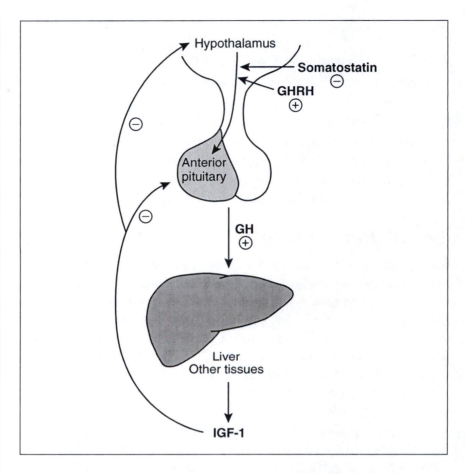

Fig. 2-7. Hypothalamic-Pituitary-Growth Axis

Both somatostatin and growth hormone-releasing hormone (GHRH) from the hypothalamus regulate growth hormone (GH) secretion. In response to GH, insulin-like growth factor-1 (IGF-1) is produced by the liver and released into the circulation. IGF-1 is also produced locally in many tissues.

pituitary somatotrophs. Gonadal hormones play a role in the neuroregulation of GH secretion at the time of puberty.

Growth hormone is secreted in adults even after linear growth stops. In addition to its growth action on bone and soft tissues, GH also affects protein, carbohydrate, and fat metabolism.

Effects of Growth Hormone

Increased	Decreased
Linear growth	Muscle glucose uptake
Bone thickness	
Soft tissue growth	
Nitrogen retention, amino acid uptake, and protein synthesis	
Fatty acid release from adipose tissue	
Insulin resistance and blood glucose	

Prolactin (PRL)

Prolactin is a 199–amino acid peptide made in the pituitary lactotrophs, which are also called mammotrophs. The regulation of prolactin secretion is unique among pituitary hormones, because PRL is secreted constitutively unless secretion is actively inhibited. Tonic inhibition of PRL is due to dopamine produced by neurons in the hypothalamus (Fig. 2-8). Dopamine action at lactotroph receptors inhibits adenylate cyclase; this inhibits both PRL synthesis and secretion. Dopamine agonists suppress PRL secretion.

> The regulation of PRL secretion is unique among pituitary hormones because dopamine from the hypothalamus is required to keep PRL secretion suppressed.

Because the hypothalamic action on PRL is inhibitory, disruption of the hypothalamus or the pituitary stalk can cause PRL levels to increase. Any dopamine antagonist increases PRL levels (e.g., phenothiazines, opiates, haloperidol). High levels of TRH in patients with hypothyroidism also increase PRL levels. When hypothyroidism is treated, PRL levels return to normal. Other pathologic processes that increase PRL secretion are listed in Table 2-3.

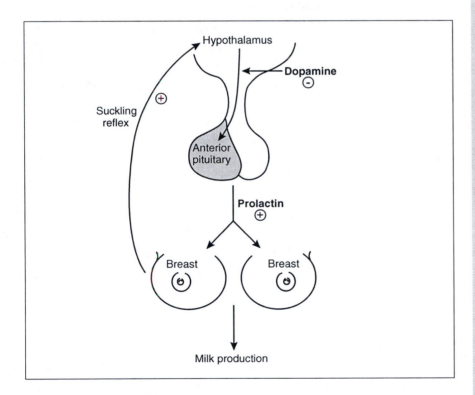

Fig. 2-8. Hypothalamic Regulation of Prolactin (PRL) Secretion

Hypothalamic dopamine inhibits pituitary PRL secretion. Suckling stimulates PRL synthesis via a neural reflex arc.

Table 2-3. Major Regulators of Prolactin (PRL) Secretion	
INCREASE PRL	**DECREASE PRL**
Pregnancy (estrogen effect), suckling, nipple stimulation, chest wall trauma, sleep, exercise, hypothyroidism (high TRH), pituitary stalk lesions, pituitary tumors, renal failure, dopamine antagonists	Dopamine and dopamine agonists

PRL production is stimulated by high estrogen levels during pregnancy and by suckling in the postpartum period. The suckling effect is mediated by neural arcs. Pituitary lactotroph hyperplasia occurs during pregnancy and lactation.

The primary physiologic actions of PRL are preparation of the breasts for lactation and stimulation of milk production postpartum. During pregnancy, PRL is one of many hormones stimulating development of the milk secretory apparatus. Lactation does not occur during pregnancy because of very high levels of estrogen and progesterone. After delivery, estrogen and progesterone levels drop, and high levels of PRL stimulated by suckling initiate lactation. Continued secretion of PRL is required if lactation is to be maintained.

CASE STUDY: CONTINUED

At his initial visit this patient had symptoms and signs of abnormal sexual function and abnormal growth of his hands, feet, nose, and jaw. The frontal bossing indicated enlargement of the frontal sinuses. His PRL level was high. GH and IGF-1 levels were also high, indicating a problem with GH regulation. His testosterone level was low. If his hypothalamic-pituitary-gonadal axis had been working normally, lack of negative feedback from testosterone should have stimulated the pituitary gland to produce high levels of FSH and LH. Since FSH and LH levels were actually low, the problem was clearly in the pituitary gland or hypothalamus, not in the testes. The combination of abnormal PRL, GH, LH, and FSH levels and his history of headaches strongly suggested a pituitary problem.

Six months after his first visit, the patient presented to his ophthalmologist for evaluation of vision problems. He had difficulty changing lanes when driving because of decreased peripheral vision. Formal visual field testing revealed a bitemporal hemianopsia. The ophthalmologist obtained a magnetic resonance imaging (MRI) scan of the head, which showed a 3.3 × 4.3 × 3.0 cm enhancing intrasellar mass. The mass extended superiorly and impinged on the optic chiasm. It also extended into the cavernous sinuses bilaterally and displaced both the carotid siphons laterally. There was some erosion of the floor of the sella. There were no calcifications or cystic areas in the mass.

PRL receptors have been found in other tissues. It is unclear what the physiologic action of PRL is at sites other than the breast. It is also not clear why men produce PRL.

Anatomic and Hormonal Effects of Pituitary Tumors

Pituitary tumors are seldom malignant and seldom metastasize. The problems they cause are related to (1) their space-occupying effects, (2) excessive hormone production, and (3) loss of function of the remaining gland.

Pituitary tumors that grow beyond the small confined area of the sella turcica can impinge on or expand into surrounding structures (Fig. 2-9) and produce significant signs and symptoms. A tumor that erodes the floor of the sella or extends into the sphenoid sinus may allow CSF to leak into the sphenoid sinus and into the nose, causing CSF rhinorrhea. Tumors extending laterally into either cavernous sinus can surround the carotid artery and produce unilateral defects in cranial nerves III, IV, $V_{1,2}$ (the ophthalmic and maxillary branches), and VI. The optic chiasm is located superiorly to the sella; in 80% of people it is directly over the gland, separated from the pituitary only by the thin fold of dura called the diaphragm sella. The hallmark of chiasmal compression by a tumor expanding upward is the visual field defect called bitemporal hemianopsia (loss of peripheral vision). The eyes

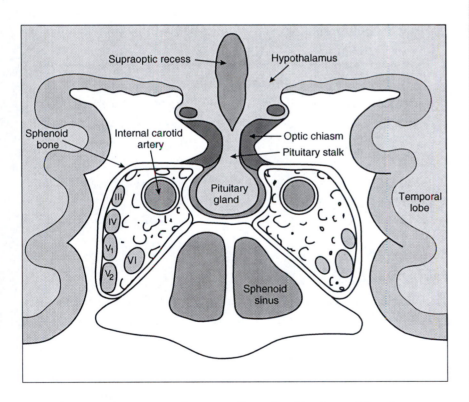

Fig. 2-9. Structures Surrounding the Pituitary Gland are Vulnerable to Expanding Pituitary tumors

may not be affected equally, and many other visual field defects, loss of visual acuity, and diplopia are also possible.

If a pituitary tumor is not producing a hormone, its space-occupying effects may be the first clues to its presence. A pituitary tumor should be considered in any patient who presents with headaches or visual changes. After the examination is complete, the presence of a pituitary tumor is best evaluated with an MRI scan. (MRI and computed tomography [CT] scans ordered for other reasons have resulted in the discovery of many pituitary tumors that might otherwise have gone undetected.) Tumors are loosely classified by size: a microadenoma is less than 10 mm in diameter; a macroadenoma is greater than 10 mm in diameter.

Hormone-secreting pituitary adenomas are thought to arise because of mutations occurring in the pituitary cells, not because of hypothalamic tumors that overproduce releasing hormones. Almost all secreting pituitary tumors are monoclonal. Approximately 90% of pituitary tumors secrete *one or more* of the anterior pituitary hormones.

Treatment of pituitary tumors involves reducing tumor size, usually by transsphenoidal surgery, or reducing tumor hormone secretion or action with a hormone antagonist or hormone receptor antagonist. A combination of treatments is often necessary. Radiation therapy can be used, but tumor destruction is very slow (may take years) and usually results in panhypopituitarism over time. Occasionally, it is necessary to remove the hormone target gland. Pituitary hormone deficiencies resulting from the tumor mass or treatment are addressed in Disorders of Pituitary Failure (below).

Pituitary Tumor	
Hormone Secretion	**Tumors Diagnosed (%)**
Prolactin	60%
GH	20%
ACTH	10%
TSH, LH, FSH	Rare
Nonfunctional	10%

PROLACTINOMAS

The classic signs of a prolactinoma in a premenopausal woman are galactorrhea (leakage of milk from the breasts) and amenorrhea or infertility. Amenorrhea occurs because hyperprolactinemia suppresses LH pulsatile secretion and perhaps GnRH pulses as well. When the gonadotropin levels are suppressed, estrogen production is lower and ovulation does not occur. The consequences are infertility and decreased libido and sexual function.

Men and postmenopausal women with prolactinomas frequently present because of symptoms created by the space-occupying effects of the tumor. Their tumors usually are larger than those in premenopausal women because premenopausal women with menstrual irregularities frequently seek medical attention sooner. Over 90% of men with prolactinomas have macroadenomas. Further evaluation often reveals impotence, loss of libido, and infertility.

The primary treatment for a prolactinoma is administration of a dopamine agonist, such as bromocriptine or cabergoline, which reduces tumor size as well as tumor secretion. Transsphenoidal surgery may also be used, but surgical cure for a prolactinoma is difficult to achieve.

GH-Producing Pituitary Adenomas

GH-producing tumors cause the syndrome called acromegaly. The prevalence of acromegaly is 5 to 6 cases per 100,000 population, so even though it is the second most common disorder of pituitary overproduction, it is still relatively rare.

Growth hormone hypersecretion is often associated with hypersecretion of other pituitary hormones, particularly prolactin.

Acromegaly derives its name from the so-called acral segments, which include the hands, feet, nose, chin, and forehead. Stimulation of growth of these bony and soft tissue segments is the hallmark of this disorder. Advanced acromegaly is characterized by spade-like hands, large feet, prognathism (prominent lower jaw), a large fleshy nose, and frontal bossing (Fig. 2-10). Progressive dental malocclusion occurs because of mandibular enlargement, and spaces form between the teeth. Often, a history of increasing hat, collar, shirt, glove, ring, and shoe sizes suggests the diagnosis. These changes occur insidiously over many years, so patients and family members often do not note them. In children GH-producing tumors cause accelerated linear growth resulting in gigantism. In adults the epiphyseal plates have already closed and further longitudinal growth is not possible. Additional symptoms and signs of acromegaly are listed in Table 2-4.

Growth hormone levels may fluctuate widely in an individual patient. This is not true of the IGF-1 level, which makes IRG-1 a more useful diagnostic measurement. Glucose-induced suppression of GH is the best test for diagnosing acromegaly. Plasma GH is measured before and 1 hour after administration of oral glucose (75–100 g). In healthy persons, GH is suppressed to less than 1 ng/mL after this glucose load.

Treatments for acromegalic patients include surgery, if the tumor is large, and a long-acting somatostatin analog such as octreotide to suppress GH secretion. The GH-receptor antagonist pegvisomant is also available. Dopamine agonists are less effective with acromegaly than with prolactinomas. These treatments reduce tumor secretion but not tumor size.

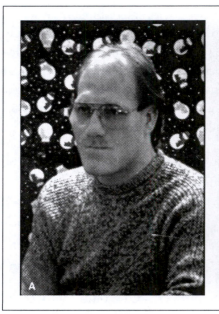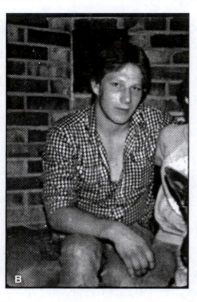

Fig. 2-10.

(A) A man with acromegaly. (B) The same man many years earlier. Note the coarsening of facial features, supraorbital prominence, and enlarged lower jaw in A compared to the normal facial features in B.

Radiation therapy can be used if all else fails, but GH suppression takes many years. A combination of treatments is usually necessary.

Patients with acromegaly have increased mortality as well as morbidity, especially due to cardiovascular disease. Mortality can be reduced to normal if IGF-1 levels and the GH response to a glucose load can be reduced to the normal range.

ACTH-Producing Pituitary Tumors

Excess ACTH production by a pituitary tumor causes the adrenal gland to secrete excess glucocorticoids and androgens. The resulting syndrome is called Cushing disease. Microadenomas account for 80% to 90% of these tumors. The clinical manifestations of Cushing disease reflect the biological effects of adrenal corticosteroids (see Chapter 5). These include central obesity, hypertension, purple abdominal striae, hirsutism, a round and plethoric face, easy bruising, glucose intolerance or diabetes, acne, and superficial fungal infections. Menstrual disorders, impotence, proximal muscle weakness, and back pain are also part of this disorder. Depression and other psychiatric disorders can also be associated with Cushing disease.

Cushing disease occurs more frequently in women than in men (female-to-male ratio 8:1). The symptoms are frequently insidious in onset. The diagnosis is established by determination of serum or urine cortisol levels and lack of suppression of cortisol levels with dexamethasone (see Chapter 5). Treatment for this disorder usually involves transsphenoidal surgery.

Table 2-4. Symptoms and Signs of Acromegaly

SKELETON

Enlarged sinuses and prominent supraorbital ridges (frontal bossing)
Enlarged lower jaw (prognathism) and widely spaced teeth
Thickened bones (including the calvarium)
Large hands and feet

CONNECTIVE TISSUE

Thickened synovium, resulting in painful joints
Large tongue and thickened tracheal cartilage, resulting in sleep apnea
Thickened vocal cords, resulting in a deeper voice
Thickened ligaments, resulting in carpal tunnel syndrome
Increased cartilage
Thick palms and soles

MUSCLES

Enlarged muscles with fiber atrophy, resulting in nerve entrapment, weakness, and fatigue

VISCERA

Enlarged brain, lungs, liver, and kidneys
Increased heart size and hypertension resulting in left ventricular hypertrophy, arrhythmias, cardiomyopathy, and congestive heart failure

SKIN

Thickened with enlarged sweat glands and excess sebum production
Increased number of skin tags

METABOLISM

Increased glucose production and insulin resistance, resulting in impaired glucose tolerance
Increased lipolysis
Increased DNA, RNA, and protein synthesis
Increased tubular resorption of phosphorous and increased urine calcium
Increased salt and water retention

OTHER HORMONE-SECRETING PITUITARY TUMORS

Pituitary tumors that secrete excess TSH are rare. They cause the classic symptoms of hyperthyroidism (see Chapter 4). Plasma levels of TSH and thyroid hormones are high. Treatment involves removing the thyroid gland or the pituitary tumor.

Gonadotropin-producing tumors are not unusual but were not recognized until recently because they secrete inefficiently and their secretion products do not produce a recognizable syndrome. Gonadotropin tumors secrete intact gonadotropins and their subunits. The α-subunit, which is common to both LH and FSH, is frequently synthesized in excess of the β-subunit, so the synthesis of the β-subunit becomes the rate-limiting factor in the formation of intact hormones. As a result, gonadotropin adenomas are recognized only if they become large enough to produce symptoms related to the space-occupying effect of the tumor.

DISORDERS OF PITUITARY FAILURE

Failure of the pituitary gland is called hypopituitarism. Failure of individual cell types causes isolated hormonal deficiencies. Failure of the entire gland is called panhypopituitarism.

Pathophysiology of Hypopituitarism
Primary pituitary disorder—loss of hormone secreting cells
Hypothalamic disorder—loss of releasing hormones
Extrinsic destruction of the hypothalamus, stalk, or pituitary gland

Table 2-5. Major Causes of Pituitary Insufficiency

Invasion	Pituitary tumor, hypothalamic, or central nervous system tumor, or craniopharyngioma
Injury	Head trauma
Infarction	Postpartum necrosis and pituitary apoplexy
Infiltration	Sarcoid and hemochromatosis
Infection	Tuberculosis
Iatrogenic	Pituitary surgery or radiation
Immune	Autoimmune hypophysitis
Idiopathic	Unknown

Specific disorders causing hypopituitarism are listed in Table 2-5. Pituitary tumors are the most common cause of hypopituitarism in adults. Impingement or compression of the anterior pituitary gland or the stalk by a large pituitary tumor can result in decreased functioning of the entire pituitary. Accidental head trauma is the leading cause of hypopituitarism seen at trauma centers.

If hypopituitarism is due to damage to the hypothalamus, all pituitary hormones may be deficient except PRL, which normally is inhibited by dopamine from the hypothalamus.

Postpartum pituitary necrosis, known as Sheehan syndrome, occurs in women who experience massive blood loss, hypovolemic shock, or both during delivery. The pituitary gland enlarges during pregnancy, and hypotension or hemorrhage creates vasospasm in the hypophyseal vessels and ischemia. A hemorrhage that occurs in a preexisting pituitary adenoma is called pituitary apoplexy. Rapid expansion of the hemorrhage causes severe headache, visual field defects, and acute hypopituitarism. This situation requires immediate surgery for decompression of the pituitary fossa.

The empty sella syndrome can also be associated with hypopituitarism. An empty sella really is not empty. The pituitary gland is flattened against the wall of the sella due to penetration or herniation of the subarachnoid space and CSF into the sella turcica. Primary empty sella syndrome due to an incompetent diaphragm sella occurs predominantly in obese, multiparous, middle-aged women who are often hypertensive. One-third of these patients demonstrate some endocrine disturbance. Secondary empty sella syndrome occurs in patients who have undergone pituitary surgery or radiotherapy for pituitary tumors.

Patients with pituitary failure are usually pale with fine skin and fine facial wrinkles. Symptoms and signs are due to failure of the target organs to produce their hormones. A precipitous drop in ACTH causes a decrease in glucocorticoids, which can lead to hypotension and cardiovascular collapse. Because this is life threatening, glucocorticoids are administered if this diagnosis is suspected, even before diagnostic testing is complete. Usually ACTH deficiency occurs gradually, causing chronic symptoms of glucocorticoid deficiency: weakness, lethargy, fatigue, nausea, arthralgias, myalgias, and vomiting (see Chapter 5). Chronic or partial ACTH deficiency may be exacerbated by an acute illness.

Hypopituitarism can also include TSH deficiency, which results in symptoms of hypothyroidism. These include fatigue, cold intolerance, constipation, dry skin, slow heart rate, and delayed drug metabolism. There is no goiter in the absence of TSH stimulation of the thyroid gland (see Chapter 4).

Deficiency of LH and FSH produces symptoms consistent with hypogonadism. Women develop amenorrhea and infertility. Men develop impotence and infertility. Both men and women experience loss of secondary sex characteristics and loss of libido (see Chapters 11 and 12). GH deficiency in children results in linear growth failure. The significance of the onset of growth hormone deficiency in adulthood is uncertain. Deficiency of PRL does not generally produce symptoms in adults except for the absence of lactation in the postpartum period.

Laboratory evaluation includes measurement of pituitary and target hormones. Both should be low. Hypothalamic hormone concentrations in the peripheral circulation are too low to measure. Further evaluation (imaging, dynamic testing) depends on the suspected cause of pituitary failure.

Laboratory Evaluation of Pituitary Insufficiency
Blood hormone levels
Hypothalamic hormones—too low to measure
Pituitary hormones—low and low-normal ranges overlap
Pituitary and target-gland hormones—measure together; both are low in hypopituitarism

---

Treatment of pituitary insufficiency usually involves replacement of target gland hormones rather than pituitary hormones, because pituitary hormones must be given in pulses, they have very short half-lives, and they are destroyed in the gastrointestinal tract. Thyroid hormone (T_4) and cortisol are used to treat TSH and ACTH deficiencies, respectively. Testosterone can be given to men with LH and FSH deficiencies. Premenopausal women are treated with estrogen and progesterone; postmenopausal women may choose not to take hormone replacement therapy (see Chapter 12). However, if fertility is desired, men and women must be treated with gonadotropins.

Children with GH deficiency must be treated with GH replacement (see Chapters 12 and 13). There is controversy about how long GH treatment should continue once GH-deficient children reach adulthood and whether patients who develop GH deficiency as adults

---

CASE STUDY: *RESOLUTION*

This patient had an enlarging pituitary adenoma producing PRL and GH. The space-occupying effects of his tumor caused his headaches, and extension of his tumor to the optic chiasm caused his bitemporal hemianopsia. The elevated GH levels resulted in typical symptoms and signs of acromegaly. Acromegaly was confirmed by a glucose suppression test. His GH level did not fall below 1 ng/mL in response to the glucose load.

His high PRL level suppressed LH pulses, which resulted in decreased testosterone production. In turn, his low testosterone levels resulted in decreased face and body hair, decreased libido, and impotence. Destruction of FSH- and LH-producing cells by the tumor may also have contributed to his low testosterone level.

Although this patient's tumor was large, it did not compress and destroy the anterior pituitary completely. Enough TSH and ACTH were being secreted to prevent hypothyroidism and adrenal insufficiency.

The patient underwent transphenoidal surgery to remove the tumor. The bitemporal hemianopsia resolved immediately. Postoperatively the PRL level remained elevated, and he was placed on a dopamine agonist, which he continues to take. His GH and IGF-1 levels have returned to normal. He needs follow-up PRL and IGF-1 levels and glucose suppression tests to be sure that the tumor is adequately resected. These tumors often recur over time, since it is difficult to remove them completely. He might require additional therapy, such as treatment with a long-acting somatostatin analog or a growth-hormone receptor antagonist in the future.

---

should be given GH replacement. Adults treated with GH have increases in lean body mass and bone mass and decreases in cholesterol and visceral fat mass. However, the magnitude of these changes is small, and other effective, less expensive treatments are available. The long-term safety of GH replacement and the effects on quality of life and morbidity and mortality are still uncertain.

Hypopituitarism is treated by replacing target organ hormones, not pituitary hormones. Pituitary hormones must be given in pulsatile fashion. They have very short half-lives, and they cannot be given orally because they are destroyed in the gastrointestinal tract.

REVIEW QUESTIONS

Directions: For each of the following questions, choose the *one best* answer.

1 A 65-year-old woman is brought to the hospital 1 week after an automobile accident. During the 2 months before the accident, she complained of headaches. She had a psychiatric disorder for which she was taking a phenothiazine. Physical examination revealed no signs of acromegaly or adrenal hormone excess or insufficiency, but she did have signs of a thyroid disorder. A magnetic resonance imaging (MRI) scan of the head and thyroid hormone, thyroid-stimulating hormone (TSH), luteinizing hormone (LH), follicle-stimulating hormone (FSH), and prolactin (PRL) levels were ordered. A high PRL level in this patient could be due to

A damage to the pituitary stalk during the accident
B stimulation of dopamine secretion by the phenothiazine
C a hypothalamic tumor producing gonadotropin-releasing hormone (GnRH)
D a pituitary tumor producing TSH

2 A 60-year-old woman complains of cold intolerance, fatigue, constipation, and dry skin. Her physician suspects hypothyroidism and wonders whether it is due to a thyroid problem or a pituitary problem. If her laboratory tests show that she has hypothyroidism due to an abnormal thyroid gland, and her pituitary gland is functioning normally, which set of laboratory test results would she be most likely to have?

A Low TSH, low thyroid hormones, and high FSH and LH
B High TSH, low thyroid hormones, and high FSH and LH
C Low TSH, low thyroid hormones, and low FSH and LH
D High TSH, low thyroid hormones, and low FSH and LH

3 A 45-year-old man is referred to his physician by his dentist because of increasing malocclusion of his teeth and an enlarging lower jaw. He has been asked to bring old photographs with him. His features are coarser than in the past, and he has oily skin, prominent supraorbital ridges, a large tongue, and very thick hands and feet. His growth hormone (GH) level is 7 ng/mL after a glucose load. He is most likely to have

A decreased lipolysis
B decreased protein synthesis
C decreased insulin action
D decreased insulin-like growth factor 1 (IGF-1) levels
E decreased gluconeogenesis

4 A 35-year-old man is undergoing an evaluation for impotence and infertility. His testicles are soft and he has less body hair than he had in the past. He complains of fatigue. Testosterone, luteinizing hormone (LH), and follicle-stimulating hormone (FSH) levels are low. An MRI scan reveals a probable craniopharyngioma (tumor arising from primitive remnants of Rathke's pouch), which is quite large. If this tumor expands further, this patient is at risk for

A impaired vision due to impingement on the optic chiasm
B bilateral defects in cranial nerves IX, X, and XII
C headaches due to shrinkage of the dura
D excess cortisol production due to Cushing disease
E low prolactin (PRL) level due to damage to the pituitary stalk

5 A 10-year-old child had radiation to the pituitary during treatment for a brain tumor 6 years ago. If radiation damage has caused loss of pituitary function, this child is most likely to experience which of the following?

A Increased cortisol production in response to stress
B Accelerated sexual maturation during puberty
C Absence of the normal growth spurt during puberty
D Development of hypothyroidism and a goiter (enlarged thyroid)

References

American Association of Clinical Endocrinologists medical guidelines for clinical practice for growth hormone use in adults and children—2003 update. *Endocr Prac* 9: 65–76, 2003.

Ben-Jonathan N, Hnasko R: Dopamine as a prolactin (PRL) inhibitor. *Endocr Rev* 22: 724–763, 2001.

Casanueva, F. Physiology of growth hormone secretion and action. *Endocrinol Metab Clin* 21: 483–517, 1992.

Cheung CC, et al: The spectrum and significance of primary hypophysitis. *J Clin Endocrinol Metab* 86: 1048, 2001.

Lamberts SWJ, de Herder WW, van der Lely AJ: Pituitary insufficiency. *Lancet* 352: 127–134, 1998.

Melmed S: Mechanisms for pituitary tumorigenesis: the plastic pituitary. *J Clin Invest* 112: 1603–1618, 2003.

Melmed S, Jackson I, Kleinberg D, Klibanski A. Current treatment guidelines for acromegaly. *J Clin Endocrinol Metab* 83: 2646–2652, 1998.

Molitch ME: Disorders of prolactin secretion. *Endocrinol Metab Clin North Am* 30: 585–610, 2001.

Tomlinson J, Holden N, Hills R, et al: Association between premature mortality and hypopituitarism. *Lancet* 357: 425–431, 2001.

Trainer PJ, Drake WM, Katznelson L, et al: Treatment of acromegaly with the growth hormone-receptor antagonist pegvisomant. *N Engl J Med* 342: 1171–1177, 2000.

3

The Posterior Pituitary, Antidiuretic Hormone, and Oxytocin

David M. Kendall, M.D.

■ CHAPTER OUTLINE ■

■ LEARNING OBJECTIVES ■

At the completion of this chapter, the student should be able to
1. describe the hypothalamic-posterior pituitary axis.
2. understand the action and regulation of the hormones secreted by the posterior pituitary.
3. describe the role of antidiuretic hormone (ADH), vascular volume, and thirst in the regulation of total body water balance.
4. identify the major hypertonic and hypotonic disorders.

CASE STUDY: *INTRODUCTION*

A 36-year-old woman with mild mental retardation and a 5-year history of bipolar affective disorder was hospitalized on the inpatient psychiatry service. She had been similarly admitted many times for agitated depression, hallucinations, and mania. The combination of psychotropic medications prescribed to her had failed to improve her condition in the past, and she was no longer taking them. Admission examination revealed a blood pressure of 110/68 mm Hg; heart rate, 84 beats/min; and temperature, 99.6°F. The neurologic examination was significant for intermittent tremor. She was minimally interactive with paranoid behavior.

During the first three days of hospitalization, she was described as "not eating well, but drinking plenty of fluid." Serum sodium (Na^+) at that time measured 140 mEq/L (normal: 135–147 mEq/dL); potassium (K^+), 3.7 mEq/L (normal: 3.5–5.0 mEq/L); blood urea nitrogen (BUN), 6 mg/dL (normal: 10–20 mg/dL); and creatinine, 0.8 mg/dL (normal: 0.8–1.4 mg/dL).

On the sixth hospital day, she was still drinking large amounts of water. Nursing notes described "large amounts of clear urine voided." Because of her ongoing paranoid behavior, she was transferred to a closed psychiatric unit where free access to fluids was not allowed.

On the ninth hospital day, the endocrinology service was asked to evaluate her excessive urination and thirst. Laboratory tests at that time revealed the following: serum Na^+, 155 mEq/L; K^+, 4.0 mEq/L; chloride (Cl^-), 115 mEq/L (normal: 95–105 mEq/L); bicarbonate (HCO_3^-), 25 mEq/L (normal: 22–28 mEq/L); BUN, 12 mg/dL; and creatinine, 0.8 mg/dL. Serum osmolality measured 312 mOsm/L (normal: 280–300 mOsm/L). Urine specific gravity was 1.005 units with urine osmolality of 156 mOsm/L (both at the low end of normal range). She had no glucose in her urine.

Introduction

The posterior pituitary gland is an extension of hypothalamic neurons, whose terminals lie closely opposed to the anterior pituitary gland. The major hormones secreted by the posterior pituitary—antidiuretic hormone (ADH) and oxytocin—are synthesized in specific hypothalamic nuclei (Fig. 3-1). ADH plays a central role in the maintenance of water balance by inhibiting diuresis. In pharmacologic amounts ADH raises vascular tone (blood pressure), so it is also known as arginine vasopressin (AVP). The term *ADH* is used in this chapter.

Antidiuretic hormone is a 9–amino acid peptide synthesized in neurons of the hypothalamus. Its release is regulated by plasma osmolality and vascular volume.

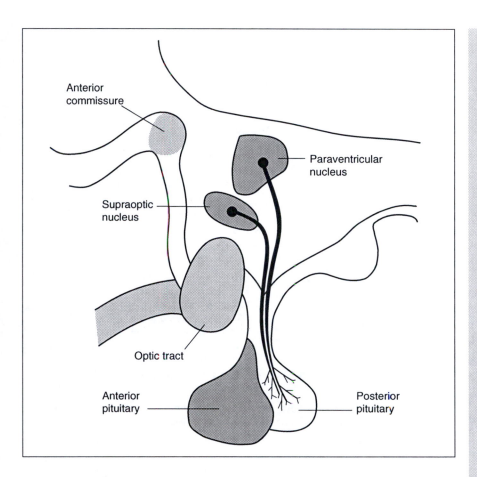

Fig. 3-1. Schematic Representation of the Hypothalamic-Posterior Pituitary Axis and Related Anatomic Structures

Neuronal cell bodies within the paraventricular and supraoptic nuclei synthesize antidiuretic hormone (ADH) and oxytocin. These hormones are stored in the neuron terminals of the posterior pituitary gland.

ADH is synthesized in the supraoptic and periventricular nuclei of the hypothalamus and then transported along neuronal projections of these nuclei into the posterior pituitary gland. It is stored in the nerve terminals of the posterior pituitary until it is released in response to changes in plasma osmolality and intravascular volume. Separate cells within these same hypothalamic nuclei are thought to synthesize oxytocin, which is also transported to nerve terminals in the posterior pituitary for storage.

Maintaining Water Balance

Water balance in humans depends on the complex interaction between water loss and water repletion. Total body water is maintained within a narrow range (defined by serum osmolality) through the balance of water ingestion and water loss in urine, feces, sweat, and water vapor. The water repletion reaction that maintains this balance is shown in Fig. 3-2.

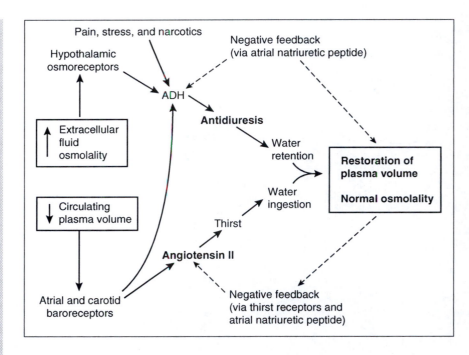

Fig. 3-2. Water Repletion

The complex interaction between vascular volume and plasma osmolality is depicted. Note that antidiuretic hormone (ADH) release is dependent on both plasma volume and plasma solute. Negative feedback suppressing ADH release is provided by atrial natriuretic peptide.

Water acquisition and water conservation are stimulated simultaneously by an increase in serum osmolality or by a decline in vascular volume. An increase in serum osmolality is sensed within osmoreceptors located in the hypothalamus just anterior to the third ventricle and near the paraventricular nuclei, which produce ADH. This results in release of ADH, which increases water retention by the kidneys (antidiuresis). An increase in serum osmolality also increases thirst, which is regulated in an unknown fashion via release of angiotensin II. Changes in vascular volume are recognized by carotid and atrial baroreceptors. Stimulation of these osmo- and baroreceptors ultimately stimulates water conservation. This coordinated water repletion reduces extracellular fluid osmolality and increases circulating blood volume. Reestablishment of normal osmolality or vascular volume stimulates release of atrial natriuretic peptide (ANP) from the atrium, which provides negative feedback to inhibit further ADH release and angiotensin II production (see Fig. 3-2).

Water balance in humans is primarily regulated by water ingestion (under the control of thirst) and water retention (under the control of ADH).

ACTION OF ANTIDIURETIC HORMONE (ADH)

ADH regulates water conservation at the level of the kidney by increasing the permeability of the renal collecting duct to water. In the absence of ADH, the renal collecting duct remains impermeable to water, and the dilute urine created in the distal nephron is excreted, resulting in free water loss. In the presence of ADH, water channels are translocated to the lumenal cell membrane. This allows water to pass freely down its concentration gradient from the tubular lumen into the hypertonic renal interstitium. The urine becomes concentrated. The concentrating effect of ADH is critically dependent upon the solute gradient across tubular cells, which is established in the renal medulla. A schematic representation of the effect of ADH on the collecting tubule is shown in Fig. 3-3.

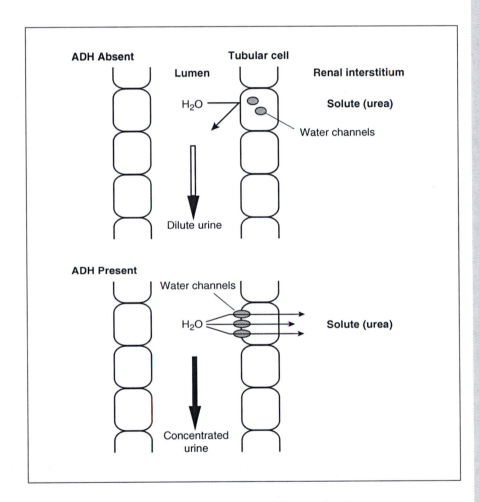

Fig. 3-3. Antidiuretic Hormone (ADH) Effect on Renal Collecting Duct

In the absence of ADH, the collecting duct is impermeable to water. The dilute urine created in the distal nephron is excreted, resulting in free water loss. If ADH is present, water channels are transposed to the tubular cell membrane and water passes freely down its concentration gradient from the collecting tubule lumen into the hypertonic renal interstitium.

The mechanism by which ADH stimulates translocation of water channels involves interaction with its V_2 antidiuretic receptors in the collecting duct, which activates specific G-proteins. This results in increased cellular adenylate cyclase activity. The increase in cellular cyclic adenine nucleotides creates downstream signals, which result in translocation of aquaporin-2 water channels from the cytoplasm of cells in the collecting duct to the lumenal surface of these cells. This permits free water to move into the cells. ADH also stimulates synthesis of aquaporin-2 water channels in the kidney, resulting in increased urine concentration of aquaporin-2.

ADH, as mentioned above, is also a potent pressor agent that acts at V_1 receptors in blood vessels walls. This increases intracellular calcium and causes vascular smooth muscle contraction to raise blood pressure. However, plasma concentrations of ADH required to increase blood pressure are many times higher than normal physiologic concentrations. There is little evidence that ADH plays a significant role in maintaining normal blood pressure in humans. Whether this pressor effect of ADH has a physiologic role in maintaining water balance is not known.

REGULATION OF ADH RELEASE

ADH is released from the posterior pituitary in response to osmotic and nonosmotic stimuli. To maintain normal plasma osmolality between 275–300 mOsm, ADH secretion must respond to small changes in plasma solute concentration (Fig. 3-4). As noted earlier, the osmotic stimulation of ADH release occurs through activation of receptors in the hypothalamus. As plasma osmolality rises and water moves out of cells, the osmoreceptors become dehydrated and ADH is released. This increase in osmolality requires an increase in *nonpermeable* solutes such as Na^+ or glucose.

The **normal threshold** for ADH release *and* for stimulation of thirst is plasma osmolality greater than 285 mOsm/L.

Nonosmotic stimulation of the posterior pituitary occurs predominantly through the sensing of intravascular volume by baroreceptors in the atria, aorta, and carotids. The relationship between blood volume, osmolality, and ADH release is such that a decrease in blood volume stimulates ADH release even if plasma osmolality is normal (or low). In dehydrated patients, low intravascular volume is a more important stimulus for water conservation than osmotic pressure.

THIRST

Regulation of the thirst response depends on many of the same factors as ADH release. Thirst is stimulated by a 2% to 3% increase in plasma tonicity. Normal serum osmolality can be maintained even in the absence of ADH if enough water is ingested. The osmotic regulation of

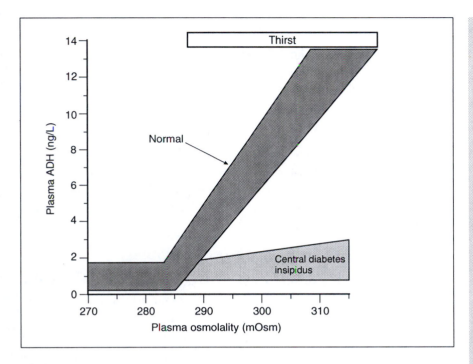

Fig. 3-4. Relationship of Plasma Osmolality to Antidiuretic Hormone (ADH) Level in Normal Humans

Increased ADH release occurs at plasma osmolality above 285 mOsm/L (dark gray). Individuals with central diabetes insipidus fail to increase ADH in response to plasma osmolality above 285 mOsm/L (light gray area).

thirst occurs through osmoreceptors in the hypothalamus, which are thought to be near the receptors that stimulate ADH release. Volume depletion detected by baroreceptors in the cardiac atria also regulates the water drinking response. Satiation of thirst occurs in response to many stimuli including normalization of osmolality and esophageal stretch. These mechanisms control the ingested volume of liquids very accurately as osmolality approaches normal.

CASE STUDY: *CONTINUED*

The patient's increased urination and thirst and her high serum Na^+ and plasma osmolality indicated a hypertonic state after she was deprived of free access to water. Her fluid restriction was lifted, and her serum Na^+ fell to the normal range within 48 hours. She continued to exhibit polydipsia and polyuria with a fluid intake of approximately 7 to 9 L/d. A review of her medical records revealed that she had been previously treated with lithium carbonate and that polydipsia and polyuria were noted at that time. A water deprivation test was ordered.

Disorders of Water Balance

Disorders of water balance can result in either hyper- or hypotonicity. Disorders related to the posterior pituitary are due to deficient or excessive secretion of ADH.

HYPERTONIC DISORDERS

Hypertonic disorders result from excess free water loss, inadequate free water intake, an impaired thirst mechanism, solute diuresis, defective ADH secretion, or defective ADH action. Major causes of hypertonic disorders are listed in Table 3-1. The ADH-related disorders result in two forms of *diabetes insipidus*.

Etiology of Diabetes Insipidus (DI)

DI is due either to a deficiency of ADH secretion from the posterior pituitary (central or neurogenic DI) or to renal insensitivity to ADH (nephrogenic DI). Water conservation in the distal collecting ducts cannot occur because ADH either is not present or is ineffective. The dilute urine created in the proximal nephron is not concentrated as it passes through the renal parenchyma, and excess free water losses occur (see Fig. 3-3).

Central (Neurogenic) Diabetes Insipidus
Decreased ADH *secretion*
Nephrogenic Diabetes Insipidus
Decreased ADH *action*

The major causes of DI are outlined in Table 3-2. Conditions associated with central DI include trauma to the pituitary stalk and posterior pituitary destruction by a number of mechanisms. Transient DI after anterior pituitary surgery is common, perhaps due to edema temporarily affecting the pituitary stalk. Permanent DI is rare after anterior pituitary surgery; the risk is higher after surgery for a hypothalamic tumor. The risk for permanent DI depends on the extent of the damage to the pituitary stalk.

Nephrogenic DI is usually due to chronic renal disease, which destroys the renal medulla concentrating gradient, or to drugs that

Table 3-1. Major Causes of Hypertonic Disorders

EXCESS FREE WATER LOSS	INADEQUATE FREE WATER INTAKE
Central diabetes insipidus (DI)	Impaired thirst
Nephrogenic DI	Inadequate access to water
Sweating	
Diarrhea	**SOLUTE DIURESIS**
Severe burns	
	Hyperglycemia
	Hypertonic intravenous infusion

Table 3-2. Major Causes of Central and Nephrogenic Diabetes Insipidus (DI)

CENTRAL (NEUROGENIC) DI	NEPHROGENIC DI
Trauma to pituitary stalk	Toxin/drug (demeclocycline, lithium, others)
Hypothalamic or pituitary surgery	Vascular (sickle cell disease)
Tumors (infiltration)	Infection (pyelonephritis)
Granulomatous disease (tuberculosis, sarcoidosis)	Infiltration (amyloid)
Ischemia (postpartum hemorrhage)	Familial (X-linked)
Infection (viral encephalitis, meningitis)	
Inflammation (autoimmune hypophysitis)	
Familial (autosomal dominant)	

Notes

inhibit ADH action, like demeclocycline and lithium. Nephrogenic DI can also be the result of rare congenital defects in the gene for the ADH V_2 receptor or abnormalities in the aquaporin-2 water channel.

The clinical picture of polyuria and thirst is the same, regardless of the cause of DI. The symptoms are described eloquently by Quain in the *Dictionary of Medicine*, which was published in 1883:

> Regarding the clinical history of polyuria, thirst and watery urine are the two prime symptoms, for there may be little wasting and the general health may be good. As long as drink is supplied in plenty, the condition of the patients is very tolerable, were it not for the broken sleep caused by the increased thirst and the desire to pass water. But any attempt to restrict the quantity of fluid gives rise to intense discomfort . . . the urine is inordinate in its quantity, and the specific gravity little above that of spring water . . . persistently at 1.001. If the drink is restricted more will be passed than is consumed by the abstraction of water from the body.

Urine volumes in excess of 6 L/24 hr can be generated. Maximal 24-hour urine volume is approximately 18 L, the total glomerular filtrate generated daily. The free water loss and increased osmolality stimulate profound thirst. If access to water is denied, hypertonicity worsens. However, if the thirst mechanism is intact, osmolality can be maintained within the normal range as long as water intake is equivalent to water loss.

Symptoms and Signs of Diabetes Insipidus

Excessive thirst
High fluid intake
High urine output
Plasma osmolality high or normal
Urine osmolality low

Differential Diagnosis of DI

DI should be suspected whenever patients present with unexplained thirst, high fluid intake, large urine volumes, and dilute urine (urine osmolality less than plasma osmolality). The initial problem in differential diagnosis usually is distinguishing DI from primary polydipsia (pathologic water drinking) or an abnormal thirst mechanism. Pathologic water drinkers ingest large volumes of water, which dilutes plasma, suppresses ADH, and results in large volumes of dilute urine.

Evaluation of patients with suspected DI begins with laboratory tests of plasma and urine osmolality (Table 3-3). Water drinkers with primary polydipsia should have decreased plasma osmolality, and patients with DI should have increased osmolality or normal osmolality if water intake is adequate. The next step in the evaluation is the water deprivation test. Patients are deprived of water in a controlled setting to avoid dangerous dehydration and surreptitious water ingestion. The patient's weight, urine volume, and urine osmolality are monitored closely until osmolality in 2 consecutive voided urine samples differs by less than 10% or the patient has lost 2% of body weight. Urine osmolality will not increase in patients with either form of DI, but should increase in patients with primary polydipsia.

To differentiate central DI from nephrogenic DI, a plasma sample for ADH measurement is obtained at the end of the water deprivation period. The patient is then given a bolus of subcutaneous aqueous vasopressin or D-desaminoarginine vasopressin (dDAVP), and urine osmolality is measured again. Patients with central or neurogenic DI will have inappropriately low plasma ADH after water deprivation but will be able to increase urine osmolality in response to the ADH injection. Patients with nephrogenic DI will have high plasma ADH in response to water deprivation but will not be able to increase urine osmolality and will not have an increase in urine aquaporin-2 after the ADH bolus.

Evaluation of Diabetes Insipidus

Plasma and urine osmolality
Water deprivation test
Plasma ADH

Table 3-3. Laboratory Studies in Cases of Polyuria: Diabetes Insipidus (DI) versus Primary Polydipsia

	CENTRAL DI	NEPHROGENIC DI	PRIMARY POLYDIPSIA
Plasma osmolality	Increased or normal	Increased or normal	Decreased
Urine osmolality	Decreased	Decreased	Decreased
Urine osmolality during H_2O deprivation	No change	No change	Increased
Urine osmolality after dDAVP	Increased	No change	Increased
Plasma ADH	Low	Normal to high	Low

Note. dDAVP = D-desaminoarginine vasopressin; ADH = antidiuretic hormone.

Treatment of DI

The treatment of DI depends on its cause. Free access to water is essential for all patients. Patients with central DI can be treated with vasopressin or one of its pharmacologic analogs, such as dDAVP, to diminish urine output and alleviate the need for chronic water drinking. dDAVP acts mainly at the V_2 receptors in the kidney, not on the V_1 receptors in blood vessels. dDAVP can be administered as a nasal spray or in tablet form. Treatment of nephrogenic DI is more difficult because exogenous ADH cannot overcome renal insensitivity to the hormone. Maintaining adequate free water intake is the principal therapy.

HYPOTONIC DISORDERS

Disorders that result in decreased serum osmolality are common (Table 3-4). These disorders result from decreased water excretion in euvolemic states, hypovolemic states that result in preservation of plasma volume at the expense of decreased serum osmolality, or excess water ingestion. Urine osmolality is inappropriately concentrated considering the hypotonic plasma.

Syndromes of Decreased Water Excretion Due to Excess ADH

The most common hypotonic disorder is the syndrome of inappropriate ADH (SIADH). Patients with SIADH have *normal vascular volume* and inappropriate ADH release in the *absence* of any osmotic stimulus. In some of these patients, nonosmotic stimuli—including pain, physical stress, and central nervous system disorders of various kinds—stimulate ADH release despite normal plasma volume and osmolality. Some tumors secrete ectopic ADH. Lung cancers and other pulmonary diseases are particularly likely to be associated with SIADH, but the syndrome occurs with many other disorders as well. Inappropriate ADH can be caused by drugs that stimulate or

---

Table 3-4. Major Causes of Hypotonic Disorders

DECREASED WATER EXCRETION (EUVOLEMIC STATES)	DECREASED WATER EXCRETION* (HYPOVOLEMIC STATES)
ADH excess due to SIADH	Congestive heart failure
Pain and physical stress	Cirrhosis
CNS infection, tumor, and trauma	Nephrotic syndrome
Ectopic tumors producing ADH	Adrenal insufficiency
Lung disease (tumor, tuberculosis, pneumonia)	Starvation
Drug-induced ADH release (opiates, analgesics, others)	
	EXCESS WATER INGESTION
	Primary polydipsia

Note. ADH = antidiuretic hormone; SIADH = syndrome of inappropriate ADH; CNS = central nervous system.
*Decreased distal solute delivery

potentiate the effects of ADH, such as narcotic analgesics, beta agonists, barbiturates, and nicotine.

Criteria for the Diagnosis of SIADH

Low plasma osmolality

Inappropriately high urine osmolality for plasma osmolality

Hyponatremia

Normal plasma volume

Normal renal and adrenal function

If ADH release and water ingestion continue unchecked, serum Na^+ concentration and plasma osmolality continue to decrease. The treatment of choice is to limit free water intake. Water restriction to 1.0 to 1.5 L/d is often necessary to maintain normal serum osmolality. If this is unsuccessful, drugs that reduce the effect of ADH at the renal tubule (e.g., demeclocycline, chlorpropamide) can be used. Sodium chloride can be given, cautiously (to avoid heart failure), if absolutely necessary.

CASE STUDY: *RESOLUTION*

A presumptive diagnosis of DI was made in this patient on the basis of her increased urination, thirst, and high serum Na^+, and plasma osmolality coupled with dilute urine. She had no history of excessive sweating, diarrhea, or burns to cause excessive water loss and nothing to suggest a solute diuresis. Plasma and urine glucose were normal, and she had not been given a solute load. Her symptoms were compatible with pathologic water drinking, but this results in hypotonicity (low plasma osmolality), not hypertonicity.

Her water deprivation test resulted in continuing urinary hypotonicity and significant free water loss with urinary volumes up to 1 L/hr. Water deprivation was stopped after she had lost 3% of her body weight. She was given a bolus of dDAVP, but there was no increase in urine osmolality or reduction in urine volume. The diagnosis of nephrogenic DI was confirmed.

Her nephrogenic DI was felt to be related to past lithium carbonate therapy. Lithium carbonate is known to cause nephrogenic DI, and symptoms can persist for many years after the drug is discontinued. The treatment of nephrogenic DI can be difficult and definitely requires that patients have free access to water to replace their water loss. It is imperative to monitor their serum osmolality, serum Na^+, and urinary water losses.

Decreased Distal Solute Delivery Causing Increased ADH

Conditions that cause intravascular volume depletion and decreased solute delivery to the distal tubules result in excess ADH release. Examples are shown in Table 3-4.

Primary Polydipsia

This pathologic condition, in which patients with psychiatric illness repeatedly ingest large amounts of fluid, results in hypotonicity with suppressed ADH levels.

Oxytocin

Oxytocin is the other major peptide hormone produced in hypothalamic nuclei and stored in the posterior pituitary. Oxytocin has two major physiologic actions in humans. It stimulates uterine contractions at the time of labor and delivery in response to distention of the reproductive tract, and it stimulates smooth muscle contraction in the breast during suckling, which results in milk let-down. Suckling and distention of the reproductive tract stimulate oxytocin release through neural pathways.

Oxytocin has a minor role in the regulation of water homeostasis. Release is stimulated by increased plasma tonicity. In pharmacologic amounts, oxytocin potentiates water retention. Severe water intoxication can occur in women who receive high doses of oxytocin to promote uterine contractions during labor.

REVIEW QUESTIONS

Directions: For each of the following questions, choose the *one best* answer.

1. In the maintenance of normal water balance, a complex process that requires integration of many signals, which of the following occurs?

   A Thirst is suppressed by hypovolemia and angiotensin II

   B Antidiuretic hormone (ADH) suppresses translocation of water channels to the surface of the collecting duct lumen

   C ADH stimulates water flow from renal interstitium to the collecting duct lumen

   D Increased plasma osmolality and loss of plasma volume elicit ADH release

Questions 2 and 3

A 26-year-old woman developed polyuria 2 days after surgical removal of a large non-hormone-producing pituitary tumor. Now her urine volume is in excess of 6 L/d, and she is drinking large amounts of water.

2 What is the most likely cause of her polyuria?

A An impaired thirst mechanism due to surgical damage
B Nephrogenic diabetes insipidus (DI)
C Central DI
D Syndrome of inappropriate ADH release (SIADH)
E Excess intravenous fluid administration

3 Unfortunately, this patient's polyuria is permanent. Urine and plasma osmolality and a water deprivation test support the diagnosis. In light of this information, which of the following statements is most likely to be true?

A Her urine osmolality is higher than her plasma osmolality
B Her water deprivation test shows no response to vasopressin
C High plasma osmolality indicates primary polydipsia
D A long-acting ADH agonist is the treatment of choice

4 A 64-year-old man was hospitalized 3 days ago for a laparotomy and cholecystectomy (gall bladder removal). He has had an uncomplicated postoperative course. He has been given intravenous fluid (5% dextrose in 0.5% normal saline) and intravenous morphine for postoperative pain control. He has no complaints other than moderate pain due to his abdominal incision. Laboratory studies include Na^+, 127 mEq/L (normal: 137–145 mEq/L) and K^+, 4.1 mEq/L (normal). Which of the following is the most likely explanation for this patient's hyponatremia?

A Excessive water ingestion
B Starvation with decreased solute delivery to the distal nephrons
C Syndrome of inappropriate ADH release
D Drug-induced suppression of ADH release

5 A 75-year-old man is being evaluated for weight loss. An ADH level is measured as part of a research protocol. His ADH level is low. This would be expected in which of the following situations?

A Ectopic ADH secretion by a tumor
B Primary polydipsia
C Nephrogenic diabetes insipidus (DI)
D Hypovolemia due to dehydration

References

Androgue HJ, Madias NE: Hypernatremia. *N Engl J Med* 342: 1493–1500 and 1581–1589, 2000.

Bichet DG: Nephrogenic diabetes insipidus. *Am J Med* 105: 431–442, 1998.

Knepper MA, Verbalis JG, Nielson S: Role of aquaporins in water balance disorders. *Curr Opin Nephrol Hypertens* 6: 499–507, 1997.

Levin ER, Gardner DG, Samson WK: Natriuretic peptides. *N Engl J Med* 339: 321–328, 1998.

Martin PY, Schrier RW: Role of aquaporin-2 water channels in urinary concentration and dilution defects. *Kidney Int* 53: S57–S62, 1998.

Quain R: Polyuria. In *A Dictionary of Medicine*. New York: Appleton, 1883, p 1239–1241.

Streeten DH, Moses AM: The syndrome of inappropriate vasopressin secretion. *The Endocrinol* 3: 353–358, 1993.

Vokes TJ, Robertson GL: Disorders of antidiuretic hormone. *Endocrinol Metab Clin North Am* 17: 456–475, 1988.

4

The Thyroid Gland

Cary N. Mariash, M.D.

■ CHAPTER OUTLINE ■

■ LEARNING OBJECTIVES ■

At the completion of this chapter, the student will:
1. understand the physiology of thyroid hormone synthesis.
2. know how feedback inhibition regulates plasma hormone concentrations.
3. be aware of the actions of thyroid hormones.
4. be able to interpret thyroid function tests.
5. identify the causes, symptoms, and signs of hyperthyroidism.
6. recognize the association of the immune system with thyroid gland dysfunction.
7. identify the causes, symptoms, and signs of hypothyroidism.

CASE STUDY: *INTRODUCTION*

The patient is a 23-year-old woman who complained of feeling extremely tired and "jumpy" for the past 4 months. She also felt short of breath and her heart "raced" whenever she exerted herself. Her symptoms had become progressively worse, and by the time of her first visit they occurred whenever she climbed a flight of stairs or carried her 2-year-old daughter from the car to the house.

She had taken medical leave from her construction job because she could not perform the strenuous tasks required. Her hands shook, and she was unable to hold a full cup of coffee without spilling it. She was irritable and argued constantly with her husband. The house always seemed hot. She lost 10 lb despite a good appetite, and her menstrual flow had become much lighter. A review of systems was positive for frequent, soft stools.

Physical examination revealed a thin woman who fidgeted continuously. Her blood pressure was 130/58 mm Hg; her pulse was 126 beats/min and regular. Her skin was warm, velvety, and moist. She had lid lag and a prominent stare. Diplopia developed during upward and outward gaze. Her thyroid gland was 3 times normal size, diffusely enlarged, and soft. A prominent bruit was present over the gland. Her cardiac examination was normal except for the tachycardia. Chest and abdominal examination was normal. Muscle strength and tone were normal. Deep tendon reflexes showed a rapid relaxation phase. Several tests were ordered.

Structure and Synthesis of Thyroid Hormones

The thyroid hormone system consists of the hormones that regulate the secretion of thyroid hormone from the thyroid gland, the thyroid gland, which secretes thyroid hormones, and the peripheral tissues that respond to thyroid hormone. The two major thyroid hormones are thyroxine (T_4) and triiodothyronine (T_3), which are iodinated amino acids (Fig. 4-1). T_4 contains four iodine molecules; T_3 contains three iodine molecules. The major secretory product of the thyroid is T_4. Approximately 15% of the T_3 produced is secreted by the thyroid; the remainder is produced in peripheral tissues by the deiodination of T_4, which results in T_3. T_3 is the physiologically active hormone.

T_4 is made within the basic functional unit of the thyroid gland, the thyroid follicle (Fig. 4-2). The follicle consists of a single layer of epithelial cells surrounding a sphere of colloid, which contains the protein thyroglobulin. T_4 is synthesized on and is covalently linked to thyroglobulin. The large capacity of thyroglobulin to store iodine-containing thyroid hormones is important, given the decreased availability of iodide in certain geographic regions of the world.

The thyroid gland concentrates iodide to levels 30 to 40 times those in plasma to maintain adequate stores for thyroid hormone

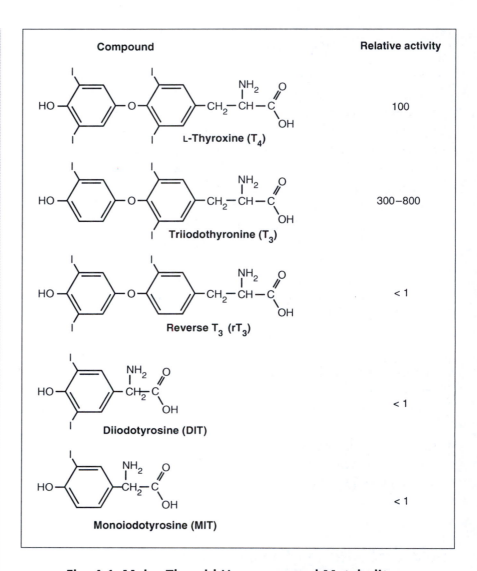

Compound	Relative activity
L-Thyroxine (T₄)	100
Triiodothyronine (T₃)	300–800
Reverse T₃ (rT₃)	< 1
Diiodotyrosine (DIT)	< 1
Monoiodotyrosine (MIT)	< 1

Fig. 4-1. Major Thyroid Hormones and Metabolites

The thyroid hormone receptor has greater affinity for triiodothyronine (T_3) than thyroxine (T_4), so the relative activity of T_3 is greater than the relative activity of T_4.

synthesis. The recommended intake of iodide to maintain thyroid hormone synthesis is 150 µg/d. Intake below 50 µg/d is inadequate. Iodide is plentiful in foods obtained from the ocean and coastal areas, but in mountain and inland areas the supply may be very low. In the United States, iodide is added to foods, salt, and vitamin preparations; therefore, iodine deficiency is rare. Some medications and contrast media contain very high concentrations of iodide.

The thyroid follicle traps inorganic iodide, transporting it against a concentration gradient. Iodide (I) is transported together with sodium (Na) by a protein called the Na/I symporter, which is located primarily in thyroid cells. During times of relative iodine insufficiency, this trapping mechanism is enhanced to assure optimal use of available iodine. Following the uptake of iodide through specific pores in the epithelial cells, the trapped iodide is oxidized to iodine by the enzyme

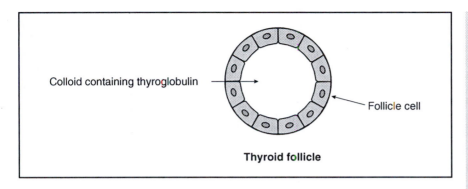

Colloid containing thyroglobulin

Follicle cell

Thyroid follicle

Fig. 4-2. Cross Section of a Thyroid Follicle

thyroid peroxidase. During this reaction, tyrosine residues on thyroglobulin are iodinated to produce monoiodotyrosine (MIT). Subsequent iodination of MIT produces diiodotyrosine (DIT). By mechanisms that are not fully understood, two DIT molecules are coupled on the thyroglobulin backbone to produce T_4. MIT and DIT can also be coupled to produce T_3. The hormones remain covalently bound to the thyroglobulin backbone; therefore, thyroglobulin in the thyroid follicle is replete with T_4, T_3, DIT, and MIT (see Fig. 4-1).

Thyroglobulin undergoes endocytosis at the apical surface of the thyroid epithelial cell and is degraded within the lysosomes of the cell. The thyroid hormones are then released from thyroglobulin and secreted into the circulation. At the same time, released MIT and DIT are deiodinated within the epithelial cell, and the iodide can be recovered. This highly efficient process assures that losses of free iodine are minimized.

Steps in Thyroid Synthesis

Iodide trapping

Organification of iodide: $I^- + peroxidase \rightarrow I^0$

Synthesis of thyroid hormones on thyroglobulin:

$I^0 + tyrosine \rightarrow MIT$

$MIT + I^0 \rightarrow DIT$

$DIT + DIT \rightarrow T_4$

$DIT + MIT \rightarrow T_3$

Proteolysis of thyroglobulin to release thyroid hormones

Removal of iodide from remaining DIT and MIT by deiodinases

Defects in any of these processes produce thyroid hormone deficiency (Table 4-1). Patients have been found with congenital defects due to abnormalities of the iodine pores, defective oxidation due to abnormal thyroid peroxidase, and inefficient iodine conservation due to deficiencies of thyroid deiodinase. Multiple defects in the two subunits of the thyroglobulin molecule are associated with defective synthesis of thyroid hormones. Finally, development of thyroid follicles must proceed normally to make adequate numbers of follicle cells.

Table 4-1. Causes of Congenital Thyroid Hormone Deficiency

Iodide deficiency

Intrathyroid defects
Defective thyroid follicle differentiation
Iodide transporter defects, thyroid peroxidase defects, thyroglobulin defects

Intrathyroid and peripheral tissue defects
Deiodinase deficiency

Recent studies have identified a number of thyroid cell–specific transcription factors that, when mutated, lead to abnormal or absent thyroid follicular cell development and congenital hypothyroidism.

The secreted hormones are eventually deiodinated in peripheral tissues to release free iodide. Since the kidney can excrete the free iodide, the kidney and the thyroid compete for iodide in the circulation. When dietary iodide is sufficient, as in most U.S. diets, the thyroid gland accumulates approximately 20% of the ingested iodide. The remainder is excreted by the kidney. However, when the iodine supply is low, the thyroid can increase the uptake and trapping of iodide. Under extreme circumstances, the thyroid can trap nearly 100% of ingested iodide. Because the thyroid gland can adapt to iodide needs, there is no need for a renal mechanism to alter clearance of iodide.

Control Mechanisms

The thyroid gland is controlled by the anterior pituitary and the hypothalamus, and they in turn are regulated by thyroid hormone feedback (Fig. 4-3). Thyroid gland function is tightly regulated by thyroid-stimulating hormone (TSH) made by the thyrotrophs in the anterior pituitary gland. TSH is composed of two highly glycosylated subunits: the α-subunit, which is common to other pituitary glycoprotein hormones, and the β-subunit, which is specific for TSH. TSH binds to its specific receptor on the surface of thyroid epithelial cells. This is followed by activation of adenylate cyclase, which increases formation of intracellular cyclic adenosine monophosphate (cAMP). A rise in intracellular cAMP stimulates most of the processes in the thyroid cell described in the previous section and results in thyroid hormone secretion.

TSH stimulates nearly all reactions required for thyroid hormone synthesis.

Secretion of TSH is regulated primarily by the pituitary T_3 level. As plasma thyroid hormone levels rise, the pituitary T_3 level rises. An increase in pituitary T_3 inhibits synthesis and secretion of TSH by inhibiting the synthesis of the messenger RNA (mRNA) for both the α- and the β-subunits of TSH.

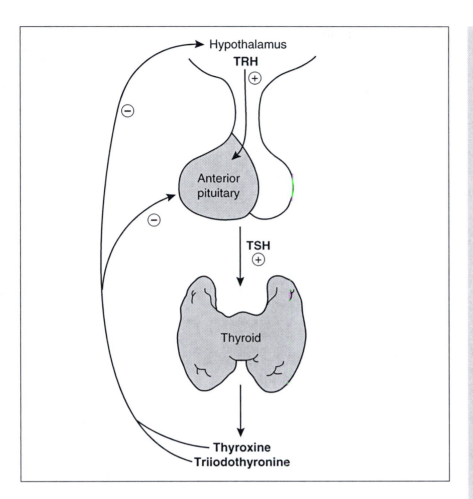

**Fig. 4-3. Hypothalamic-Pituitary-Thyroid Gland
Feedback Control Loops**

Thyrotropin-releasing hormone (TRH) from the hypothalamus stimulates release of thyroid-stimulating hormone (TSH) from the pituitary. TSH stimulates secretion of thyroxine (T_4) and triiodothyronine (T_3) from the thyroid gland. Circulating T_4 goes to the liver and other tissues where it is converted to T_3. T_3 inhibits hypothalamic secretion of TRH and pituitary secretion of TSH. $+$ = stimulatory; $-$ = inhibitory.

Control of Thyroid Hormone Synthesis
Level of iodide for hormone synthesis
Activity of deiodinases
Negative feedback regulation of hypothalamic-pituitary-
    thyroid axis

TSH activity is also regulated by thyrotropin-releasing hormone (TRH), a cyclic tripeptide made from a larger precursor in the hypothalamus. TRH is released from the hypothalamus into the hypothalamic-pituitary portal system, which conveys it to the pituitary thyrotrophs. TRH plays an important role in modulating the pituitary response to feedback by T_3. When TRH secretion is increased, the pituitary set point for feedback inhibition by T_3 is raised, making the pituitary less sensitive to T_3 inhibition. Conversely, when TRH is low, the pituitary is more sensitive to T_3 inhibition. TRH regulates both the acute release of TSH from the pituitary and glycosylation of the TSH molecule, which is required for TSH bioactivity.

Functions of TRH

Regulates pituitary sensitivity to T_3 feedback

Stimulates acute TSH release

Regulates glycosylation of TSH

Synthesis and release of TRH are regulated by negative feedback inhibition by T_3. When plasma T_3 levels are elevated, hypothalamic TRH content is reduced, and when plasma T_3 levels are low, the content of hypothalamic TRH is high.

Hormone Transport and Metabolism

Thyroid hormones are relatively water insoluble, so they are transported in the plasma bound to carrier proteins. The three major carrier proteins are thyroxine-binding globulin (TBG), albumin, and transthyretin. The relative distribution of thyroxine on these proteins is approximately 70%, 10%, and 20%, respectively. T_3 also circulates bound to proteins, primarily to TBG and albumin. Approximately 99.99% of thyroxine and 99.9% of T_3 are bound. Bound hormones are in equilibrium with free hormones in plasma. Only the small amount of unbound (free) hormone is available to move into the interstitial tissue fluid and ultimately into individual cells. Tissues respond to the concentration of free hormone, not the concentration of total thyroid hormone. The feedback inhibition discussed above refers to the free hormone concentration. A change in binding protein concentration alters the concentration of total plasma hormone, but the level of free hormone changes only transiently.

Major Plasma Carrier Proteins for Thyroid Hormones

Thyroxine-binding globulin (TBG)

Transthyretin (prealbumin)

Albumin

Inside cells, thyroid hormones are metabolized further. The *outer ring* of T_4 is 5'-deiodinated to produce the more potent T_3 (3,5,3'-triiodothyronine). This reaction occurs mostly in peripheral tissues, catalyzed by deiodinase enzymes. There are several deiodinases, which are unusual enzymes because they contain selenium. Type I deiodinase, which occurs mostly in liver and kidney but also in muscle, thyroid, and other tissues, provides T_3 to the plasma. Type I deiodinase activity is decreased by fasting and some drugs. Type II deiodinase is found primarily in the brain, adipose tissue, and the pituitary gland. Activity of type II deiodinase increases when the circulating T_4 level is low and decreases when the circulating T_4 level is high. This regulation maintains normal levels of T_3 within the nervous system and allows the pituitary and hypothalamus to respond to T_4 feedback from the thyroid gland.

Sources of T_3

Thyroid gland, 15%
Peripheral tissue T_4 to T_3 conversion, 85%

Deiodinases are also involved in the inactivation and degradation of thyroid hormones. Type III deiodinase removes iodine from the 5 position on the *inner* ring of T_4 to produce inactive 3,3',5'-triiodothyronine (reverse T_3, or rT_3) [see Fig. 4-1]. rT_3 can be deiodinated further by type I 5'-deiodinase to 3,3'-diiodothyronine (T_2). Continued deiodination of T_3 and T_2 leads to other inactive products. The iodine is recirculated for use by the thyroid gland or excreted in the urine. Other degradative processes include conjugation of T_4 with glucuronic acid or sulfate. The conjugated products are excreted in the bile.

EFFECTS OF ILLNESS ON THYROID HORMONE METABOLISM

Peripheral metabolism of thyroid hormones undergoes major changes in the presence of starvation, anorexia, carbohydrate deprivation, untreated diabetes mellitus, or nonthyroid systemic illness. In the presence of these illnesses, type I deiodinase is inhibited, and conversion of T_4 to T_3 is decreased, resulting in a low circulating T_3 level. Since degradation of rT_3 to T_2 is also decreased, the concentration of rT_3 is high. It is unclear whether the fall in the serum T_3 level is deleterious, protective, or simply represents an epiphenomenon. The lower concentration of T_3 should result in reduced energy expenditure in the setting of starvation or illness. TSH levels are usually normal, unless the patient is receiving glucocorticoids or dopamine, which suppress TSH. Thyroid hormone replacement is not indicated, as studies to date have failed to show any benefit from efforts to restore thyroid hormone levels to normal. Hormone levels return to normal when the illness subsides.

Thyroid Hormone Action

Thyroid hormone action at the cellular level is initiated by the binding of thyroid hormone to a specific nuclear receptor. The hormone-receptor complex binds to specific response elements on DNA. There are three thyroid hormone receptor proteins (α_1, β_1, β_2), which are the products of two different genes. The distribution of these receptors differs among different tissues, and the response of the tissues to thyroid hormone depends on the relative occupancy of the receptors by thyroid hormone. The receptors preferentially bind T_3, which is why

T_3 is more active than T_4. Once bound to the receptor, T_3 regulates the expression of different genes in different tissues.

Thyroid hormones exert major effects on growth and development. The role of thyroid hormone in prenatal development is still uncertain, but the absence of thyroid hormone in the early postnatal period is devastating. Thyroid hormone deficiency in the first few months of life leads to irreversible abnormalities in brain development. Prolonged and severe thyroid hormone deficiency in early infancy results in cretinism, which is characterized by marked mental retardation and short stature. If hypothyroidism develops later in childhood, growth is delayed, but normal growth can be restored by thyroid hormone replacement therapy.

Role of T_3 in Development
Normal postnatal brain development
Normal growth

Thyroid hormone increases oxygen consumption and heat production. This can be measured as changes in resting (basal) metabolic rate. At the cellular level, the increase in metabolic rate is associated with changes in many metabolic processes, including an increase in sodium–potassium adenosine triphosphatase (Na^+–K^+-ATPase) in liver and skeletal muscle, increases in lipid synthesis and lipid oxidation, and increases in protein synthesis and protein degradation. The effects on lipids and protein represent futile cycles in which there is no net change in end product (such as lipid content) at the expense of increased oxygen consumption and heat production.

Oxygen consumption and heat production are also regulated by conditioning, diet, genetics, and other hormones. The net result reflects the interaction of these factors and the thyroid hormone status. Thyroid hormone influences many other physiologic processes, including glucose absorption, insulin requirements, sensitivity to catecholamines, and the rate of drug metabolism (all increased in hyperthyroidism and decreased in hypothyroidism). Some effects of thyroid hormone on specific organ systems are listed in Table 4-2.

Functions Increased by T_3

Oxygen consumption	Protein synthesis
Heat production	Protein degradation
Metabolic rate	Drug metabolism
Lipid synthesis	Catecholamine sensitivity*
Lipid oxidation	Glucose absorption*
Cholesterol synthesis and degradation	Gluconeogenesis*

*Important only in hyperthyroidism

Table 4-2. Effects of Thyroid Hormone on Organ Systems

ORGAN SYSTEM	HORMONE EXCESS	HORMONE DEFICIENCY
Heart	Increased heart rate, increased contractility	Decreased heart rate, decreased cardiac output
Vascular	Vasodilatation, widened pulse pressure	Vasoconstriction, hypertension
Skin	Warm, smooth, and moist	Rough and dry
Gastrointestinal	Increased motility and absorption	Decreased motility
Skeletal	Increased bone turnover	Decreased bone turnover
Neuromuscular	Hyperactivity, rapid muscle relaxation, muscle weakness	Lethargy, slow muscle relaxation
	Increased muscle contraction	

Thyroid Function Testing

Symptoms and signs of thyroid hormone excess and deficiency are often not specific and can be confused with those of other disorders. Appropriate thyroid function testing provides an accurate assessment of the thyroid status of the patient, defines the pathogenesis of the dysfunction, and helps to assess the response to treatment.

Early investigators at the turn of the 20th century established a relationship between the rate of oxygen consumption under basal conditions and thyroid status. For several decades, measurement of the basal metabolic rate (BMR) was the only objective test for thyroid function. In the 1940s, measurement of protein-bound iodine (PBI)

CASE STUDY: CONTINUED

The patient presented with heat intolerance, weight loss, palpitations, increased heart rate, vasodilatation (causing the warm, smooth, moist skin), increased gastrointestinal motility, and neuromuscular hyperactivity (irritability, hyperactivity, lid lag, stare, tremor, and rapid relaxation of deep tendon reflexes), suggesting excessive thyroid hormone action on many organ systems. In order to confirm this diagnosis and to evaluate the cause and severity of her thyroid disease, laboratory tests were performed. These included measurements of circulating thyroid hormone levels, antibodies indicating autoimmune thyroid disease, the ability of the thyroid gland to take up iodide, and the distribution of iodine within the gland. These studies revealed a high free T_4, high T_3, a high titer of thyroid-stimulating immunoglobulin, and high radioactive iodine uptake. A thyroid scan showed an enlarged gland with diffuse uptake in a homogenous pattern.

and radioiodine uptake by the thyroid represented major advances in assessing thyroid function. However, the BMR and PBI are influenced by many factors other than thyroid status, and these tests are no longer used to assess thyroid function.

THYROID-PITUITARY AXIS HORMONES IN BLOOD

Total and Free Serum T_4 and Free T_4 Index

Since the late 1960s, tests for the level of circulating T_4 have been based on the interaction of T_4 with antibodies directed to the T_4 molecule. Measurement of total serum T_4 is one of the classic tests of clinical thyroid status.

The level of total T_4 does not always reflect the actual thyroid status of the patient. The total T_4 level is a mixture of free T_4 (FT_4) [the active form] and T_4 attached to binding proteins. If binding protein concentrations are high or low, total T_4 will be high or low, reflecting the amount of T_4 bound, but the FT_4 may be within normal limits. For example, in pregnancy total T_4 is high because the increase in estrogen stimulates increased production of TBG, and TBG clearance is decreased. FT_4 concentrations are normal. Some clinically euthyroid individuals have high levels of total T_4 all of their lives due to genetic overproduction of TBG. Families with a propensity toward increased transthyretin or an abnormal albumin that binds more than normal amounts of T_4 also have high total T_4 levels but normal FT_4 levels.

Conversely, patients treated with androgens and individuals with genetic underproduction of TBG have low levels of total T_4, normal levels of FT_4, and no symptoms of hypothyroidism. Table 4-3 lists conditions associated with altered plasma protein-binding due to changes in TBG.

Since the total T_4 level does not always indicate the true thyroid status, it is necessary to assess the level of circulating FT_4. The FT_4 concentration can be measured by equilibrium or nonequilibrium dialysis (techniques to assess the fraction of free hormone) or by ultrafiltration.

Table 4-3. Major Conditions Associated with Changes in Thyroxine-Binding Globulin (TBG)

INCREASED BINDING	DECREASED BINDING
Pregnancy ($\uparrow$ TBG synthesis, $\downarrow$ TBG clearance)	Nonthyroid illness[a]
Estrogen treatment ($\uparrow$ TBG synthesis, $\downarrow$ TBG clearance)	Testosterone treatment ($\downarrow$ TBG synthesis, $\uparrow$ TBG clearance)
Acute hepatitis (damaged cells release TBG)	Hereditary decrease in TBG
Hereditary increase in TBG	Hyperthyroidism ($\uparrow$ catabolism of TBG)
Hypothyroidism ($\downarrow$ catabolism of TBG)	

[a] Decreased protein synthesis, increased protein loss (malnutrition, nephrotic syndrome, others).

Reliable measurements of FT_4 have become more widely available and are being used instead of the indirect tests, which measure the strength of T_4 binding to plasma proteins.

Indirect tests provide an estimate of the FT_4 level, or free T_4 index (FT_4I), by measuring the binding of radiolabeled thyroid hormone to resin, charcoal, or antibody that has been added to serum. This measurement makes it possible to determine the relative strength of plasma protein-binding. The FT_4I is calculated by multiplying the total T_4 concentration by the measurement of relative plasma protein-binding. This corrects the total T_4 concentration for abnormalities of binding proteins. The FT_4I is an excellent approximation of true thyroid status except in patients with severe illness or very abnormal binding protein. In these situations it is better to obtain a direct measurement of the FT_4 level.

Total and Free Serum T_3

Total serum T_3 and free T_3 (FT_3) levels can be measured or estimated by methods similar to those used for total and free T_4 levels. Since T_3 is the active hormone, one would predict that the serum FT_3 level would be the best test of hormone action at the cellular level. However, the plasma FT_3 concentration may not reflect the tissue T_3 concentration accurately because local tissue T_3 concentrations are greatly influenced by local tissue conversion of T_4 to T_3. This may establish a tissue-to-plasma T_3 gradient that is specific for each organ. Also, the plasma half-life of T_3 is much shorter than that of T_4, and diurnal factors affect plasma measurements.

The major indication for determination of serum T_3 levels is suspected hyperthyroidism. In patients with early Graves disease or a toxic adenoma, secretion of T_3 is increased even more than the secretion of T_4. In these patients, the serum concentration of T_3 can be high while the serum concentration of T_4 remains within the normal range.

In the hypothyroid state, the fall in serum T_4 stimulates deiodinase activity, leading to a compensatory increase in the conversion of T_4 to T_3. In the very early stages of hypothyroidism, T_3 values may still be within the normal range. Serum TSH levels together with serum FT_4 or FT_4I are better tests for diagnosis of early thyroid failure.

Serum TSH

The radioimmunoassay for circulating TSH was introduced in the 1960s. The earliest TSH assays could measure accurately only the elevated levels of TSH in the hypothyroid state. However, progressive improvements in the immunoassays have made it possible to measure the level of TSH in the euthyroid range and to measure the low level of TSH due to negative feedback to the hypothalamus and pituitary in patients with hyperthyroidism.

The TSH level in euthyroid individuals ranges from approximately 0.5 to 5 μU/mL. However, clinical manifestations of hypothyroidism are difficult to demonstrate until TSH levels rise to 10 μU/mL or higher. Symptoms of hyperthyroidism do not generally become evident until the TSH level falls below 0.05 µU/mL. Finding abnormal TSH levels in patients who are asymptomatic may warrant careful follow-up rather than immediate treatment, but each situation should be evaluated on its clinical merits. The TSH assay is particularly helpful for following the results of treatment of hypothyroidism and hyperthyroidism.

The TSH level is low or low-normal if hypothalamic or pituitary disease is present. It is not clear why the TSH level is not uniformly low in pituitary insufficiency. The diagnosis of pituitary hypothyroidism can be made by finding a low FT_4I or FT_4 level in addition to deficits of other pituitary hormones. Radiographic studies can demonstrate structural damage in the pituitary-hypothalamic system.

The sensitive **TSH assay** has become the single most useful clinical test of thyroid function.

Thyroid Function Testing Patients with Nonthyroid Disease

Problems in the interpretation of thyroid function tests arise in patients with catabolic nonthyroid disease. The level of circulating thyroid hormones is depressed in patients with severe illness. Recent studies from intensive care units (ICUs) have shown that the lower the level of T_4, the higher the mortality rate. The level of T_3 is also low in these patients. Low T_3 concentrations also occur with a very high prevalence in patients who are dieting or who have only minor disease. These changes in T_4 and T_3 are generally not accompanied by alterations in steady-state levels of serum TSH. In this setting, a decreased level of FT_4 and FT_3 or a low FT_4I or FT_3I cannot be used to make the diagnosis of primary hypothyroidism. A substantial elevation of TSH above the normal range is essential for making the diagnosis.

Serum Thyroglobulin

Thyroglobulin is mostly contained in the colloid within thyroid follicles, but low concentrations of thyroglobulin can be detected in serum from euthyroid individuals. Serum thyroglobulin is increased in various forms of thyroiditis when the protein escapes from a damaged thyroid gland. The level is also elevated in patients with hyperthyroidism who have thyroid overactivity, in patients with large goiters, and in patients with metastatic thyroid carcinomas. Patients with thyroid carcinomas who have undergone near total or total ablation of the thyroid gland have very low levels of thyroglobulin unless they have metastatic disease. A subsequent rise in serum thyroglobulin indicates a recurrence.

High RAIU	Low RAIU
Graves disease	Thyroiditis
Multinodular goiter	After ingestion of exogenous thyroid hormone
Toxic nodule	After ingestion of iodide-containing medications
TSH-producing tumors	After administration of iodide-containing contrast material
	Ectopic thyroid tissue

RADIOACTIVE IODINE UPTAKE (RAIU)

The RAIU by the thyroid remains a useful test of thyroid function. A tracer dose of radioactive iodine is administered orally, and the amount of tracer located in the thyroid gland is measured 6 or 24 hours later. The normal range for RAIU depends on dietary iodine intake. The RAIU is higher in areas where usual dietary iodine intake is low and is lower in areas where the usual iodine intake is high. RAIU is increased in hyperthyroid states such as Graves disease or toxic multinodular goiter, where thyroid hormone synthesis is increased. However, RAIU is low in patients with thyroiditis who are hyperthyroid due to the release of stored hormone from damaged cells. The injured or inflamed gland cannot take up iodine. RAIU is low in patients taking exogenous thyroid hormone whose TSH levels are suppressed. RAIU is also low following ingestion of drugs or administration of contrast material containing iodide because the thyroid gland is saturated with iodine.

Causes of Nontoxic Goiter

Iodine deficiency
Genetic defects in thyroid hormone synthesis
Drugs or chemicals impairing thyroid hormone synthesis
Goitrogens in the diet

TESTS OF THYROID AUTOIMMUNITY

Thyroid-Stimulating Immunoglobulin

This assay is useful in the diagnosis of Graves disease, a form of hyperthyroidism caused by endogenously generated autoantibodies to the TSH receptor. When immortalized rat thyroid cells or hamster cells expressing human TSH receptor are exposed to serum containing these antibodies, cAMP is generated. The presence of such antibodies in the patient's serum is the hallmark of the disorder.

Antithyroid-Peroxidase and Antithyroglobulin Antibodies

These antibodies are elevated in patients with chronic lymphocytic thyroiditis (Hashimoto disease) and reflect the autoimmune basis of this disorder. They do not cause the thyroid disease but are markers of thyroid damage. Continued elevation of these antibodies may foreshadow progressive reduction in thyroid function. Patients with increased titers of these antibodies need periodic evaluation for hypothyroidism.

THYROID IMAGING

A radioactive iodine (^{123}I) or technetium scan provides information about the size and functioning areas of the thyroid gland. Functioning thyroid nodules that take up the isotope are called "hot" nodules; nonfunctioning or poorly functioning areas of the thyroid that take up little isotope are called "cold" areas. A tracer dose of ^{131}I, which has a longer half-life than ^{123}I, is used for total body scanning for thyroid cancer metastases.

Thyroid ultrasound is used primarily to follow changes in the size of thyroid nodules and for differentiating cystic from solid nodules. Computed tomography (CT) scanning, magnetic resonance imaging (MRI), and positron emission technology (PET) are used to follow thyroid malignancies.

THYROID CYTOLOGY

The fine needle aspiration biopsy of thyroid nodules is simple, well tolerated, and provides a small amount of material for screening thyroid nodules for malignant cells. It is approximately 90% accurate in the hands of an experienced cytologist.

Thyroid Hormone System Disorders

GOITER

Goiters are enlargements of the thyroid gland that arise because of increased stimulation of the thyroid gland by TSH or by thyroid-stimulating immunoglobulins, resulting in multiplication of follicle epithelial cells and eventually new follicles. Other growth factors may also contribute.

Diffuse simple or nontoxic goiters may develop in response to inadequate synthesis of thyroid hormone. TSH secretion then increases and induces diffuse thyroid hyperplasia. Some areas outgrow their blood supply and become necrotic and then fibrotic, as other new areas are becoming hyperplastic. Some follicles become autonomous; their growth is no longer dependent on TSH. Eventually, the goiter becomes filled with nodules of different sizes and varying capacity for thyroid hormone synthesis. The diffuse goiter has been transformed into a multinodular goiter. If the goiter becomes large enough, patients may complain of neck pressure and difficulty swallowing. Treatment with

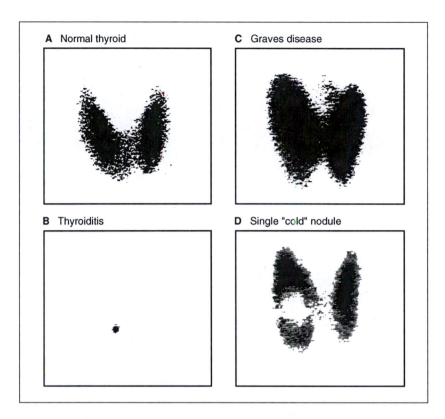

A Normal thyroid

C Graves disease

B Thyroiditis

D Single "cold" nodule

Fig. 4-4. Radioactive Iodine Scans

(A) Iodine uptake in a normal thyroid gland. (B) Little or no iodine uptake in a patient with thyroiditis. Only the marker indicating the sternal notch is seen. (C) An enlarged thyroid gland with increased iodine uptake in a homogeneous pattern in a patient with Graves disease. (D) An area of decreased iodine uptake in a solitary "cold" nodule in the right lobe of the thyroid gland.

T_4 to suppress TSH into the normal range may cause these goiters to regress, but autonomous areas and necrotic, hemorrhagic, or fibrotic areas do not respond. Sometimes surgery is necessary for cosmetic reasons or symptom relief.

Patients with these goiters are euthyroid if thyroid hyperplasia compensates for the defect in thyroid hormone synthesis and their FT_4, FT_4I, and TSH levels are normal. If the increased follicle growth is not enough to compensate for the defect in hormone synthesis, patients are hypothyroid. These goiters can also be associated with hyperthyroidism if autonomous follicle growth is accompanied by excessive thyroid hormone secretion. In these cases, the nontoxic goiters have been transformed into toxic multinodular goiters (see Toxic Multinodular Goiter, below).

THYROTOXICOSIS

Thyrotoxicosis results from the actions of excess thyroid hormone from any cause on peripheral tissues. The terms *thyrotoxicosis* and *hyperthyroidism* often are used interchangeably, but *hyperthyroidism*

Table 4-4. Causes of Thyrotoxicosis

	RAIU	IODINE SCAN
Graves disease	High	Diffuse uptake
Toxic multinodular goiter	High	Patchy uptake
Toxic adenoma	High	Hot nodule
Thyroiditis	Low	Little uptake
Subacute granulomatous (de Quervain thyroiditis)		
Chronic lymphocytic (Hashimoto thyroiditis)		
Acute bacterial thyroiditis		
Radiation-indued thyroiditis		
Exogenous thyroid hormone	Low	Little uptake
Thyroid hormone pills		
Meat contaminated with thyroid tissue		
Rare causes of thyrotoxicosis		
TSH-secreting pituitary adenoma	High	Diffuse uptake
Metastatic thyroid cancer	High	Uptake in metastases
Ectopic thyroid tissue (struma ovarii)	High	Uptake in pelvis only
Trophoblastic tumor	High	Diffuse uptake

Note. RAIU = radioactive iodine uptake; TSH = thyroid-stimulating hormone.

Notes

refers specifically to overproduction of thyroid hormone by the thyroid gland. Major causes of thyrotoxicosis are listed in Table 4-4.

Common symptoms of thyrotoxicosis include hyperactivity, nervousness, fatigue, palpitations, excessive sweating, hyperdefecation, and heat intolerance. Menstruating women often have decreased menstrual flow or oligomenorrhea, possibly resulting from abnormal follicle-stimulating hormone (FSH) and luteinizing hormone (LH) pulses due to excess thyroid hormone. Signs of thyrotoxicosis include weight loss despite a good appetite (if the increase in caloric intake does not match the increase in caloric expenditure), lid lag and stare due to spasm of the upper eyelid, sinus tachycardia, atrial fibrillation, warm and moist skin, fine tremor of the outstretched hands, muscle weakness, and muscle wasting.

These symptoms and signs reflect the effects of excess thyroid hormone on several organ systems (Table 4-5). For example, excessive sweating is due to increased total body heat production (from liver and muscle) accompanied by increased cardiac output (heart contractility and heart rate), vasodilatation (peripheral vascular system), and increased sympathetic tone to the sweat glands (nervous system).

The combination of nervousness, tachycardia, sweating, lid lag, stare, and tremor suggests catecholamine excess. Plasma epinephrine levels are normal, but their effects may be increased. Beta blockers suppress the symptoms but do not treat the underlying disease. It is likely that excess thyroid hormone affects the heart and brain directly, independent of the adrenergic nervous system.

Table 4-5. Signs and Symptoms of Thyrotoxicosis

ORGAN SYSTEM	SIGNS AND SYMPTOMS
General	Fatigue, hyperactivity, and nervousness Heat intolerance and weight loss
Cardiovascular	Palpitations and rapid heart rate Increased cardiac output Atrial fibrillation
Gastrointestinal	Increased appetite and hyperdefecation
Musculoskeletal	Muscle weakness and muscle wasting Increased bone turnover and bone loss
Nervous	Hyperkinesia Lid lag and stare Fine tremor Rapid relaxation of deep tendon reflexes
Reproductive	Oligomenorrhea
Skin	Smooth, warm, and moist Excessive sweating
Growth (childhood)	Rapid growth Accelerated bone maturation

Typical Presentation of Thyrotoxicosis

Young patients: symptoms and signs of catecholamine excess
Elderly patients: apathetic hyperthyroidism

In older patients, manifestations of thyrotoxicosis are often very subtle. These patients may present with weight loss, fatigue, lethargy, and depression rather than signs of catecholamine excess. This presentation is called *apathetic hyperthyroidism*. This diagnosis should be considered in elderly patients who develop a new mood disorder.

Thyrotoxicosis can be treated with the antithyroid drugs methimazole or propylthiouracil. These are sulfonamide derivatives that inhibit oxidation and organic binding of thyroid iodide. Drug treatment must often be continued for many years, and the incidence of permanent remission is low (35%). Major side effects of these drugs include rash, a hepatitis-like reaction, and agranulocytosis (in approximately 1/1000 patients).

Patients can also be treated with radioactive iodine since iodine is selectively taken up by the thyroid gland without causing significant damage to other tissues. It is difficult to destroy enough thyroid tissue to restore the euthyroid state without causing hypothyroidism. At least 50% of patients successfully treated with radioactive iodine eventually require thyroid hormone supplementation.

Surgical treatment (subtotal thyroidectomy) can be performed after patients have been made euthyroid with antithyroid drugs.

Potential complications include damage to the recurrent laryngeal nerve with vocal cord paralysis and hoarseness, and damage to the parathyroid glands resulting in hypoparathyroidism. If too little thyroid tissue is removed, patients remain hyperthyroid; if too much is removed, patients develop hypothyroidism.

Treatment Options for Thyrotoxicosis

Antithyroid drugs
Radioactive iodine
Partial thyroidectomy

GRAVES DISEASE

Graves disease, an autoimmune disorder, is the most common cause of hyperthyroidism. It occurs in approximately 0.5% of the population and is more common in women than men. T lymphocytes become sensitized to thyroid antigens and stimulate B cells to produce antibodies. Nearly all patients with Graves disease have a high titer of an immunoglobulin of the IgG class that is directed against the TSH receptor. Interaction of the autoantibody with the TSH receptor stimulates the release of thyroid hormone from the thyroid gland. The autoantibody acts like TSH to stimulate the thyroid cell but does not cross-react with TSH in TSH immunoassays. This autoimmune disease often runs in families, with a very high concordance among monozygotic twins. The prevalence of Graves disease is higher in Caucasians who carry the human leukocyte antigens (HLA) HLA-B8 and HLA-DRw3, indicating that part of the genetic predisposition to Graves disease is linked to the HLA complex.

The autoantibody causes excess production of T_4 and T_3 independent of TSH. TSH is suppressed by high levels of T_3 and T_4 because the normal feedback regulation of the pituitary remains intact. The stimulatory action of the Graves immunoglobulin causes the thyroid gland to take up a large fraction of radioactive iodine in spite of the suppressed TSH. A radioactive iodine scan shows diffuse iodine uptake throughout an enlarged gland.

Graves disease is of particular concern during pregnancy because the IgG readily crosses the placenta and can stimulate the fetal or neonatal thyroid gland. If a woman with a history of Graves disease has a positive Graves IgG titer prior to delivery, her physician should be concerned about possible neonatal hyperthyroidism.

A smooth, diffuse goiter is almost always present although it may be difficult to palpate in elderly patients. Vascularity of the thyroid gland is increased, and a bruit may be heard over the goiter. Other specific signs include Graves eye signs (Graves ophthalmopathy) and a rare dermopathy known as pretibial myxedema.

Graves ophthalmopathy can be demonstrated in nearly all patients with Graves disease if sensitive tests are used. Lymphocytes directed to an unknown antigen infiltrate into the orbital tissues, especially the eye muscles. Lymphocyte infiltration is associated with production of cytokines and inflammation. The infiltration and inflammation produce congestion and swollen eye muscles. This causes forward displacement of the eyeball (proptosis), protrusion of the globe because there is no room in the bony orbit for additional tissue and fluid, and periorbital edema. The protrusion is known as exophthalmos (Figures 4-5 and 4-6). Eventually the eye muscles can become fibrotic. This leads to diplopia, which is most common on upward, outward gaze due to involvement of the inferior rectus muscle. Excessive intraorbital pressure can cause optic nerve compression and blindness in severe cases that are not treated appropriately.

Dermopathy occurs in only 2% to 3% of patients. The skin becomes markedly thickened over the pretibial areas due to the accumulation of glycosaminoglycans. Patients with Graves disease can also have separation of the fingernails from their beds (onycholysis).

Hallmarks of Graves Disease

Smooth diffuse goiter	High FT_3 and FT_4
Graves ophthalmopathy	Suppressed TSH
Dermopathy (rare)	High RAIU

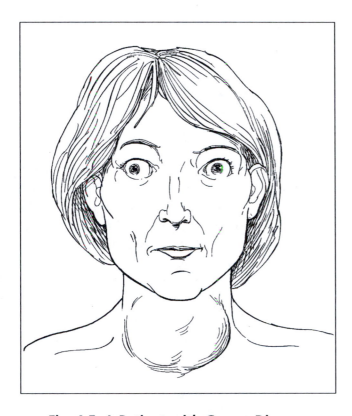

Fig. 4-5. A Patient with Graves Disease

Note the presence of exophthalmos and evidence of weight loss and goiter.

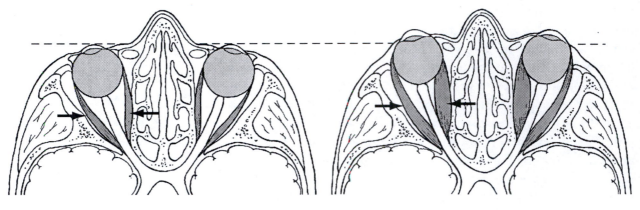

A. Normal   B. Graves' ophthalmopathy

Fig. 4-6. Graves Ophthalmopathy

Computed tomographic scans of the orbits in a normal subject (panel A) and in a patient with Graves opthalmopathy (panel B). Note the enlarged extraocular muscles in panel B. The *arrows* point to an enlarged medial rectus muscle. In panel A the *arrows* point to a normal lateral rectus muscle.

Notes

Treatment of Graves disease is directed toward reducing secretion of thyroid hormone. There is no way to target immune suppression for Graves IgG, and general immune suppression is unwarranted unless the ophthalmopathy is severe. If symptoms of thyrotoxicosis are severe, β-adrenergic blockade can be used until an antithyroid drug, radioactive iodine, or surgery has treated the underlying disease. The ophthalmopathy may not respond to the treatment for thyrotoxicosis, and patients with ophthalmopathy should be treated by ophthalmologists. Severe eye disease may require glucocorticoid therapy, external x-ray therapy, or surgery.

TOXIC MULTINODULAR GOITER

Toxic multinodular goiter (also called Plummer disease) usually occurs in patients older than 50 years of age. These patients often have a long history of a benign goiter and normal thyroid tests. Hyperthyroidism develops gradually and is usually less severe than that seen in Graves disease. The precise mechanism that leads to autonomous function of multiple nodules is unknown. In some cases, the hyperthyroidism is precipitated by the ingestion of large quantities of iodide, especially iodide-containing drugs like amiodarone and contrast dye.

The goiter may extend substernally, making it difficult to appreciate the full size of the gland. FT$_4$, FT$_3$, and the radioactive iodine uptake are high, and the TSH level is suppressed. A radioactive iodine scan reveals diffuse patchy uptake, with the more active areas taking up iodine more intensely. Treatment options for multinodular goiters are the same as those for Graves disease: antithyroid drugs, radioactive iodine, or surgery.

Toxic Adenoma (toxic nodule)

This condition is similar to multinodular goiter except that a single nodule accounts for the hyperthyroidism. Recent reports indicate that some of these nodules represent a clonal expansion of cells in which a somatic mutation in the TSH receptor has occurred. The mutation is associated with activation of the receptor in the absence of TSH. The excess thyroid hormone secreted by the nodule results in suppression of TSH.

A radioactive iodine scan reveals a single "hot" toxic nodule. These patients may be ideal candidates for radioactive iodine treatment. Since most of the gland is suppressed and will not take up the radioactive iodine, only the nodule is destroyed. After destruction of the nodule, TSH is no longer suppressed, and the rest of the gland can resume normal function. The incidence of hypothyroidism following radioactive iodine treatment for a toxic nodule is much lower than the incidence of hypothyroidism after similar treatment for Graves disease.

Thyroiditis

Several forms of thyroiditis are associated with thyrotoxicosis, which is caused by the release of stored thyroid hormone from a damaged gland. *Painful, subacute thyroiditis* (also called de Quervain thyroiditis and granulomatous thyroiditis) is an inflammatory disorder often associated with a viral infection. In addition to a painful, tender thyroid gland, patients have systemic symptoms such as fever, muscle aches, and a high erythrocyte sedimentation rate (ESR).

FT_4 and FT_3 are high and TSH is suppressed. However, since the thyroid gland is damaged, radioactive iodine uptake is very low. A radioactive iodine scan would reveal very little uptake throughout the gland. As the gland becomes depleted of stored hormone, circulating levels of T_3 and T_4 drop, and the suppressed TSH level begins to rise. Patients may then pass through a hypothyroid phase until the gland recovers and the patients return to euthyroidism.

No treatment is needed for the hyperthyroidism, which is self-limited, but β-adrenergic blockers can alleviate some of the symptoms. Aspirin is used for relief of fever and muscle aches. Glucocorticoid therapy may be necessary if the inflammation is severe.

Chronic lymphocytic thyroiditis (Hashimoto thyroiditis) is an autoimmune disease that is usually associated with hypothyroidism (see Hypothyroidism) but can also be associated in its early phase with transient hyperthyroidism. Autoimmune destruction of the thyroid gland leads to release of preformed hormone and transient hyperthyroidism. During the hyperthyroid phase, TSH and radioactive iodine uptake are suppressed. Many of these patients have ongoing destruction of the thyroid gland, leading to eventual hypothyroidism.

Acute bacterial thyroiditis and *radiation thyroiditis* can cause hyperthyroidism. The mechanism of hyperthyroidism is the same as the other forms of thyroiditis: release of preformed hormone from a damaged gland. These forms of thyroiditis are rare.

EXCESS THYROID HORMONE INGESTION (THYROIDITIS FACTITIA)

This condition can be self-induced, usually by patients trying to lose weight, or can be due to overtreatment of hypothyroidism. There is no goiter, since TSH is suppressed by exogenous hormone. Both ingestion of exogenous thyroid hormone and thyroiditis are associated with a high FT_4, low TSH, and suppressed radioactive iodine uptake. However, thyroiditis usually causes an elevation of serum thyroglobulin, which is released from the damaged gland. The thyroglobulin level is normal or low after exogenous hormone ingestion because TSH and endogenous hormone release are suppressed.

An epidemic of exogenous hyperthyroidism due to hamburger made from neck muscle contaminated with thyroid tissue was reported several years ago. Ground meat containing neck muscle can no longer be sold for human consumption.

OTHER CAUSES OF THYROTOXICOSIS

Other forms of thyrotoxicosis listed in Table 4-4 are very rare and can be difficult to diagnose. Hyperthyroidism caused by a TSH-producing tumor is distinguished by a high TSH level. In all other forms of thyrotoxicosis, TSH is suppressed. Metastatic thyroid carcinoma is occasionally able to produce enough thyroid hormone to cause thyrotoxicosis. Women with struma ovarii have mild thyrotoxicosis due to oversecretion of thyroid hormones by thyroid tissue within an ovarian teratoma. The ovarian thyroid tissue takes up iodine, but since TSH is suppressed, thyroid tissue does not. A trophoblastic tumor (hydatidiform mole) produces human chorionic gonadotropin (HCG), which has some TSH-like activity. If tumor production of HCG is very high, the thyroid gland is stimulated to overproduce its hormones.

Hypothyroidism

Hypothyroidism is the syndrome that results from a lack of thyroid hormone action on tissues and organ systems. Hypothyroidism can be classified as primary hypothyroidism, which results from failure of the thyroid gland; secondary hypothyroidism, which is due to pituitary failure; or tertiary hypothyroidism, which is caused by disorders of the hypothalamus. There are rare cases of hypothyroidism due to peripheral resistance to thyroid hormones. Affected individuals have abnormal thyroid hormone receptors or postreceptor defects.

The consequences are most severe when hypothyroidism presents in infancy. Untreated neonatal hypothyroidism results in irreversible cretinism. This syndrome includes mental retardation, growth failure, puffy hands and face, and often deaf-mutism. Hypothyroidism that develops later in childhood is associated with slowed mentation, retardation of bone development, decreased longitudinal growth, and delayed sexual maturation, which are reversible with treatment of the hypothyroidism.

CASE STUDY: *CONTINUED*

The individual signs and symptoms in this patient can be associated with a number of different diseases, but the overall constellation of signs and symptoms clearly indicate thyrotoxicosis. The differential diagnosis of the causes of thyrotoxicosis is relatively limited in this case. A soft, diffusely enlarged, nontender goiter suggests Graves disease rather than a multinodular goiter or a single hyperfunctioning nodule. Graves disease is the most common cause of hyperthyroidism, especially in a young woman. Excess exogenous thyroid hormone is unlikely because exogenous hormone would suppress TSH, and she would not have a goiter.

Lid lag and stare can be seen with thyrotoxicosis of almost any cause. They reflect the increased sympathetic tone associated with thyrotoxicosis. However, the diplopia with movement of the eye to the upper-outer quadrant indicates restriction of the inferior rectus muscle due to lymphocytic infiltration, which is specific for Graves ophthalmopathy.

The diagnosis of thyrotoxicosis was confirmed by the laboratory tests. She had elevated FT_4 and FT_3 levels. Her low TSH level showed that normal feedback inhibition was intact and that the excess thyroid hormone was independent of the pituitary and hypothalamus. The elevated radioactive iodine uptake showed that the source of excess thyroid hormone was from the thyroid gland, and the diffuse homogenous uptake over the enlarged gland indicated Graves disease. The diagnosis was confirmed by the elevated level of thyroid-stimulating immunoglobulin, the IgG responsible for the development of Graves thyroid disease.

She was treated with ^{131}I to destroy some of her thyroid tissue after a pregnancy test confirmed that she was not pregnant (radioactive iodine crosses the placenta). Two months later she felt much better and returned to her construction job. She did not return for follow-up because she felt well and did not think that further visits were necessary.

Two years after treatment she experienced symptoms again. She felt fatigued, her skin had become unusually dry, she was constipated, and her menses had been irregular and unusually heavy for several months. She returned for further evaluation.

Type of Hypothyroidism	Site of Defect
Primary hypothyroidism	Thyroid gland
Secondary hypothyroidism	Pituitary gland
Tertiary hypothyroidism	Hypothalamus
Thyroid hormone resistance	Peripheral tissues

Hypothyroidism can develop slowly and insidiously, and early symptoms are often nonspecific. As the disease progresses, more than 50% of patients complain of lethargy, fatigue, mental slowness, depression, cold intolerance, muscle aches, constipation, and dry, coarse skin. The most common physical findings are a delayed relaxation phase of deep tendon reflexes due to delayed muscle contraction, and cool, dry, coarse skin due to vasoconstriction. Additional symptoms and signs are listed in Table 4-6.

Hyperthyroidism causes weight loss, but hypothyroidism is not a common cause of obesity. Patients with hypothyroidism rarely gain more than 10% of their premorbid weight, and the weight gain is primarily due to accumulation of glycosaminoglycans and interstitial edema, not adipose tissue (Fig. 4-7). The interstitial edema may account, in part, for the association of hypertension with hypothyroidism. Hypothyroidism results in delayed absorption of nutrients and drugs, slower metabolism of drugs and anesthetics, decreased catabolism of LDL cholesterol, and decreased clearance of circulating enzymes. Aspartate aminotransferase (AST), alanine aminotransferase (ALT), and especially creatine kinase (CK) levels can be elevated.

Major deposition of glycosaminoglycans and interstitial edema in patients with hypothyroidism is referred to as **myxedema**.

Table 4-6. Signs and Symptoms of Hypothyroidism

ORGAN SYSTEM	SIGNS AND SYMPTOMS
General	Fatigue, lethargy, and cold intolerance
Cardiovascular	Slow heart rate and enlarged heart, decreased cardiac output, pericardial effusion, hypertension
Gastrointestinal	Constipation
Nervous	Slow speech, delayed relaxation of deep tendon reflexes; depression, mental retardation (neonatal, untreated), dementia (especially in the elderly)
Musculoskeletal	Muscle cramps
Circulatory	Anemia
Renal	Impaired water excretion and mild hyponatremia
Reproductive	Ovulatory failure, irregular menses and menorrhalgia, oligospermia, decreased libido
Skin	Cool, dry, and coarse skin; puffy face
Interstitial tissue	Accumulation of glycosaminoglycans, capillary leak, and loss of albumin
Growth (childhood)	Delayed bone age and short stature

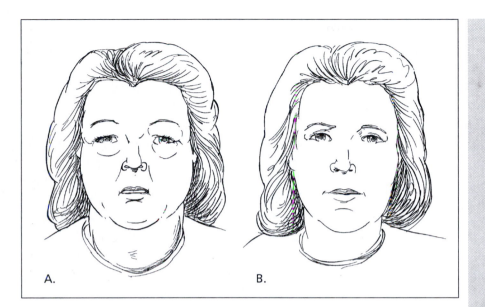

Fig. 4-7. Patient with Hypothyroidism before (A) and after (B) Treatment

Very severe, untreated hypothyroidism results in weakness, hypothermia, hypoventilation, water retention, hyponatremia, hypoglycemia, bradycardia, pericardial effusion, shock, depression, and severe stupor (sometimes called myxedema coma).

PRIMARY HYPOTHYROIDISM

Primary hypothyroidism is characterized by a low FT_4 or FT_4I and a low or low-normal FT_3 or FT_3I. The TSH level is high, as the pituitary gland responds to the low level of circulating thyroid hormones. Major causes of primary hypothyroidism are listed in Table 4-7.

Table 4-7. Causes of Hypothyroidism

TYPE OF HYPOTHYROIDISM	CAUSES

Primary hypothyroidism	Autoimmune disease
	    Chronic lumphocytic thyroiditis (Hashimoto thyroiditis)
	    Antibodies inhibiting the TSH receptor
	Gland destruction
	    Surgery
	    Radioactive iodine
	    External radiation
	Dietary goitrogens
	Drugs
	Iodine deficiency
	Congenital defects

Secondary hypothyroidism	pituitary disease
Tertiary hypothyroidism	Hypothalamic disorders

Note. TSH = thyroid-stimulating hormone.

Chronic Lymphocytic Thyroiditis (Hashimoto thyroiditis)

This disease, the most common cause of hypothyroidism in the United States, is due to autoimmune destruction of the thyroid gland. The specific thyroid antigens that activate the T lymphocytes and lead to destruction of the thyroid are unknown. Hashimoto disease is associated with the production of specific antibodies directed against thyroglobulin and thyroid peroxidase, but the evidence suggests that these antibodies are the result rather than the cause of thyroid damage. They are useful markers of Hashimoto thyroiditis, and their presence in high titers helps to confirm the diagnosis.

Destruction of the thyroid gland occurs slowly over the course of many years. As the gland is destroyed and the serum T_4 level falls, a compensatory rise in the serum TSH level often allows the serum T_3 level to remain normal, and the patient to remain symptom free. The constellation of a low T_4 level, an elevated TSH level, and a normal T_3 level is known as the "failing gland" syndrome. Although the patients are clinically euthyroid during this phase, the rise in TSH and the lymphocytic infiltration of the thyroid gland can produce very firm goiters that can become quite large. Patients who develop overt hypothyroidism have low FT_4 and FT_3 and high TSH levels. Radioactive iodine uptake is low.

Hashimoto thyroiditis and Graves disease are autoimmune diseases. They may be familial, they are associated with specific HLA haplotypes, and they may be associated with autoimmune destruction of other endocrine glands. Some patients have features of both Graves disease and Hashimoto disease (a condition known as Hashitoxicosis).

Antibodies to the TSH Receptor

Antibodies to the TSH receptor have been found in some patients. These autoantibodies are inhibitory, not stimulatory like the antibodies to the receptor associated with Graves disease, and they lead to thyroid gland atrophy.

Thyroid Ablation

Another common cause of hypothyroidism is ablation of the thyroid gland secondary to surgery or radioactive iodine therapy. Radioactive iodine damages thyroid cell DNA. Hypothyroidism may develop over several weeks or may take as long as 30 years. External radiation to the neck can also destroy the thyroid gland.

Subacute Thyroiditis (resolving phase)

Patients in the resolving phase of subacute thyroiditis may develop hypothyroidism (see above). This is usually temporary, but some patients fail to recover fully and remain hypothyroid.

Dietary Goitrogens and Drugs

Foods such as cassava, cabbage, bamboo shoots, and sweet potatoes contain compounds that interfere with the synthesis of thyroid hormones in the thyroid. Foods grown in soils that contain natural goitrogens or goitrogens from industrial wastes may accumulate enough of these compounds to cause goiters and hypothyroidism. Medications can also do this. Lithium, for example, inhibits thyroid hormone synthesis. Drugs that contain excess iodine, like amiodarone, cause hypothyroidism in some patients. The antithyroid drugs propylthiouracil and methimazole, which interfere with thyroid hormone synthesis, also produce hypothyroidism.

Iodine Deficiency

This is a common cause of hypothyroidism worldwide, although it is rare in the United States, where many foods and salt are supplemented with iodide. Because there is no underlying destruction of the thyroid gland, the associated rise in TSH leads to the development of a goiter. If the iodine deficiency persists for many years, the goiter may remain even after successful iodine replacement.

Congenital Defects

A number of congenital defects of the thyroid gland are associated with decreased synthesis or secretion of thyroid hormones and hypothyroidism (see Table 4-1). In response to low thyroid hormone levels, pituitary secretion of TSH increases and causes development of a goiter. Administration of iodine may exacerbate the defect in thyroid hormone synthesis or secretion. Congenital hypothyroidism can also be due to congenital absence of a thyroid gland.

SECONDARY AND TERTIARY HYPOTHYROIDISM

Primary pituitary or hypothalamic disease can result in TSH insufficiency and secondary and tertiary hypothyroidism, respectively. Usually this is associated with other pituitary hormone deficiencies. The thyroid gland does produce some thyroid hormone in the absence of TSH, so secondary hypothyroidism is usually not severe. The serum TSH level is low or low-normal and is not a reliable marker for hypothyroidism. In these patients, the diagnosis is based on symptoms and signs of hypothyroidism, a low FT_4, and evidence (clinical, laboratory, x-ray) of other defects in pituitary function.

THERAPY OF HYPOTHYROIDISM

Primary hypothyroidism is almost always treated by administration of T_4. The plasma half-life of T_4 is 7 to 10 days, so daily administration of replacement hormone does not cause large fluctuations in the plasma concentration of T_4. Peripheral tissue conversion of T_4 to T_3 supplies the active hormone. The dose of T_4 is increased gradually until the serum TSH level is within the normal range. Adjustments in the dosage should be made at 4 to 6 week intervals, after steady-state concentrations of the hormone are attained. Doses for patients with ischemic heart disease may need to be adjusted more slowly.

Secondary hypothyroidism is also treated with replacement of T_4. In these patients, the serum TSH level cannot be used to titrate the replacement dose of hormone. Rather, the physician must rely on changes in signs and symptoms while monitoring the serum FT_4 or FT_4I. Most patients' TSH levels will be appropriately replaced when the FT_4 is near the upper limits of normal.

CASE STUDY: *RESOLUTION*

When the patient returned to the clinic her blood pressure was 140/90, her heart rate was 55, and her temperature was 97.2°F. Her skin was dry and her hair was thinning. She had no lid lag, but diplopia was still present. She had no goiter. Her heart sounds were normal but distant. Deep tendon reflexes showed a marked delay in the relaxation phase.

Laboratory tests revealed a low FT_4 level. The TSH level was 90 µU/mL (normal: 0.4–5.5). The electrocardiogram (ECG) showed sinus bradycardia and low voltage. Her total cholesterol level was higher than before.

The patient's symptoms and signs suggested hypothyroidism. Insufficient thyroid hormone causes bradycardia; vasoconstriction resulting in cool, dry, coarse skin; decreased bowel motility; and delayed muscle relaxation. Hypertension, distant heart sounds, and ECG showing low voltage are due to accumulation of fluid in interstitial spaces, resulting in pericardial fluid accumulation and decreased vascular compliance. Menstrual changes are due to failure of ovulation, possibly due to inadequate luteinizing hormone and progesterone production, resulting in endometrial proliferation and excessive breakthrough bleeding (see Chapter 12). Metabolic processes, including cholesterol catabolism, are decreased in patients with hypothyroidism.

The low FT_4 level confirms the hypothyroidism. A high TSH level shows that the hypothyroidism is due to failure of the thyroid gland and that the pituitary-hypothalamic feedback axis is intact. The patient's hypothyroidism was most likely due to destruction of her gland by previous radioiodine therapy. This is consistent with the absence of a goiter despite a high TSH level. Patients treated with radioiodine need continuing follow-up because of the high incidence of subsequent hypothyroidism. She was treated with thyroxine replacement.

REVIEW QUESTIONS

Directions: For each of the following questions, choose the *one best* answer.

1 A 20-year-old university student came to the clinic because she had been unable to concentrate for several months and her test scores had fallen significantly. Her appetite had increased, she had trouble sleeping because her apartment was too hot, and she was awakened by palpitations. Physical examination revealed the following: a heart rate of 120 beats/min, slight lid lag, a smooth goiter, and warm, moist skin. Hyperthyroidism was suspected and several tests were ordered. Which of the following results was most consistent with Graves disease?

A Low free thyroxine (FT_4), low triiodothyronine (T_3), and low thyroid-stimulating hormone (TSH)

B High T_3, low TSH, and high radioactive iodine uptake (RAIU)

C High FT_4, high TSH, low RAIU

D High TSH, high RAIU, and low thyroid-stimulating immunoglobulin

2 Eighteen years later the patient returns to the clinic. She is now 38 years old and feels older than her age. She complains of fatigue and dry skin, and her menses are more infrequent and heavier than usual. Physical examination reveals that her pulse is 58 beats/min, her thyroid gland is not palpable, and her deep tendon reflexes show a slow relaxation phase. Laboratory tests reveal the following: TSH, 58 µU/mL (normal: 0.4–5.0 µU/mL) and low FT_4. Her chart confirms that she was treated with radioactive iodine for Graves disease 18 years ago and had normal thyroid tests for several years after treatment. Which of the following is the most likely diagnosis?

A Recurrent hyperthyroidism

B Chronic lymphocytic thyroiditis

C Graves ophthalmopathy

D Pituitary failure (secondary hypothyroidism)

E Hypothyroidism due to previous radioactive iodine therapy

3 A fourth-year medical student is on an international medicine rotation in a remote mountain region. The student notices that many of the local residents have large goiters. According to local residents, the goiters developed after a new commercial mining operation opened. The student wonders if the mining operation is discharging a chemical into the town's water supply that inhibits release of T_4 and T_3 from thyroidal thyroglobulin. If this hypothesis is correct, which of the following test results would one expect?

A A high TSH level because the circulating FT_4 level is low

B A high serum FT_4 level because the thyroid is large and full of thyroglobulin

C A low TSH level because the excess intrathyroidal T_4 inhibits the release of thyrotropin-releasing hormone (TRH)

D A high serum T_3 level and a low TSH level because of increased intrathyroidal conversion of T_4 to T_3

4 A 29-year-old woman comes to the clinic complaining of lack of energy, occasional headaches, muscle aches, and irregular menses. She takes no medications or over-the-counter products. She appears depressed. Physical examination reveals a heart rate of 60, dry skin, mild periorbital edema, a thyroid gland that is difficult to palpate, and delayed deep tendon reflex relaxation. A pregnancy test is negative. Laboratory testing reveals low FT_4 and low TSH. Her differential diagnosis should include

A autoimmune thyroiditis with a low T_3

B a large pituitary tumor with low gonadotropin levels

C a hypothalamic lesion resulting in high TRH and low T_3

D unreported thyroxine ingestion to lose weight

5 A male patient has lost weight despite having a good appetite. His eyes have become more prominent (proptosis), and he has developed double vision (diplopia). Further examination reveals tachycardia, lid lag, stare, goiter, proximal muscle weakness, tremor, and rapid relaxation of deep tendon reflexes. The physician suspects

A decreased cardiac contractility and vasoconstriction

B reduced lipid, protein, and bone turnover

C increased metabolic rate and heat production

D infiltration of extraocular muscles by malignant cells

6 A 66-year-old man complains of fatigue. He has mild weight loss and his heart rate has increased over the past 3 years. Physical examination reveals an enlarged, bilaterally irregular, nontender thyroid gland that is slowly increasing in size. His FT_4 level has been increasing slowly, and his TSH level has dropped below the normal range. Further evaluation would most likely reveal

A a strong family history of thyroid disease

B increased patchy uptake of radioactive iodine

C increased iodine uptake by a toxic nodule

D low radioactive iodine uptake due to thyroiditis

E hyperthyroidism due to thyroid cancer

References

Boyages SC: Iodine deficiency disorders. *J Clin Endocrinol Metab* 77: 587–591, 1993.

Braverman LE: The physiology and pathophysiology of iodine and the thyroid. *Thyroid* 11: 405, 2001.

Ekholm R: Biosynthesis of thyroid hormones. *Int Rev Cytol* 120: 243–288, 1990.

Francois D, Burgi H, Chen ZP, et al: World status of monitoring iodine deficiency disorders control programs. *Thyroid* 12: 915–924, 2002.

Freake HC, Oppenheimer JH: Thermogenesis and thyroid function. *Ann Rev Nutr* 15: 263–291, 1995.

Klein I, Ojamaa K: Thyroid hormone and the cardiovascular system. *N Engl J Med* 344: 501–509, 2001.

LiVolsi VA: The pathology of autoimmune thyroid disease: a review. *Thyroid* 4: 333–339, 1994.

Pearce EN, Farwell AP, Braverman LE: Thyroiditis. *N Engl J Med* 348: 26, 2003.

Singer PA, Cooper DS, Levy ES, et al: Treatment guidelines for patients with hyperthyroidism and hypothyroidism. *JAMA* 273: 808–812, 1995.

Staub J-J, Althaus BU, Engler H, et al: Spectrum of subclinical and overt hypothyroidism: effect on thyrotropin, prolactin and thyroid reserve, and metabolic impact on peripheral target tissues. *Am J Med* 92: 631–642, 1992.

Toft AD: Clinical practice. Subclinical hyperthyroidism. *N Engl J Med* 345: 512–516, 2001.

Wiersinga WM, Bartalena L: Epidemiology and prevention of Graves' ophthalmopathy. *Thyroid* 12: 855–860, 2002.

5

The Adrenal Cortex

John P. Bantle, M.D., and Nacide G. Ercan-Fang, M.D.

▓ CHAPTER OUTLINE ▓

▓ LEARNING OBJECTIVES ▓

At the completion of this chapter, the student will:

1. understand how the adrenal hormones cortisol, aldosterone, and dehydroepiandrosterone (DHEA) are produced and regulated.
2. be able to describe the biologic effects of cortisol, aldosterone, and dehydroepiandrosterone.
3. understand the most important tests of adrenal function.
4. be familiar with commonly used pharmacologic adrenal steroid preparations.
5. understand the major disorders of adrenal insufficiency and adrenal hormone excess.

CASE STUDY: *INTRODUCTION*

A 16-year-old boy first noted easy fatigability during high-school summer vacation. By the following November, he had to stop and rest after climbing two flights of stairs. He found himself exhausted after his school day and usually went to bed upon arriving home from school. He was frequently nauseated and occasionally vomited. His weight had decreased 8 lb since the summer.

In December he was hospitalized due to weakness. He was unable to get out of bed without assistance, experienced continuous nausea and intermittent vomiting, and was noted to have episodes of confusion and disorientation. Physical examination was remarkable for blood pressure of 90/70 mm Hg supine and 60/40 mm Hg upright. He had a "dark" complexion, but his examination otherwise was normal. Laboratory tests revealed a low serum sodium (Na^+) level and a high serum potassium (K^+) level. His physician told his parents that he might not live beyond Christmas. A diagnostic test was performed.

Adrenal Physiology

The adrenal glands are located just above the kidneys. They are triangular in shape and are composed of an outer cortex and an inner medulla. Although the cortex and the medulla are contained within the same capsule, they are derived from different tissues and function as separate entities. The adrenal medulla is an extension of the sympathetic nervous system and is discussed in Chapter 6. The adrenal cortex produces three types of steroid hormones: glucocorticoid hormones, so called because of their influence on glucose metabolism; mineralocorticoids, which regulate Na^+ and K^+ balance; and dehydroepiandrosterone (DHEA), which can be converted into androgens.

Major Adrenal Cortex Hormones

Glucocorticoid: cortisol (hydrocortisone)
Mineralocorticoid: aldosterone
Androgen: dehydroepiandrosterone (DHEA)

The adult adrenal cortex is composed of three zones. The outer zona glomerulosa produces aldosterone and is regulated primarily by the renin-angiotensin system. The thicker middle zona fasciculata, with its columns of cells, and the compact innermost zona reticularis produce cortisol and androgens and are regulated by ACTH from the pituitary gland as described below.

STEROID HORMONE BIOSYNTHESIS AND REGULATION

Secretion of cortisol and adrenal androgens is regulated by the hypo-thalamic-pituitary-adrenal axis (Fig. 5-1). The hypothalamic and pituitary components of this axis are corticotropin-releasing hormone (CRH) and ACTH.

Corticotropin-Releasing Hormone

CRH is a 41–amino acid peptide produced in the hypothalamus. It is also present in other areas of the brain, the pancreas, and the intestine. Its purpose in these areas is not understood. CRH produced in the hypothalamus is secreted into the portal vessels reaching the pituitary. CRH stimulates adrenocorticotropic hormone synthesis and secretion by the pituitary.

Stress of all kinds (e.g., major illness, surgery, injury, exercise, hypo-glycemia, starvation) *increases* CRH secretion. CRH is under negative feedback control from cortisol, which *decreases* CRH synthesis and secretion.

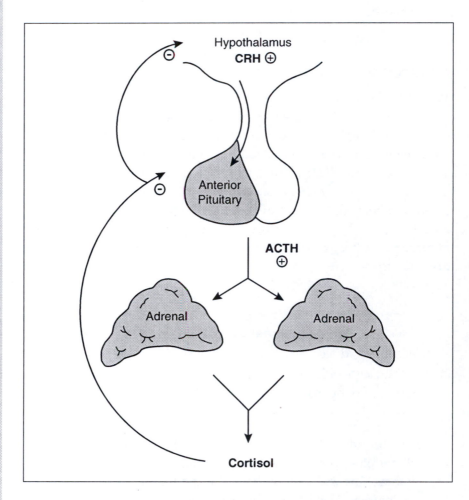

Fig. 5-1. Regulation of Adrenal Cortisol Secretion by the Hypothalamic-Pituitary-Adrenal Axis

CRH = corticotropin-releasing hormone; ACTH = adrenocorticotropic hormone; + = stimulation; − = negative feedback inhibition.

Regulators of ACTH Secretion

CRH pulses
Superimposed stress (via CRH)
Negative feedback from cortisol

Adrenocorticotropic Hormone

ACTH is produced by pituitary corticotrophs, which comprise about 15% of pituitary cells and are clustered in the central pituitary. ACTH is a 39–amino acid peptide derived from a larger precursor molecule called pro-opiomelanocortin. Pro-opiomelanocortin is cleaved to yield ACTH and β-lipotropin, which are secreted together.

ACTH is secreted in pulses with a diurnal rhythm superimposed upon the pulses. The highest plasma ACTH concentrations occur in the early morning (4:00–6:00 AM); the lowest ACTH concentrations occur at night. This diurnal rhythm is abolished by stress, which causes increased ACTH secretion at all times of the day or night. ACTH has a half-life in the circulation of less than 10 minutes.

ACTH *stimulates* the adrenal glands to secrete cortisol. In turn, cortisol *inhibits* ACTH synthesis and secretion by negative feedback. ACTH also stimulates adrenal aldosterone secretion, but the renin-angiotensin system is the primary regulator of aldosterone. ACTH, β-lipotropin, or one of their subfragments stimulates melanocytes to produce melanin and thereby increase skin pigmentation.

Biosynthesis of Cortisol and Adrenal Androgens

Pituitary ACTH binds to specific receptors on the surface of adrenal cortical cells and is the primary regulator of adrenal cortisol production. This receptor binding activates adenyl cyclase, leading to an increase in cyclic adenosine monophosphate (cAMP). cAMP then activates protein kinases, which initiate ACTH action.

Acutely, ACTH stimulates removal of the 6-carbon side chain from cholesterol to form pregnenolone, which is the first and rate-limiting step in cortisol synthesis (Fig. 5-2). This effect occurs minutes after ACTH secretion by the pituitary. Chronically, ACTH stimulates the formation of all enzymes involved in steroid synthesis.

ACTH is also the primary regulator of adrenal androgen production. Although adrenal androgens like DHEA and androstenedione are produced in substantial amounts, they are considerably less potent than the gonadal androgen testosterone.

Biosynthesis of Aldosterone

Aldosterone secretion is under the primary control of the renin–angiotensin system. Renin is a proteolytic enzyme produced by the juxtaglomerular (JG) cells of the kidney. The JG cells surround glomerular afferent arterioles. The substrate for renin is angiotensinogen, which is converted by renin into angiotensin I. Angiotensin I is

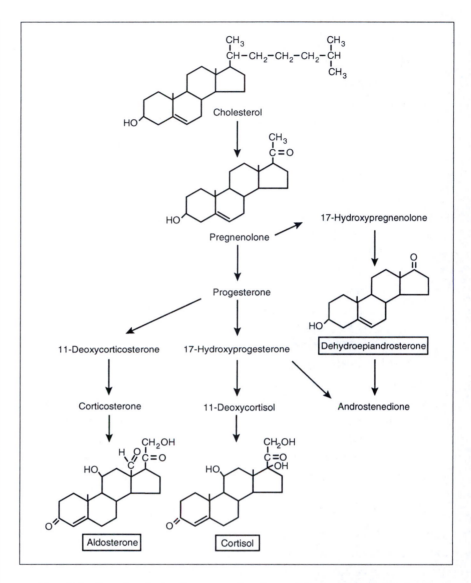

Fig. 5-2. Synthetic Pathways of Adrenal Steroid Production

These pathways lead to three products: cortisol (glucocorticoid), aldosterone (mineralocorticoid), and dehydroepiandrosterone (androgen precursor).

converted to angiotensin II by angiotensin-converting enzyme, which is present primarily in the pulmonary vascular endothelium. Angiotensin II stimulates adrenal aldosterone secretion; it is also a potent pressor that acts directly on arteriolar smooth muscle. Adrenal aldosterone secretion is stimulated by:

1. reduced renal afferent arteriolar pressure (stimulates renin secretion by the JG cells). The increased secretion of aldosterone results in renal sodium retention and expansion of extracellular fluid volume, which tends to raise blood pressure.
2. increased sympathetic nervous system activity.
3. increased serum K^+, which stimulates aldosterone secretion directly.
4. ACTH, which also stimulates aldosterone secretion directly.

Stimulators of Aldosterone Secretion

Renin-angiotensin system

Sympathetic nervous system

Increased serum K$^+$

ACTH

Figure 5-2 summarizes the synthetic pathways for adrenal steroid production. Note that there are three major pathways leading to cortisol, aldosterone, and adrenal androgens such as DHEA and androstenedione.

STEROID HORMONE TRANSPORT IN BLOOD

After cortisol is secreted into the bloodstream, approximately 90% becomes protein bound. Cortisol's primary transport protein is cortisol-binding globulin (CBG). However, cortisol is in dynamic equilibrium between protein-bound and free forms. It is the free cortisol that is able to leave the vascular compartment, enter cells, and initiate hormone actions. Aldosterone and androgens are also bound to transport proteins.

MECHANISM OF ACTION OF ADRENAL STEROID HORMONES

Adrenal cortex hormones are typical steroid hormones. Free cortisol molecules in the circulation enter cells of target tissues and bind to specific glucocorticoid receptor proteins present in the cytosol. The binding of cortisol to its receptor causes a modification in the receptor molecule, changing it to a protein with high affinity for DNA. This process is called activation. The cortisol-receptor complex then moves to the nucleus (translocation) and binds to specific sites on specific genes. This binding causes increased transcription of specific RNA sequences and synthesis of specific proteins. These proteins become the mediators of the biologic effects of cortisol.

Binding of the cortisol-receptor complex to other specific genes results in decreased transcription of RNA sequences and decreased translation of the related proteins. Thus, cortisol causes an increase in the synthesis of certain proteins and a decrease in the synthesis of other proteins. The mechanism of action of cortisol is summarized in Fig. 5-3.

BIOLOGIC EFFECTS OF ADRENAL HORMONES

Cortisol

Cortisol is the principal glucocorticoid hormone of the adrenal cortex. It promotes the conversion of amino acids to glucose (gluconeogenesis) in the liver by stimulating enzymes of the gluconeogenic pathway. Cortisol also increases protein catabolism, which increases the supply of amino acids for gluconeogenesis. Cortisol inhibits glucose uptake by muscle and fat, resulting in insulin resistance. Cortisol promotes glycogen deposition by stimulating the enzymes required

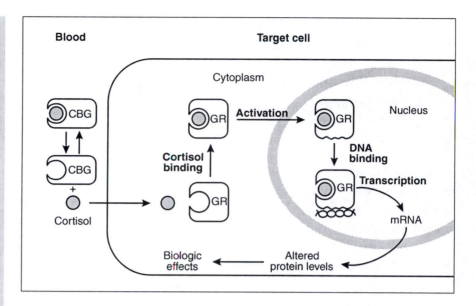

Fig. 5-3. Mechanism of Cellular Cortisol Action

CBG = cortisol-binding globulin; GR = glucocorticoid receptor.

for glycogen synthesis, but the net effect of cortisol is to increase the blood glucose concentration. In adipose tissue, cortisol stimulates lipolysis, which releases free fatty acids into the circulation. Free fatty acids supply energy for muscle and other non-glucose-dependent tissues.

Major Metabolic Effects of Cortisol

Carbohydrate metabolism
Increased gluconeogenesis
Increased insulin resistance
Increased blood glucose
Increased glycogen synthesis

Fat metabolism
Increased lipolysis and free fatty acids

Protein metabolism
Increased protein breakdown
Increased urinary nitrogen excretion

When cortisol is present in excess as a result of stress, adrenal hyperfunction, or pharmacologic administration, it has many additional effects. It stimulates appetite, causing increased energy intake and weight gain. Cortisol suppresses inflammation and immune function, the primary reasons why cortisol and its analogs are used pharmacologically. Cortisol suppresses bone formation and has catabolic effects on bone, connective tissue, and muscle, which result in loss of bone mass, poor wound healing, easy bruising, loss of muscle mass, and weakness. Cortisol inhibits linear growth in children. Excess cortisol can also alter mood, sometimes resulting in euphoria, insomnia, and even psychosis.

Major Biologic Effects of Increased Cortisol

Weight gain and truncal obesity

Na^+ and water retention

Suppressed inflammation

Suppressed immune system

Inhibited fibroblasts, loss of connective tissue, thin skin, easy bruising, abdominal striae, impaired wound healing

Growth failure in children

Decreased calcium absorption

Osteoblast inhibition

Bone loss

Altered mood, behavior, and cognition

Cortisol has mineralocorticoid activity. It binds very well to the mineralocorticoid receptor, the same receptor that binds aldosterone. However, in the kidney, most cortisol is converted to inactive cortisone by the enzyme 11β-hydroxysteroid dehydrogenase type 2. Excess cortisol increases blood pressure due to increased salt and water retention.

Aldosterone

Aldosterone is the principal adrenal mineralocorticoid. It exerts its effects by binding to mineralocorticoid receptors, particularly in the kidney. It promotes Na^+ retention by reducing urinary sodium excretion by the distal renal tubule and collecting ducts. Aldosterone also increases urinary K^+ and hydrogen ion (H^+) excretion.

DHEA and Other Adrenal Androgens

These are weak androgens. They do not have any known important effect in adult males because of the presence of more potent testicular androgens such as testosterone. However, adrenal androgens are important in the maintenance of female axillary and pubic hair and perhaps libido. If present in excess, adrenal androgens can cause hirsutism (abnormal facial and body hair) and masculinization of females and prepubertal males.

Tests of Adrenal Function

PLASMA HORMONE LEVELS

Although it is possible to measure plasma levels of ACTH and a wide variety of adrenal cortical hormones, such measurements are often not very helpful. Many of these hormones are secreted in pulses with a diurnal rhythm and demonstrate substantial variation with time of day. In addition, hormones such as ACTH and cortisol are secreted in response to stress, so their concentrations can fluctuate substantially. Cortisol, in particular, is best measured under defined conditions such as after ACTH stimulation or dexamethasone suppression (discussed further below). Aldosterone secretion is dependent in large part on Na^+ intake; thus it is also best measured under defined conditions. Tests of adrenal function are listed in Table 5-1.

Plasma levels of androgens may be helpful in cases of apparent androgen excess in boys and girls or women. DHEA and its metabolite dehydroepiandrosterone-sulfate (DHEAS) are the adrenal androgens usually measured. When a congenital enzyme defect is suspected, measuring the serum level of the precursor just prior to the block, can help make the diagnosis. For instance, measurement of 17-hydroxy-progesterone can be used to make the diagnosis of 21-hydroxylase deficiency.

URINARY STEROID EXCRETION

Urinary steroid excretion is often measured to assess adrenal cortex hormone production. Non–protein-bound cortisol in blood is filtered by the kidney and excreted unchanged in the urine. Conditions in which free cortisol is increased in blood result in increased urine free cortisol (UFC). UFC is determined after collection of a 24-hour urine specimen and is expressed per gram of urinary creatinine. Measuring urinary steroids over 24 hours gives an integrated picture of hormone production over the course of the entire day. Expressing the result per gram of creatinine takes into account body muscle mass and the possibility that the patient has provided a 24-hour urine collection that is not complete. UFC is measured by high performance liquid

---

Table 5-1. Tests of Adrenal Function

Plasma Hormone Levels	Localizing ACTH Overproduction
ACTH	CRH stimulation test
Cortisol	High-dose dexamethasone suppression
Aldosterone	
17-Hydroxyprogesterone	**Adrenal Insufficiency**
11-Deoxycortisol	ACTH stimulation tests
Dehydroepiandrosterone	
Dehydroepiandrosterone sulfate	**Pituitary Insufficiency**
Androstenedione	Metyrapone test
	CRH stimulation test
Urine 24-Hour Steroid Excretion	
Urine free cortisol	**Aldosterone Overproduction**
	Aldosterone suppression test
Screening for Cushing Syndrome	Plasma renin activity
Urine free cortisol	
1 mg (overnight) dexamethasone suppression test	
2-day (low-dose) dexamethasone suppression test	

chromatography or gas chromatography combined with mass spectrometry, or, less specifically, by a radioimmunoassay for cortisol in urine.

Cortisol Underproduction (Adrenal Hypofunction)

ACTH Stimulation Tests

These tests assess the ability of the adrenal cortex to increase cortisol secretion in response to ACTH. Three ACTH stimulation tests are used: the 4-hour ACTH stimulation test, the rapid ACTH stimulation test, and the low-dose ACTH stimulation test.

The 4-hour test is performed as follows: at approximately 8:00 AM, a plasma sample for cortisol is obtained. For the next 4 hours, a high dose of synthetic ACTH (cosyntropin 250 µg) is infused intravenously. At approximately noon, a second plasma sample for cortisol is obtained. In a normal individual, plasma cortisol will increase to a value greater than 17 to 18 µg/dL after ACTH infusion. In someone with adrenal insufficiency, the adrenal glands do not respond normally and the increase in plasma cortisol is subnormal.

Sometimes a shortened version of the ACTH stimulation test is done for screening purposes. In this "rapid" ACTH stimulation test, a bolus of ACTH is administered intravenously, and plasma cortisol is checked 60 minutes later. If the rapid test is abnormal, the 4-hour ACTH test should be performed to establish the diagnosis of adrenal insufficiency.

In the low-dose ACTH stimulation test, ACTH is given intravenously at a physiologic dose (cosyntropin 1 µg). This test may be helpful in distinguishing more subtle defects in cortisol secretion due to chronic pituitary disease, where the sluggish adrenal response is due to lack of ACTH stimulation (secondary adrenal insufficiency).

Hypothalamic-Pituitary-Adrenal Function

After pituitary surgery or trauma, or a period of pituitary suppression by exogenous steroids, it is sometimes necessary to determine whether the pituitary can produce enough ACTH for times of stress. In the past, the cortisol response to the stress of insulin-induced hypoglycemia was used to test ACTH secretion. This involved some risk, so induced hypoglycemia has been replaced by the metyrapone and CRH stimulation tests.

Metyrapone Test

Metyrapone blocks the last step in cortisol synthesis. If the hypothalamus and pituitary are able to respond to the low cortisol level by increasing production of CRH and ACTH, there will be an abrupt increase in 11-deoxycortisol, the immediate precursor of cortisol. This tests the entire hypothalamic-pituitary-adrenal axis. Patients must be monitored carefully when cortisol is low.

CRH Stimulation Test

An intravenous infusion of CRH is used to elicit an ACTH response.

CORTISOL OVERPRODUCTION

Urine Free Cortisol (UFC)

As indicated above, UFC is increased under conditions of cortisol over-production due to pituitary or adrenal disease. However, other conditions such as depression, anxiety, severe obesity, alcoholism, and poorly controlled diabetes can also produce higher than normal levels of UFC. Additional tests to assess the hypothalamic-pituitary-adrenal axis are needed (Table 5-2).

Loss of Cortisol Diurnal Rhythm

Normal ACTH pulses are highest in the early morning, and plasma cortisol normally is highest between 7:00 and 8:00 AM. As ACTH pulses diminish, cortisol levels become progressively lower throughout the day and evening, with a nadir around midnight. Loss of this diurnal rhythm is one of the earliest signs of cortisol overproduction. A high *midnight plasma cortisol* level obtained from an unstressed, sleeping patient indicates cortisol overproduction, but this is not a practical test for outpatients. The saliva cortisol concentration is closely correlated with the plasma cortisol level, and *bedtime salivary cortisol* can be collected at home using a special sampling tube. A higher than normal level indicates cortisol overproduction. This has the potential to be a useful screening test. These tests are not valid for patients who normally do not sleep at night or who are traveling from other time zones.

Dexamethasone Suppression Tests

Dexamethasone is a long-acting cortisol analog that suppresses ACTH secretion but is not measured in the assay for cortisol. Failure of dexamethasone to suppress ACTH and cortisol levels indicates cortisol overproduction.

Table 5-2. Evaluation of Suspected Cushing Syndrome

TEST	PITUITARY CAUSE	ADRENAL CAUSE	ECTOPIC ACTH
PLASMA OR URINE FREE CORTISOL			
Plasma ACTH	High or high-normal	Suppressed	High or very high
Low-dose dexamethasone	No suppression	No suppression	No suppression
High-dose dexamethasone	Suppression	No suppression	No suppression
CRH stimulation	Response	No response	Variable
IMAGING RESULTS			
MRI pituitary	Adenoma	Negative	Negative
MRI/CT adrenals	Negative or hyperplasia	Mass or masses	Negative or hyperplasia

Note. ACTH = adrenocorticotropic hormone; CRH = corticotropin-releasing hormone; MRI = magnetic resonance imaging; CT = computed tomography.

One-mg Overnight Dexamethasone Suppression Test. One mg of dexamethasone is administered orally at 11:00 PM. At 8:00 AM the next day, a blood sample is obtained to determine the plasma cortisol level. In a healthy individual, plasma cortisol should be suppressed to less than 1.8 µg/dL. There are almost no false negative results; patients who suppress normally do not have cortisol overproduction. However, stress of any kind can cause a false positive result. Patients with malnutrition, malabsorption, obesity, depression, renal failure, and many other medical conditions may not suppress plasma cortisol normally, probably because the associated stress increases ACTH secretion. If the overnight dexamethasone suppression test is abnormal under these conditions, the 2-day (low-dose) dexamethasone suppression test can be used.

Two-Day (low dose) Desamethasone Suppresstion Test. Dexamethasone 0.5 mg is taken orally every 6 hours for 8 doses, and plasma cortisol is measured 2 or 6 hours after the last dose. Failure of dexamethasone to suppress ACTH and cortisol indicates cortisol overproduction (Table 5-2).

Dexamethasone-CRH. This test is cumbersome and is used only when other test results are equivocal. Dexamethasone is given to suppress the pituitary just as in the 2-day (low-dose) dexamethasone test. This is followed by intravenous CRH, and then plasma ACTH and cortisol are measured. A higher than normal cortisol response to CRH despite previous dexamethasone suppression indicates cortisol overproduction.

ACTH OVERPRODUCTION

If testing reveals excess cortisol production, a morning ACTH level should be measured. If the ACTH level is low (<10 pg/mL), cortisol production is independent of ACTH, and an adrenal gland tumor is likely. Adrenal tumor cortisol suppresses pituitary production of ACTH by negative feedback.

If the ACTH level is not suppressed, excess cortisol is most likely due to an ACTH-secreting pituitary tumor or to ectopic ACTH produced by a nonpituitary tumor such as a lung carcinoma. Additional tests must be done to determine the source of the ACTH.

CRH Stimulation Test

The plasma ACTH response to intravenous CRH is measured. Pituitary tumors are more likely to contain CRH receptors and to respond to CRH than are ectopic ACTH-producing tumors.

High-Dose Dexamethasone Suppression Test

Pituitary tumors producing ACTH are more likely than ectopic ACTH tumors to be suppressed by very large doses of dexamethasone. After a baseline plasma cortisol or UFC is obtained, 2 mg of dexamethasone is given every 6 hours for 2 days, or 8 mg of dexamethasone is given at night, with measurement of plasma cortisol the following morning or UFC the following day. If the cortisol is decreased by at least 50% from baseline, the source of ACTH is more likely to be a pituitary tumor (Table 5-2).

Pituitary Magnetic Resonance Imaging (MRI)

Pituitary MRI may reveal an adenoma, but these tumors are often hard to detect, and at least 10% of healthy people between the ages of 20 and 40 have incidental (benign, non-hormone-producing) pituitary nodules on MRI.

Inferior Petrosal Sinus Sampling (IPSS)

Blood leaving the anterior pituitary via pituitary veins collects first in the cavernous sinus on the same side and then reaches the inferior petrosal sinus on the same side. A skilled radiologist may be able to sample the blood in the petrosal sinuses after CRH is given. A large increase in ACTH on one side compared to the other indicates that the excess ACTH is produced by a pituitary tumor on that side.

ALDOSTERONE OVERPRODUCTION

A patient who has hyperaldosteronism should have a high plasma aldosterone level, and the sodium and water retention caused by the high aldosterone should suppress plasma renin activity. Therefore, high plasma aldosterone in the presence of low plasma renin activity indicates hyperaldosteronism. Hyperaldosteronism can also be assessed by the aldosterone suppression test. Normal saline is infused into the patient for 4 hours. This expands the extracellular volume, which should suppress plasma renin, thereby suppressing aldosterone. Patients with hyperaldosteronism do not have normal suppression of aldosterone in response to volume expansion.

Commonly Used Pharmacologic Adrenal-Steroid Preparations

Because cortisol (hydrocortisone) is the principal naturally occurring glucocorticoid, it is the preferred drug for treatment of adrenal insufficiency. Hydrocortisone replacement is given in divided doses, usually two-thirds in the morning and one-third at noon or in the early afternoon in an attempt to mimic the natural diurnal rhythm of cortisol secretion. Cortisone is also used to treat adrenal insufficiency, but cortisone must be converted in vivo to cortisol by 11β-hydroxylation before it becomes biologically active. This conversion is not complete, so cortisone is slightly less potent per unit weight than is cortisol.

Cortisol replacement provides considerable mineralocorticoid activity, but patients with adrenal insufficiency may require additional mineralocorticoid replacement to maintain salt and water balance. This can be provided by potent, synthetic fluorinated mineralocorticoids such as fludrocortisone.

Glucocorticoids are frequently prescribed for their anti-inflammatory and anti-immune properties rather than for treatment of adrenal insufficiency. In these situations pharmacologic rather than physiologic doses are required. Prednisone and dexamethasone are synthetic glucocorticoid analogs used to treat a wide variety of medical conditions.

Cortisol in large doses would have the same anti-inflammatory and anti-immune effects but would also have unwanted mineralocorticoid activity. When large doses of prednisone or dexamethasone are used chronically to treat a disease process, serious side effects are likely. These include opportunistic infections, hypertension, unmasking of latent diabetes mellitus, loss of bone mass (osteoporosis), psychiatric disorders, and growth retardation in children. Thus, the lowest effective dose of glucocorticoid should be used. Table 5-3 provides a summary of commonly used steroid preparations.

Disorders of the Adrenal Glands

PRIMARY ADRENAL INSUFFICIENCY (ADDISON DISEASE)

Adrenal insufficiency is rare, with a prevalence of 4 to 6 cases per 100,000 people. Until recently, tuberculosis was probably the most common cause of adrenal insufficiency. Now the most common cause is bilateral destruction of the adrenal glands by autoimmune adrenalitis. This is often associated with other autoimmune endocrine disorders such as type 1 diabetes mellitus, chronic lymphocytic thyroiditis, and vitiligo (patches of white, totally depigmented skin). Vitiligo is due to an autoimmune process that attacks melanocytes and can be a clue to the presence of autoimmune adrenalitis. Autoimmune adrenalitis is more common in women, as are other autoimmune endocrine disorders.

Major Diseases of the Adrenal Cortex

Adrenal insufficiency
Adrenal hyperfunction
Hyperaldosteronism
Congenital adrenal hyperplasia

Tuberculosis still is the major infectious cause of primary adrenal insufficiency. Adrenal gland destruction due to cytomegalovirus occurs as part of the acquired immunodeficiency syndrome (AIDS).

Table 5-3. Commonly Used Pharmacologic Steroid Preparations

NAME	RELATIVE GLUCO-CORTICOID POTENCY	RELATIVE MINERALO-CORTICOID POTENCY	DURATION OF BIOLOGIC ACTIVITY
Cortisol (hydrocortisone)	1	1	<12 hours
Cortisone	0.8	0.8	<12 hours
Prednisone*	4–5	0.25	24 hours
Dexamathasone*	30–40	Negligible	48 hours
Fludrocortisone* (Florinef)	Negligible	14	24 hours

* Not naturally occurring

Other causes of primary adrenal insufficiency include treatment with antifungal drugs (e.g., ketoconazole), adrenal hemorrhage, metastatic carcinoma, and surgical removal of the adrenal glands.

Major Causes of Adrenal Insufficiency

Autoimmune adrenalitis
Infection
Hemorrhage
Metastases
Surgery

Fatigue and weakness are common in patients with primary adrenal insufficiency, and adrenal insufficiency should always be considered in patients with unexplained weight loss. Nausea, anorexia, and abdominal pain are common symptoms, and women often have amenorrhea.

Primary Adrenal Insufficiency

Symptoms and Signs	Patients (%)
Weakness, fatigue	99
Hyperpigmentation	98
Unexplained weight loss	97
Anorexia, nausea, vomiting	90
Hypotension (blood pressure <110/70 mm Hg)	88
Hyponatremia (low serum Na^+)	88
Hyperkalemia (high serum K^+)	64

Hyperpigmentation occurs frequently because the high levels of ACTH, β-lipotropin, or one of their subfragments that occur in response to the low level of cortisol are responsible for stimulation of melanocytes and increased production of melanin. Hyperpigmentation is present everywhere but is particularly prominent over pressure points, such as elbows and knees. The buccal mucosa and palmar creases are other places to look for hyperpigmentation. The degree to which a change in pigmentation is detectable depends on the underlying skin pigment of the patient.

Hypoglycemia may also be present. Hyponatremia and hyperkalemia are caused by aldosterone deficiency and are accompanied by orthostatic hypotension.

Patients are treated with cortisol (hydrocortisone). They also usually require a mineralocorticoid such as fludrocortisone. Women with adrenal insufficiency also may benefit from treatment with dehydroepiandrosterone, which increases a sense of well-being and libido.

SECONDARY (PITUITARY) ADRENAL INSUFFICIENCY

Adrenal insufficiency can be due to inadequate secretion of ACTH by the pituitary gland. Pituitary insufficiency can be caused by pituitary tumors, postpartum pituitary infarction (see Chapter 12), pituitary irradiation or surgery, head trauma, or withdrawal of long-term exogenous glucocorticoid therapy that has suppressed pituitary ACTH production. It may take months after withdrawal of exogenous glucocorticoid for ACTH production to recover after chronic suppression.

Symptoms and signs are similar to those of primary adrenal insufficiency *except* that patients exhibit pallor instead of hyperpigmentation (Table 5-4). ACTH and β-lipotropin secretion are low, and melanocyte stimulation is decreased. Usually there are no electrolyte abnormalities because the renin-angiotensin-aldosterone system remains intact. Patients lose axillary and body hair if both ACTH and gonadotropin secretion are defective and total androgen production is low.

Diagnosis of secondary adrenal insufficiency is indicated by low plasma cortisol and ACTH levels, and low urine free cortisol. Other pituitary hormone deficiencies are almost always present. Patients are treated with cortisol, but fludrocortisone is usually not necessary

Table 5-4. Primary vs. Secondary Adrenal Insufficiency

MANIFESTATIONS	PRIMARY	SECONDARY
Hyperpigmentation	Yes	No
Pallor	No	Yes
Low Na$^+$	Yes	No
High K$^+$	Yes	No
Hypotension	Yes	No
Cortisol level	Low	Low
ACTH level	High	Low

because the renin-angiotensin-aldosterone axis should be intact. The underlying pituitary disorder must also be treated, and other hormone deficiencies should be corrected, if present.

ACUTE ADRENAL CRISIS

Individuals with a normal hypothalamic-pituitary-adrenal axis respond to stress (e.g., infection or surgery) with acute increases in CRH, ACTH, and cortisol. Patients receiving treatment for adrenal insufficiency must compensate by increasing their dose of cortisol above the usual maintenance level during stress. If they do not, they may present with acute adrenal crisis: a combination of extreme weakness, dehydration, hypotension, fever, nausea, vomiting, and hypoglycemia, which can be fatal if untreated. They must be given high doses of cortisol, intravenous fluids, and glucose; the cause of the underlying stress must also be treated.

Symptoms and Signs of Adrenal (Addisonian) Crisis
Volume depletion
Hypotension and shock
Fever
Nausea and vomiting
Weakness
Hypoglycemia

Patients with undiagnosed adrenal insufficiency can present for the first time in adrenal crisis. Those who have been on chronic glucocorticoid therapy for immunosuppression or suppression of inflammation can also present with adrenal crisis if their glucocorticoid dose is discontinued abruptly. Their hypothalamic-pituitary-adrenal axis will be suppressed and unable to resume cortisol production acutely.

ADRENAL HYPERFUNCTION (CUSHING SYNDROME)

Cortisol excess due to any cause results in a characteristic constellation of symptoms and signs that is referred to as *Cushing syndrome*. Long-term use of pharmacologic doses of exogenous glucocorticoids (cortisol, prednisone, dexamethasone) prescribed for treatment of chronic inflammation or immune suppression is most often the cause. CRH and ACTH production are suppressed by the high plasma exogenous glucocorticoid concentration.

ACTH-producing pituitary tumors cause bilateral adrenal hyperplasia and excess cortisol secretion. Cushing syndrome due to an ACTH-producing pituitary tumor is referred to specifically as Cushing *disease*. ACTH production by pituitary tumors remains partially responsive to feedback inhibition by high doses of glucocorticoids (see Dexamethasone Suppression Tests).

Major Causes of Cushing Syndrome

Exogenous glucocorticoids (cortisol, prednisone, dexamethasone)

ACTH-producing pituitary tumors

Cortisol-secreting adrenal adenoma or adrenal carcinoma

Ectopic ACTH production by nonpituitary tumors

Ectopic CRH production by nonhypothalamic tumors

ACTH production by nonpituitary neoplasms such as carcinomas of the lung (ectopic ACTH) is less likely to be regulated by CRH or to respond to feedback inhibition by high-dose dexamethasone. CRH production by nonhypothalamic neoplasms (ectopic CRH) stimulates excess pituitary ACTH production, resulting in bilateral adrenal hyperplasia. This is rare. Adrenal adenomas or carcinomas can produce cortisol without ACTH stimulation. CRH and ACTH production are suppressed by the high cortisol levels.

Patients with Cushing syndrome lose the classic diurnal rhythm of cortisol secretion. Their cortisol levels are high day and night. Symptoms and signs of cortisol excess (Table 5-5) include weight gain with a typical body habitus due to fat deposition in the face (round face or "moon" facies), neck, and trunk, especially the abdomen. Excess connective tissue catabolism results in purple abdominal striae (stretch marks with visible subcutaneous blood vessels), pink cheeks, and easy bruising. Weakness and muscle wasting due to protein catabolism are common. Osteoporosis (loss of bone mass) due to suppressed bone formation, decreased calcium absorption, and increased urinary calcium excretion results in vertebral compression fractures and other fractures. Women develop hirsutism and amenorrhea due to excess adrenal androgen production. Growth retardation occurs in children. Hypertension and hypokalemia result from the mineralocorticoid activity of cortisol. Hyperglycemia and sometimes overt diabetes are due to increased gluconeogenesis and insulin resistance.

Table 5-5. Cushing Syndrome

SYMPTOMS AND SIGNS	NUMBER OF PATIENTS
Weight gain, round facies, truncal obesity	97%
Weakness	87%
Hypertension (blood pressure >150/90 mm Hg)	82%
Hirsutism (in women)	80%
Amenorrhea	77%
Purple cutaneous striae	67%
Ecchymoses	65%
Osteoporosis	Common
Hyperglycemia	Common
Growth retardation (in children)	

Patients with tumors producing ectopic ACTH are often very ill from the underlying neoplasm, and weight loss and weakness are common. ACTH levels are very high, resulting in hyperpigmentation. Hypertension and hypokalemia are often the prominent problems in these patients. These tumors progress rapidly, and there is usually not enough time for the other manifestations of glucocorticoid excess to develop.

If the physical examination suggests Cushing syndrome, UFC and an evening cortisol level should be measured and the 1 mg dexamethasone suppression test should be performed. If screening tests confirm Cushing syndrome, a morning ACTH level is obtained to determine the cause. High cortisol and low (suppressed) ACTH suggest an adrenal tumor. Adrenal MRI or computed tomography is likely to show an adrenal mass. If ACTH is not suppressed, tests should be done to determine whether the excess ACTH is produced by a pituitary or nonpituitary tumor (Fig. 5-4).

Differential Diagnosis of Cushing Syndrome

Diagnosis	ACTH	Cortisol
Pituitary tumor	High	High
Ectopic ACTH	High	High
Adrenal tumor	Low	High
Exogenous cortisol	Low	High
Exogenous prednisone or dexamethasone	Low	Low

Treatment of Cushing syndrome depends on the cause. An ACTH-producing pituitary adenoma (Cushing disease) can often be removed by transsphenoidal pituitary adenomectomy. An adrenal adenoma or carcinoma can be treated with adrenal surgery. Tumors producing ectopic ACTH are treated surgically or with chemotherapy. If tumors causing Cushing syndrome cannot be controlled with surgery or chemotherapy, cortisol synthesis can be blocked pharmacologically with aminoglutethimide or ketoconazole.

When Cushing syndrome is caused by exogenous glucocorticoid, the dose should be reduced, if possible. Patients treated with cortisol will have high cortisol and low ACTH levels due to feedback inhibition; those treated with prednisone or dexamethasone will have low ACTH and cortisol levels.

PRIMARY HYPERALDOSTERONISM (CONN SYNDROME)

Hyperaldosteronism accounts for hypertension in about 1% of hypertensive patients. Excess production of aldosterone is most often due to an adrenal adenoma or bilateral adrenal hyperplasia. The cause or causes are unknown. Cortisol production remains normal. Hypertension is usually the only clinical sign. Unexplained hypokalemia is often an important diagnostic clue.

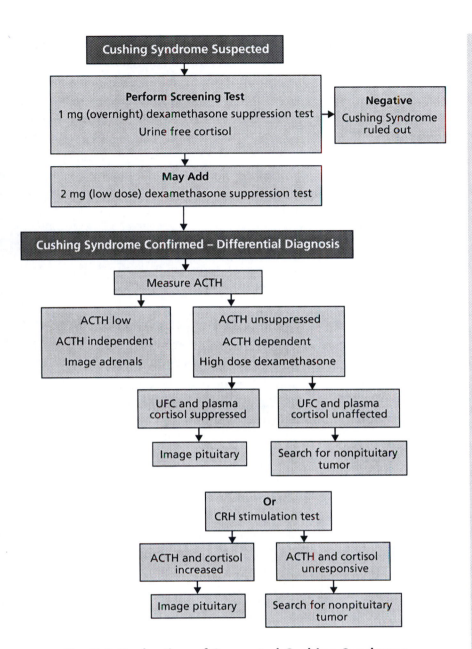

Fig. 5-4. Evaluation of Suspected Cushing Syndrome

If the history and physical examination suggest cortisol overproduction, the 1 mg (overnight) dexamethasone screening test is preformed. If this is negative, Cushing syndrome is ruled out. If the test is positive, it is necessary to refer the patient to an endocrinologist or to proceed with further testing. ACTH = adrenocorticotropic hormone; UFC = urine free cortisol; CRH = corticotropin-releasing hormone.

Signs of Hyperaldosteronism

Hypertension
Hypokalemia
Suppressed plasma renin activity
Abnormal aldosterone suppression

Serum potassium, plasma aldosterone, and plasma renin activity are measured to make the diagnosis. Plasma renin activity should be suppressed because the high aldosterone level causes sodium retention and expansion of plasma volume. A high plasma aldosterone level with a plasma aldosterone to plasma renin activity ratio >20 suggests hyperaldosteronism. The aldosterone suppression test is abnormal. An abdominal CT scan can be obtained to determine if an adenoma is present.

An adrenal adenoma can be removed surgically. If this is not possible, the hypertension and hypokalemia can be treated with spironolactone, an aldosterone antagonist, or eplerenone, another aldosterone antagonist with fewer side effects. An aldosterone antagonist is the treatment of choice when hyperaldosteronism is due to bilateral adrenal hyperplasia.

CONGENITAL ADRENAL HYPERPLASIA DUE TO 21-HYDROXYLASE DEFICIENCY

Congenital adrenal hyperplasia (CAH) is due to an inborn error of metabolism with a specific deficiency in one of the enzymes involved in cortisol synthesis. The most common is a deficiency in 21-hydroxylase. Because of the deficiency in the 21-hydroxylase enzyme,

---

CASE STUDY: *RESOLUTION*

When the patient was hospitalized 1 month later for further evaluation, he said that he felt 100% normal. He was noted to be hyperpigmented and his blood pressure was 125/75 mm Hg.

Physical examination and laboratory tests suggested that this was primary adrenal insufficiency, not secondary adrenal insufficiency. Hyperpigmentation indicated that ACTH was high, and the initial hypotension, low sodium, and high potassium suggested concomitant aldosterone deficiency. This would be expected with adrenal destruction but not with ACTH deficiency because aldosterone is regulated primarily by the renin-angiotensin system, not ACTH. There was no evidence of tuberculosis or other infection, and the cause of his adrenal insufficiency was thought to be autoimmune adrenalitis.

He was placed on maintenance therapy with cortisol (hydrocortisone) and fludrocortisone and has had a normal productive life. He was instructed to increase his maintenance dose of cortisol when he became ill. Several years later he developed chronic lymphocytic thyroiditis, providing additional support for an autoimmune cause of his adrenal insufficiency.

Many years after his medical close call, this patient is married with two children, is the full-time manager of an automobile dealership, and enjoys running approximately 20 miles per week.

there is a block in cortisol production. This causes a compensatory increase in ACTH secretion and intense stimulation of the adrenal cortex. With this stimulation, it is often possible to produce adequate amounts of cortisol. However, cortisol precursors proximal to the block are produced in large quantities. As depicted in Fig. 5-5, excess 17-hydroxyprogesterone and other precursor steroids are shunted into the androgen pathway and result in increased adrenal androgen secretion.

Symptoms and signs of CAH include masculinization of external genitalia in female infants, precocious sexual development of male infants, and rapid early growth but final short stature due to premature closure of the epiphyses (see Chapters 13 and 14). In some cases where there is also a block in aldosterone production, there is excessive urinary Na$^+$ loss. This usually presents in early infancy as an adrenal crisis. Women with adult-onset CAH may develop hirsutism, oligomenorrhea, and infertility.

The diagnosis is made by measuring a serum 17-hydroxyprogesterone level, which should be very high. Patients with CAH are treated with enough cortisol, prednisone, or dexamethasone to suppress ACTH secretion, thereby preventing excess androgen production.

INCIDENTAL ADRENAL MASS

As abdomen and pelvis imaging procedures have improved in resolution and quality, more and more images are being ordered. Many patients are found to have a completely unexpected adrenal mass.

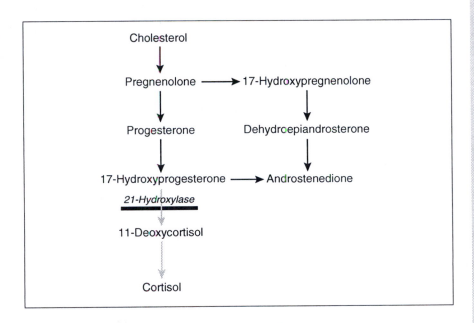

Fig. 5-5. Adrenal Steroid Production in Congenital Hyperplasia Due to 21-Hydroxylase Deficiency

Because of the block in cortisol production and the increased adrenocorticotropin (ACTH) stimulation that results, 17-hydroxyprogesterone and other precursors accumulate and are shunted into the androgen pathway.

These patients often have no symptoms and signs to suggest an adrenal disorder. Most of these masses are benign, especially those smaller than 6 cm. However, it is important to make sure that these masses are not producing excess cortisol, aldosterone, adrenal androgens, or hormones of the adrenal medulla (see Chapter 6).

REVIEW QUESTIONS

Directions: For each of the following questions, choose the *one best* answer.

1 A 27-year-old man with adrenal insufficiency is being treated with cortisol. He can expect cortisol to do which one of the following?

A Increase corticotropin-releasing hormone (CRH) secretion
B Increase adrenocorticotropic hormone (ACTH) secretion
C Increase conversion of amino acids to glucose
D Increase inflammation and wound healing
E Increase sensitivity to insulin in muscle

2 A 43-year-old woman complains of fatigue, intermittent vomiting, and weight loss of 15 lb. Physical examination is remarkable for blood pressure of 100/60 mm Hg supine and 80/40 mm Hg standing. She has a large patch of white, depigmented skin on the right side of her neck. Her serum sodium (Na^+) level is low and her potassium (K^+) level is high. Her diagnostic evaluation should include which of the following tests?

A Midnight plasma cortisol
B Adrenocorticotropic hormone (ACTH) stimulation test
C Aldosterone suppression test
D One-mg (overnight) dexamethasone suppression test
E High-dose dexamethasone suppression test

Questions 3 and 4

3 A 40-year-old woman complains of fatigue, weight gain of 30 lb, cessation of menstruation, and recent growth of dark facial, chest, and abdominal hair. Physical examination is remarkable for a blood pressure of 160/95 mm Hg, a round face, obesity, hirsutism involving the face and trunk, multiple ecchymoses, and purplish abdominal striae. Which of the following tests should be the next step in her evaluation?

A Corticotropin-releasing hormone (CRH) stimulation test
B Adrenocorticotropic hormone (ACTH) stimulation test
C Aldosterone suppression test
D One-mg (overnight) dexamethasone suppression test
E High-dose dexamethasone suppression test

4 After screening tests indicate that she has Cushing syndrome, the morning plasma ACTH level is measured and found to be high. After CRH stimulation, her ACTH and cortisol levels are increased. After high-dose dexamethasone, her plasma cortisol level is decreased by 75%. What is the most likely cause of this patient's Cushing syndrome?

A A pituitary tumor producing adrenocorticotropic hormone (ACTH)
B A lung carcinoma producing ectopic ACTH
C An adrenal adenoma
D An adrenal carcinoma
E Surreptitious use of the medication prednisone

5 A 47-year-old man with diabetic nephropathy and end-stage renal disease received a kidney transplant 4 months ago. His post-transplant immunosuppressant medications include prednisone, 15 mg twice daily. Renal function is now normal. Evaluation of his hypothalamic-pituitary-adrenal axis would most likely yield which of the following results?

A Decreased plasma adrenocorticotropic hormone (ACTH), increased plasma cortisol, increased urine free cortisol
B Decreased plasma ACTH, increased plasma cortisol, decreased urine free cortisol
C Increased plasma ACTH, increased plasma cortisol, increased urine free cortisol
D Increased plasma ACTH, decreased plasma cortisol, decreased urine free cortisol
E Decreased plasma ACTH, decreased plasma cortisol, decreased urine free cortisol

6 A 42-year-old man is discovered to have hypertension during a routine examination. He takes no medications. Physical examination is normal except for blood pressure of 156/95 mm Hg. Several additional blood pressure readings are elevated. Laboratory evaluation demonstrates normal renal function but low serum potassium (K^+). Further evaluation should include which of the following?

A Plasma cortisol
B Plasma adrenocorticotropic hormone (ACTH)
C Plasma renin activity and aldosterone
D Plasma 17-hydroxyprogesterone
E Plasma 11-deoxycortisol

References

Arlt W, Callies F, van Vlijmen JC, et al: Dehydroepiandrosterone replacement in women with adrenal insufficiency. *N Engl J Med* 341: 1013–1020, 1999.

Notes

Arnaldi G, Angeli A, Atkinson AB, et al: Diagnosis and complications of Cushing's syndrome: a consensus statement. *J Clin Endocrinol Metab* 88: 5593–5602, 2003.

Chrousos GP: The hypothalamic-pituitary-adrenal axis and immune-mediated inflammation. *N Engl J Med* 332: 1351–1362,1995.

Cooper NS, Stewart PM: Corticosteroid insufficiency in acutely ill patients. *N Engl J Med* 348: 727–724, 2003.

Cutler GB, Laue L: Congenital adrenal hyperplasia due to 21-hydroxylase deficiency. *N Engl J Med* 323: 1806–1813, 1990.

Ghose RP, Hall PM, Bravo EL: Medical management of aldosterone-producing adenomas. *Ann Int Med* 131: 105–108, 1999.

Grinspoon SK, Biller BMK: Laboratory assessment of adrenal insufficiency. *J Clin Endocrinol Metab* 79: 923–931, 1994.

Raff H, Findling JW: A physiologic approach to diagnosis of the Cushing syndrome. *Ann Int Med* 138: 980–991, 2003.

White PC: Disorders of aldosterone biosynthesis and action. *N Engl J Med* 331:250–258, 1994.

6

The Adrenal Medulla

J. Michael Gonzalez-Campoy, M.D., Ph.D.

■ CHAPTER OUTLINE ■

■ LEARNING OBJECTIVES ■

At the completion of this chapter, the student will:
1. understand the embryological origin of the adrenal medulla.
2. know the hormones released from the adrenal medulla and the physiologic stimuli for secretion.
3. be aware of the effects of catecholamines.
4. understand the clinical measurements of adrenal medullary function.
5. understand the consequences of catecholamine excess.
6. understand the evaluation and management of a suspected pheochromocytoma.

CASE STUDY: *INTRODUCTION*

At age 27, Kim R. began complaining of heat intolerance, excessive sweating, palpitations, and occasional headaches. These symptoms came in paroxysms and often lasted for days. Despite careful consideration, she could not identify any precipitating events. At times her symptoms were accompanied by chest pain, abdominal pain, nausea, vomiting, and pallor. Her physician documented an elevated blood pressure, but this was attributed to anxiety.

Ms. R. continued to experience episodic symptoms. Four years later, at the age of 31, she again sought medical care and was found to have an elevated blood glucose. She was given a diagnosis of diabetes and was encouraged to follow a weight reduction diet.

Embryologic Origin of the Adrenal Medulla

There are two adrenal glands, one superior to each kidney. Each adrenal gland consists of two morphologically and functionally distinct endocrine tissues: the outer cortex and the inner medulla. The adrenal cortex secretes steroid hormones and is the subject of Chapter 5.

The adrenal medulla is derived embryologically from pheochromoblasts, which migrate from the neural crest. During differentiation pheochromoblasts give rise to modified neuronal (gland) cells, not neurons. After birth, extra-adrenal pheochromoblast derivatives degenerate, and adrenomedullary cells mature. These mature cells turn brown when treated with oxidizing agents and are therefore referred to as *chromaffin* cells. Chromaffin cells are confined to the adrenal medulla and the paraganglia of the sympathetic nervous system.

Hormones of the Adrenal Medulla

CATECHOLAMINE SYNTHESIS

The adrenal medulla secretes amine hormones and may be considered a modified sympathetic ganglion whose cell bodies do not send out nerve fibers, but rather release hormones into the circulation. The two major amines released from the adrenal medulla are *epinephrine* and *norepinephrine*. *Dopamine* is also released, but in smaller quantities. Together, this group of compounds constitutes the catecholamines. They all contain a catechol ring (i.e., six-sided carbon ring with two adjacent hydroxyl groups). They also contain an amine group. Figure 6-1 shows the biochemical structures of the major catecholamines; tyrosine, their common precursor; and their major metabolites. The rate-limiting enzyme in the catecholamine synthesis cascade is tyrosine hydroxylase, which converts tyrosine to dihydroxyphenylalanine (dopa).

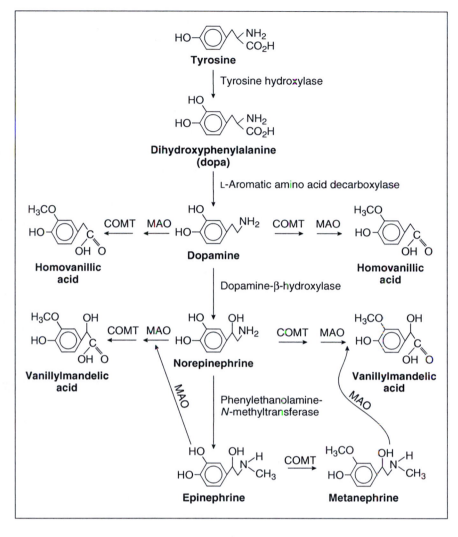

Fig. 6-1. Catecholamine Synthetic and Metabolic Pathways

The conversion of tyrosine to dopa is the rate-limiting step in catecholamine synthesis. MAO = monoamine oxidase; COMT = catechol-O-methyltransferase.

Adrenal Medulla Catecholamine Hormones

Epinephrine
Norepinephrine
Dopamine

The adrenal medulla contains large amounts of the enzyme *phenylethanolamine N-methyltransferase (PNMT)*, which catalyzes the conversion of norepinephrine to epinephrine. High glucocorticoid concentrations arriving via the adrenal cortico-medullary portal system induce PNMT activity. Thus, the normal adrenal secretion of epinephrine is four times more than that of norepinephrine. (Basal circulating levels of norepinephrine are higher due to neurotransmitter release by postganglionic sympathetic neurons, not to secretion by the adrenal medulla). The secretion of dopamine is negligible by comparison.

The adrenal medulla is functionally an amplifier of the sympathetic nervous system. The adrenal medulla is innervated by preganglionic sympathetic axons, which use acetylcholine (ACh) as a neurotransmitter. ACh depolarizes the chromaffin cells by increasing plasma membrane permeability to sodium (Na^+). This results in an influx of calcium (Ca^{2+}), a rise in the cytoplasmic Ca^{2+} level, and the exocytotic release of catecholamines. Adenosine triphosphate (ATP), enkephalins, chromogranins, neuropeptide Y, and dopamine β-hydroxylase are released from the exocytotic vessels at the same time.

The **adrenal medulla** is an amplifier for the sympathetic nervous system.

SIGNALS FOR CATECHOLAMINE RELEASE

Anything that stimulates sympathetic outflow from the central nervous system (CNS) leads to increased catecholamine release seconds to minutes later from storage granules in the adrenal medulla. Major conditions associated with changes in catecholamine release from the adrenal medulla are listed in Table 6-1. Significant changes in circulating adrenal medulla hormone concentrations occur primarily in response to stress, such as a change in intravascular volume or marked hypoglycemia (blood glucose <50 mg/dL). In most of these situations secretion of epinephrine increases more than secretion of norepinephrine. The hormones circulate as free hormones or are loosely bound to plasma protein.

Table 6-1. Major Conditions Affecting Plasma Catecholamine Levels

CATECHOLAMINES INCREASED	CATECHOLAMINES DECREASED
Change in posture (supine to standing)	Change in posture (standing to supine)
Low intravascular volume	Bilateral adrenal hemorrhage
Hypoglycemia	Bilateral adrenal damage
Severe illness	Bilateral adrenalectomy
Emotional stress	
fear (initiating fight or flight response)	
rage	
Tumors	
pheochromocytoma	
paraganglioma	

Major Signals for Catecholamine Release

Decreased blood pressure
Decreased blood volume
Decreased blood glucose
Severe illness
Severe emotional stress

Catecholamine-Receptor Interaction

Catecholamines released from the adrenal medulla and cate-cholamines released from sympathetic nerve endings bind to the same family of receptors, which are located on cell membranes throughout the body. Five different types of receptors have been identified for epinephrine and norepinephrine: the α-adrenergic receptors, α_1 and α_2, and the β-adrenergic receptors, β_1, β_2, and β_3. Three α_1 and three α_2 receptor subtypes have also been identified. Epinephrine is slightly more active than norepinephrine at α_2 receptors, but they have similar potency at β_1 receptors. Epinephrine is much more potent than norepinephrine at β_2 receptors. The adrenergic receptors are part of the dual innervation of most tissues, with parasympathetic or cholinergic receptors representing the other half. Adrenergic and cholinergic effects on tissues often oppose each other.

Receptor:Hormone Affinity

α_1, α_2:epinephrine > norepinephrine
β_1:epinephrine = norepinephrine
β_2:epinephrine >>> norepinephrine

Receptor-binding by catecholamines triggers a complex series of intracellular events. The catecholamine-receptor complex associates with membrane-bound G-proteins, which in turn activate intracellular effector molecules commonly termed second messengers. Beta-adrenoreceptor activation results in the generation of the second messenger cyclic adenosine monophosphate (cAMP). Stimulation of adrenoreceptors results in the activation of either phospholipase C or cAMP and may also directly affect Ca^{2+} and potassium (K^+) channels. A significant change in the number of catecholamine receptors obviously affects the response elicited by the hormones.

Four dopamine receptor types have been characterized. By convention the CNS dopaminergic receptors are denoted as D_1, D_2, D_3, and D_4; the peripheral dopaminergic receptors are DA_1, DA_2, DA_3, and DA_4. All known dopamine receptors are coupled to adenylate cyclase via G-proteins. DA_1 and D_1 activate stimulatory Gs-proteins and also adenylate cyclase. DA$_2$ and D$_2$ activate inhibitory Gi-proteins and inhibit adenylate cyclase.

ACTIONS OF EPINEPHRINE AND NOREPINEPHRINE

Norepinephrine and epinephrine secreted by peripheral sympathetic nerves act as local regulators of glucose and fat metabolism, visceral function, cardiovascular responses, and response to stress. Since the adrenal medulla secretes these hormones into the circulation rather than locally, the responses are more general. Tables 6-2 and 6-3 list the major effects of adrenergic stimulation on various tissues and metabolism. A fully activated sympathetic response is called the "fight-or-flight" response, since the hormones increase skeletal muscle blood flow and contraction at the expense of blood flow to visceral organs and skin. The accompanying increase in glycogenolysis, gluconeogenesis, and lipolysis provides the fuel for the increased oxygen consumption required.

ROLE OF DOPAMINE

Although dopamine is a critical neurotransmitter in the CNS and plays a crucial role in the modulation of prolactin release from the pituitary gland, dopamine action on peripheral tissues is much less important than epinephrine and norepinephrine action. Dopamine is the most abundant free catecholamine in the urine. The kidneys synthesize it from levodopa (L-dopa), and renal excretion of dopamine exceeds its renal clearance. This is not true of the other catecholamines.

Table 6-2. Major Physiological Effects of Increased Epinephrine and Norepinephrine

ORGAN	RECEPTOR TYPE	EFFECT
Skeletal muscle	β_2	Increased contractility
Heart	β_1	Increased heart rate, conduction velocity, contractility
Arterioles	α (norepinephrine effect) β_2 (epinephrine effect)	Constriction (abdominal viscera) Vasodilatation (skeletal muscle)
Lungs	β_2	Bronchodilatation
Stomach, intestine	α_1, β_2	Decreased motility, increased sphincter contraction
Gallbladder	β_2	Relaxation
Kidney	β_1	Increased renin causing increased blood pressure
Ureter	α	Increased motility
Urinary bladder	β α	Detrusor relaxation Sphincter contraction
Uterus	β_2	Relaxation
Penis	α	Ejaculation
Skin	α	Increased pallor and sweating (palms)
Posterior pituitary	β_1	Increased antidiuretic hormone secretion causing decreased urine output

Table 6-3. Major Metabolic Effects of Increased Epinephrine

ORGAN	EFFECT
Liver	Increased gluconeogenesis and glycogenolysis
Skeletal muscle	Increased glycogenolysis
Adipose tissue	Increased lipolysis
Overall	Increased oxygen consumption and thermogenesis

Major Actions of Catecholamines

↑ Blood glucose

↑ Lipolysis

↑ Skeletal muscle blood flow and contractility

↑ Heart rate, contractility and cardiac output

↑ Blood pressure

↓ Visceral blood flow

↓ GI tract motility

↓ Urine output

CATECHOLAMINE METABOLISM AND DISPOSAL

Secreted catecholamines have a short half-life of a few minutes. Catecholamines secreted by sympathetic nerves are usually taken up again and metabolized in sympathetic nerve terminals. Adrenal medulla hormones are mostly metabolized to inactive compounds by the enzymes catechol-O-methyltransferase (COMT) and monoamine oxidase (MAO) to metanephrine and normetanephrine or to vanillyl-mandelic acid (VMA) by less specific monoamine oxidation (see Figure 6-1) in peripheral tissues such as liver and kidney. Catecholamines and metanephrines can be conjugated with sulfate ion. Free and conjugated catecholamines and their metabolites circulate in plasma and are excreted in the urine. Since catecholamines are secreted in bursts in response to changing situations, plasma concentrations are highly variable and a single blood level may not provide an accurate picture of catecholamine secretion. In clinical practice, measurement of catecholamine levels, particularly total metanephrine, in a timed urine collection is useful. A 24-hour urine collection indicates the total daily production of catecholamines. Blood for plasma levels must be collected when a patient is fasting and supine with an indwelling cannula in place for at least 20 minutes. Table 6-4 indicates the normal concentrations of catecholamines and their major metabolites in plasma and urine and shows the effects of upright posture on plasma epinephrine and norepinephrine concentrations.

Table 6-4. Normal Plasma and Urine Values of Catecholamines in Adults

	PLASMA	URINE (24 HOUR)
Norepinephrine	70–750 pg/mL (supine) 200–1700 pg/mL (standing)	15–80 µg
Epinephrine	<110 pg/mL (supine) <140 pg/mL (standing)	0–20 µg
Dopamine	<30 pg/mL (supine) <30 pg/mL (standing)	65–400 µg
Metanephrines		<1.3 mg
Vanillylmandelic acid (VMA)		<9 µg/mg creatinine

Notes

ADRENOMEDULLIN

Adrenomedullin (AM) is a regulatory peptide identified in a human chromaffin cell tumor that has been located in various human tissues including the adrenal gland, heart, lung, kidney, and aorta. AM is generated from a larger 185–amino acid prehormone through consecutive enzymatic cleavage and amidation, ultimately resulting in a 52–amino acid biologically active peptide. AM is a vasodilatory agent and a natriuretic factor. It acts through specific receptors identified in heart, lung, spleen, liver, muscle, and spinal cord. Upon interaction

CASE STUDY: CONTINUED

The patient's symptoms and signs of hypertension, headaches (perhaps due to episodic hypertension), increased sweating and palpitations (increased cardiac contractility), and hyperglycemia are not specific when considered alone, but they should suggest epinephrine excess when taken together. Two years later, her symptoms increased in frequency and severity. Her blood pressure was elevated at 180/100 mm Hg. She was referred to an endocrinologist for further evaluation.

Her medical history was otherwise unremarkable. She had no history of illicit drug use. She denied regular use of any over-the-counter medications. Her maternal grandfather had undergone surgery for a "gland" tumor.

On physical examination her blood pressure while seated was 192/104 mm Hg measured on the right arm. Her heart rate was 92 beats/min and regular. Her head, ears, eyes, nose, throat, lungs, heart, abdomen, and pelvis were normal. Neurologic and peripheral vascular examinations were also normal. Her thyroid gland was normal in size, and there were no nodules. She had no cutaneous lesions, ecchymoses, cafe-au-lait spots, or mucosal neuromas. A 24-hour urine metanephrine level was 1856 µg. Her 24-hour urine epinephrine and fractionated plasma free metanephrine levels were also high.

with its receptor, AM activates adenylate cyclase and modulates Ca^{2+} flux in target cells.

The precise physiologic role of AM is yet to be defined. Individuals with congestive heart failure (CHF) exhibit progressively more elevated levels of AM, which correlate with the clinical severity of their disease, and AM may play a role in the cardiovascular abnormalities associated with sepsis. In addition to its vasodilatory effects in the periphery and natriuretic actions in the kidney, AM is an inhibitor of ACTH secretion by pituitary cells. AM inhibits insulin secretion, and hyperinsulinemia stimulates AM secretion, but the role of AM in glucose metabolism remains unclear.

Pheochromocytoma

DEFINITIONS

Pheochromocytoma is a catecholamine-secreting tumor of chromaffin cells arising from the adrenal medulla. *Paraganglioma* is a catecholamine-secreting tumor of chromaffin cells arising from the sympathetic paraganglia. In the literature, these terms are used interchangeably, and pheochromocytoma denotes any catecholamine-secreting tumor of neural crest origin. These tumors are described as either adrenal or extra-adrenal pheochromocytomas.

Catecholamine-Secreting Tumors of Chromaffin Cells
Pheochromocytoma: tumor arising from adrenal medulla
Paraganglioma: tumor arising from sympathetic paraganglia

INCIDENCE

Pheochromocytoma is a rare tumor. The incidence rate is approximately 1 in 100,000 person years. It is found in less than 0.1% of patients with hypertension, the hallmark of the disease. The peak prevalence is in the third through the fifth decades, but it may occur in any age group. There is no race or sex predisposition.

Over 90% of pheochromocytomas are located in the abdomen; 85% to 90% of these arise within the adrenal glands. Pheochromocytomas are sometimes described by the "rule of 10." Approximately 10% to 15% are extra-adrenal. Approximately 10% of pheochromocytomas are bilateral and multicentric. Approximately 10% of pheochromocytomas are malignant (more likely if extra-adrenal), with metastases most often to regional lymph nodes, liver, bone, lung, and the CNS. Malignant pheochromocytomas are more likely to be greater than 6 cm in size.

Most paragangliomas (extra-adrenal pheochromocytomas) are non-hormone-secreting tumor masses in the head and neck regions. The most common locations for hormone-secreting paragangliomas are

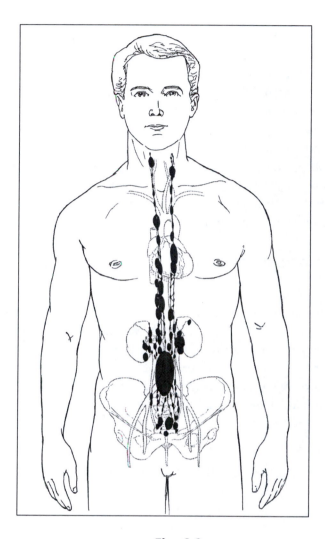

Fig. 6-2.

The anatomic distribution of paragangliomas (extra-adrenal pheochromocytomas) reported in the literature.

around the abdominal aorta and the aorta bifurcation, in the bladder wall, and in the chest. Figure 6-2 shows the reported locations of paragangliomas.

Familial pheochromocytoma is inherited as an autosomal dominant trait either alone or as part of the multiple endocrine neoplasia type 2 syndromes (MEN-2A and MEN-2B) and von Hippel-Lindau (VHL) disease. MEN-2 is associated with mutations in RET proto-oncogene, causing activation of the receptor tyrosine kinase. VHL disease is associated with inactivating mutations in a VHL tumor suppressor gene which regulates normal degradation of proteins. Familial pheochromocytomas are also associated with several neurocutaneous disorders, including neurofibromatosis, ataxia-telangectasia, tuberous sclerosis, and Sturge-Weber syndrome. Autosomal dominant familial paraganglioma is associated with mutations in the genes encoding a subunit of succinate dehydrogenase, part of mitochondrial complex II, which

Table 6-5. Familial Disorders Associated with Pheochromocytoma

Multiple endocrine neoplasia type 2A
  Pheochromocytoma, medullary carcinoma of the thyroid, hyperparathyroidism
Multiple endocrine neoplasia type 2B
  Pheochromocytoma, mucosal neuromas, hyperparathyroidism (rare)
von Hippel-Lindau disease
Neurofibromatosis
Ataxia-telangectsia
Tuberous sclerosis
Sturge-Weber syndrome

regulates oxygen sensing and signaling. Table 6-5 summarizes the pathological conditions associated with pheochromocytoma and highlights the need for taking a thorough family history in the evaluation of these patients.

SIGNS AND SYMPTOMS

Patients have symptoms related to excess circulating catecholamines. The hallmark of pheochromocytoma is either paroxysmal hypertension or sustained hypertension that is often labile and resistant to treatment. Other signs and symptoms classically associated with pheochromocytoma are headache, sweating, palpitations, chest or abdominal pain, pallor, anxiety, and glucose intolerance (Table 6-6). Some patients have postural hypotension due to altered sympathetic vascular regulation, especially in tumors secreting predominantly epinephrine or dopamine. The classic triad of sudden severe headache, diaphoresis, and palpitations carries a high degree of specificity (94%) and sensitivity (91%) for pheochromocytoma in a hypertensive population. The absence of all three symptoms makes the diagnosis of pheochromocytoma extremely unlikely. Paroxysmal attacks may be triggered by a variety of stimuli, which are summarized in Table 6-7. Again, a careful review of the medical and family history is essential.

DIAGNOSIS

The diagnosis of pheochromocytoma depends on the demonstration of excessive amounts of catecholamines or their metabolites in urine or plasma. A 24-hour urine collection for fractionated and total metanephrines is a good screening test for pheochromocytoma.

Table 6-6. Major Symptoms and Signs of Pheochromocytoma

Hypertension: sustained or paroxysmal	Tremor
Headache	Pallor
Sweating	Hyperglycemia
Palpitations	Nausea, vomiting, abdominal pain
Anxiety, nervousness	

Table 6-7. Major Stimuli Causing Paroxysmal Catecholamine Release

Activity: postural change, exertion, sexual intercourse
Meals, alcohol, smoking
Urination, straining at stool
Emotional stress
Physical trauma and pain
General anesthesia, barbiturates
Hormones/drugs: glucagon, adrenocorticotropic hormone (ACTH), histamine

Patients with paroxysmal symptoms should start the urine collection with the onset of the spell. If suspicion for pheochromocytoma is high, 24-hour urine concentrations of epinephrine, norepinephrine, and dopamine and fractionated plasma free (not conjugated) metanephrines are obtained. If these levels are twofold above normal, or urine total metanephrine levels exceed 1300 pg, studies to localize the tumor are done. Some medications—particularly antidepressants, acetaminophen, alcohol, opiates, smoking—and major physical stressors such as myocardial infarction, stroke, heart failure, and renal failure interfere with laboratory measurements.

Major Tests for Pheochromocytoma
Diagnosis
24-hour urine metanephrines (first choice)
24-hour urine epinephrine, norepinephrine, and dopamine
Fractionated plasma free metanephrines
Clonidine suppression test
Localization
Adrenal-abdominal magnetic resonance imaging (MRI) [first choice] *or*
Adrenal-abdominal computerized tomography (CT) scan
^{131}I-meta-iodobenzylguanidine

Cases in which screening tests are equivocal warrant a clonidine suppression test. Clonidine is a centrally active α_2-agonist. In individuals with essential hypertension, in whom increased catecholamine secretion is due to neurogenic stimulation rather than a tumor, 0.3 mg of orally administered clonidine suppresses catecholamine release, and plasma catecholamines decrease to less than 500 pg/mL. Patients with pheochromocytoma fail to suppress catecholamine release. Other diagnostic tests that should be considered in patients in whom MEN-2A is suspected include a plasma calcitonin level to exclude medullary thyroid cancer and plasma parathyroid hormone (PTH) and Ca^{2+} levels to exclude hyperparathyroidism.

If biochemical studies confirm the diagnosis of pheochromocytoma, imaging studies are necessary to determine whether the tumor is adrenal or extra-adrenal. Magnetic resonance imaging (MRI) is preferable to computed axial tomography (CAT) scanning for locating very small or extra-adrenal tumors. Scintigraphic localization with ^{131}I-meta-iodobenzylguanidine (MIBG) can be used when CAT scanning or MRI imaging is inconclusive.

MANAGEMENT

Definitive treatment of pheochromocytoma is surgical resection. Preoperative α- and β-adrenergic blockade is indicated to control blood pressure and reduce the risk of postoperative hypotension. α-adrenergic blockade with phenoxybenzamine is started 7 to 10 days before surgery. β-blockade to control tachycardia is instituted after α-blockade is achieved, because unopposed α-stimulation as a consequence of β-blockade could lead to increased vasoconstriction and even worse hypertension. Calcium channel blockers, which block nor-epinephrine-induced Ca^{2+} transport into vascular smooth muscle, are also used to control blood pressure before surgery. Postoperative hypotension following removal of vasoconstricting tumor hormones requires intravascular volume expansion. To check for recurrence, 24-hour urine catecholamines and metanephrines should be measured 2 weeks after surgery and then annually for 10 years. If familial pheochromocytoma is suspected, genetic counseling and genetic testing should be considered.

CASE STUDY: *RESOLUTION*

Kim R.'s symptoms and signs, high urine metanephrines and cate-cholamines, and high fractionated plasma free metanephrines indicated that she had a pheochromocytoma. She had no signs of a neuroectodermal disorder, but her family history of a "gland" tumor made it imperative to rule out MEN-2. Her plasma calcitonin, PTH, and Ca^{2+} values were all within the normal range. Her grandfather's hospital records were eventually located and indicated that a pheochromocytoma had been removed.

Magnetic resonance imaging (MRI) of her abdomen revealed a 5×5.3 cm right adrenal mass. She was treated with the α-blocker phenoxybenzamine for 10 days before surgery, and a β-blocker was added 3 days before surgery. The tumor was removed successfully, and a brief period of postoperative hypotension was easily managed with intravenous fluids. The tumor was indeed a pheochromocytoma. Two weeks after surgery her urine metanephrine levels were normal. Her hyperglycemia also resolved after the tumor was removed. She was referred for genetic counseling in view of probable familial pheochromocytoma. The presence of hypertension accompanied by paroxysmal headaches and palpitations over a period of years should have prompted an evaluation for pheochromocytoma much earlier.

REVIEW QUESTIONS

Directions: For each of the following questions, choose the *one best* answer.

1 Catecholamine levels are high in a 60-year-old man who has just had a severe myocardial infarction. Which of the following physiologic responses is most likely to result from his increased catecholamine secretion?

   A Decreased lipolysis to reduce his circulating free fatty acids
   B Increased glycogen synthesis to increase fuel stores in his myocardium
   C Hyperglycemia due to increased gluconeogenesis and glycogenolysis
   D Decreased oxygen consumption to protect his remaining myocardium

2 A 44-year-old man suddenly finds himself in a terrifying situation inducing both fear and rage. His appropriate catecholamine response elicits

   A increased urine output
   B increased blood flow to muscle and less to viscera
   C increased blood flow to skin so that he can remain cool
   D decreased cardiac output and heart rate to help him remain calm

Questions 3-6

A 20-year-old woman comes to the physician's office with a history of paroxysmal hypertension, palpitations, headache, and profuse sweating. Her father died from thyroid cancer, and a paternal aunt has hypercalcemia and hypertension.

3 What would be the most appropriate first step in evaluating this woman?
   A Draw blood for measurement of free T_4 and TSH levels and order a radioactive iodine uptake and scan
   B Obtain an electrocardiogram and, if it is normal, treat her hypertension with a β-adrenergic blocker
   C Collect urine for 24 hours starting at the onset of a paroxysm and measure levels of metanephrines, epinephrine, and norepinephrine
   D Refer this woman for psychiatric evaluation for her anxiety

4 In view of this woman's family medical history, the physician would be most likely to measure serum levels of

   A calcitonin, calcium, and glucose
   B glucagon, insulin, and cholesterol
   C thyroid hormone, adrenomedullin, and phosphorous
   D nerve growth factor, gastrin, and renin

5 The woman's test results are consistent with a pheochromocytoma. After a careful history and physical examination, her physician would be most likely to order

A surgical exploration of the adrenal glands
B magnetic resonance imaging (MRI) or computed tomography (CT) screening
C surgical exploration of the thyroid and parathyroid glands
D a clonidine suppression test

6 Surgery to remove this woman's pheochromocytoma is scheduled, and her hypertension is treated appropriately preoperatively. After surgery, management is likely to include all of the following EXCEPT

A genetic counseling
B measurement of 24-hour urine metanephrines
C testing for calcitonin overproduction
D treatment with a diuretic to promote salt and water loss

References

Bravo EL: Pheochromocytoma. *Cardiol Rev* 10: 44–50, 2002.

Dluhy RG: Pheochromocytoma—death of an axiom. *N Engl J Med* 346: 1486–1487, 2002.

Eng C, Clayton D, Schuffenecker I, et al: The relationship between specific RET proto-oncogene mutations and disease phenotype in multiple endocrine neoplasia type 2: international RET mutation consortium analysis. *JAMA* 276: 1575–1579, 1996.

Erickson D, Kudva YC, Ebersold MJ, et al: Benign paragangliomas: clinical presentation and treatment outcomes in 236 patients. *J Clin Endocrinol Metab* 86: 5210–5216, 2001.

Lenders JW, Pacak K, Walther MM. et al: Biochemical diagnosis of pheochromocytoma: which test is best? *JAMA* 287: 1427–1434, 2002.

Neumann HPH, Berger DP, Sigmund G, et al: Pheochromocytomas, multiple endocrine neoplasia type 2, and von Hippel-Lindau disease. *N Engl J Med* 329:1531, 1993.

Neumann HPH, Bausch B, McWhinney SR, et al: Germ-line mutations in nonsyndromic pheochromocytoma. *N Engl J Med* 346: 1459–1466, 2002.

Pacak K, Linehan Wm, Eisenhofer G, et al: Recent advances in genetics, diagnosis, localization and treatment of pheochromocytoma. *Ann Int Med* 134: 315–329, 2001.

Sawka AM, Jaeschke R, Singh RJ, Young WF Jr: A comparison of biochemical tests for pheochromocytoma: measurement of fractionated plasma metanephrines compared with the combination of 24-hour urinary metanephrines and catecholamines. *J Clin Endocrinol Metab* 88: 553–558, 2003

7

Calcium-Regulating Hormones and Metabolic Bone Disease

Catherine B. Niewoehner, M.D.

■ CHAPTER OUTLINE ■

■ LEARNING OBJECTIVES ■

At the completion of this chapter, the student will:
1. recognize the importance and major sites of calcium regulation.
2. know the major hormones regulating calcium homeostasis and their mechanisms of action
3. understand the causes, consequences, evaluation, and management of hypercalcemia.
4. understand the causes, consequences, evaluation, and management of hypocalcemia.
5. recognize the causes and consequences of vitamin D deficiency.
6 understand the risk factors, consequences, and prevention of osteoporosis.
7. be aware of Paget disease of bone.

Calcium and Phosphorus Homeostasis

Calcium is critically important for a wide range of body functions. Extracellular calcium is essential for blood clotting, nerve and muscle membrane excitability, and maintaining the skeletal system. Intracellular calcium regulates hormone secretion, neuron activation, and muscle contraction, and calcium ions are cofactors for enzymes and act as intracellular second messengers. Calcium homeostasis is jealously guarded, and the extracellular calcium concentration normally changes very little (a few percent) over an entire lifetime (Table 7-1)

Table 7-1. Calcium and Phosphorus Levels in Plasma and Bone

MEASUREMENT	CALCIUM	PHOSPHOROUS
Total plasma concentration (mg/dL)	8.6–10.2	2.5–4.5
Total plasma concentration (mmol/L)	2.1–2.5	0.8–1.4
Plasma ionized concentration (mg/dL)	4.1–4.7	2.1–3.8
plasma ionized concentration (mmol/L)	1.0–1.2	0.68–1.2
Bound to plasma proteins	45%	15%
Percent of total body stores in bone	99%	85%

despite major fluctuations in dietary calcium, calcium entering and leaving the skeleton, renal calcium excretion, and the extra demands of pregnancy and lactation. The cytosolic calcium concentration can change dramatically due to release of calcium from intracellular stores or influx of extracellular calcium, but it is generally maintained at a level 10,000 times lower than the extracellular calcium.

Problems for Calcium Homeostasis

Narrow normal range for extracellular calcium

Extracellular:intracellular calcium concentration gradient ~10,000:1

Extra calcium requirement for growth, pregnancy, and lactation

Preserving circulating calcium without excessive bone loss

Phosphorous is distributed more widely than calcium. It is required for generation of high-energy bonds (e.g., in ATP), is a component of phospholipids in all membranes, and regulates enzyme action and protein function by phosphorylation of proteins. Both calcium and phosphorous are required to form hydroxyapatite $(Ca_{10}[PO_4]_6[OH]_2)$, the major mineral of bone. The extracellular concentration of phosphorous is less tightly regulated than the calcium extracellular concentration, and the normal plasma concentration can vary by almost 100% (Table 7-1). The levels of calcium and phosphorous are often regulated together, sometimes in opposite directions. A low calcium × phosphorous product (<20 mg/dL or 0.7 mmol/L) indicates a major deficiency; a high calcium × phosphorous (>70 mg/dL or 2.2 mmol/L) increases the propensity for deposition of insoluble $CaPO_4$ in soft tissues.

Phosphorous is widely available in foods and most of the ingested phosphorous (70%–80%) normally is absorbed from the small bowel. The kidneys play the major role in protecting the plasma phosphorous concentration in the face of dietary deficiency.

Calcium traffic is more complex. It is more difficult to obtain adequate calcium from the diet because calcium is less ubiquitous than

Table 7-2. Optimal Daily Calcium Intakes (mg/d)

Infants (birth–6 mo)	400
Infants (6–12 mo)	600
Children (1–5 yr)	800
Children (6–10 yr)	800–1200
Adolescent /young adult (11–24 yr)	1200–1500
Adult men	1000
Premenopausal adult women	1000
Postmenopausal women taking estrogen	1000
Pregnant/lactating women	1200–1500
Pregnant/lactating women below age 19	1600
Postmenopausal women not taking estrogen	1500
Elderly (over age 65)	1500

Note. Intakes recommended by National Institutes of Health Consensus Conference, 1994.

phosphorous, and absorption of calcium from the small bowel is less efficient. The optimum dietary calcium intake varies markedly with age (Table 7-2). Infants and adolescents require extra calcium for rapid growth. Pregnant women also require extra calcium, especially in the last trimester when the fetal skeleton develops. Lactating women require extra calcium to replace the calcium secreted in breast milk. These groups absorb dietary calcium very efficiently, particularly when calcium intake is low. Postmenopausal women and the elderly require more calcium because they do not absorb dietary calcium as well, and their renal losses are greater.

Dairy products are the best source of dietary calcium intake unless lactose intolerance is a problem. Fish with bones, nuts, and green vegetables are also good sources, but the amounts required can be rather daunting (Table 7-3). Dietary calcium can be augmented with oral calcium supplements (Table 7-4), if necessary. The calcium content and cost of these supplements differ markedly. Calcium carbonate is absorbed better if it is taken with meals.

Table 7-3. Dietary Sources of Calcium (mg)

Dairy		Fish	
Milk (8 oz)	300	Salmon (canned, + bones, 2 oz)	120
Yogurt (8 oz)	350	Sardines (canned, 2 oz)	220
Yogurt (low fat, 8 oz)	425		
Cottage cheese (1 cup)	150	**Nuts**	
Ice cream (1 cup)	175	Almonds (1 cup)	200
Cheese (1 oz)	150–250	Peanuts (1 cup)	200
Vegetable		**Other**	
Kale (1 cup)	200	Tofu (raw, firm, 1/2 cup)	250
Collards (cooked, 1/2 cup)	180	Orange juice (supplemented, 8 oz)	300
Broccoli (cooked, 1/2 cup)	90	Cereal (supplemented, 3/4 cup)	150–300

Table 7-4. Calcium Content of Oral Calcium Supplements

TYPE	AMOUNT (%)
Calcium carbonate	40
Tricalcium phosphate	39
Calcium phosphate dibasic	31
Calcium citrate	21
Calcium lactate	13
Calcium gluconate	9

Calcium homeostasis for a healthy, young adult in calcium balance is shown in Fig. 7-1. Only 55% of plasma calcium is available for active metabolism because 45% is bound to protein, mostly to albumin (Table 7-1). Most of the ionized calcium that is filtered by the kidneys is reabsorbed in the proximal tubules. Additional resorption in the distal tubules is highly regulated by hormones. Most of the calcium in the body is contained in the skeleton. Only 1% of skeletal calcium is readily exchangeable with plasma, but this constitutes a major calcium reserve that can be used to maintain the plasma calcium concentrations when needed. Calcium entry and exit from the skeleton are highly regulated by the hormones described below.

Major Sites of Calcium Regulation
Absorption from the gastrointestinal tract
Reabsorption from the kidney
Resorption from bone

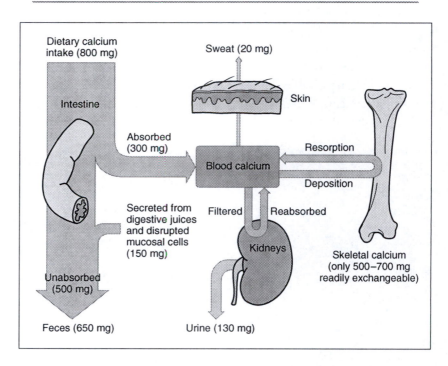

Fig. 7-1. Calcium Balance Maintenance on Dietary Intake of 800 Mg Calcium/Day

Hormonal Regulators of Calcium Balance

The two most influential hormones affecting calcium balance are PTH and $1,25(OH)_2D$. The roles of calcitonin and parathyroid hormone-related protein (PTHrP) in normal human physiology are uncertain, but calcitonin is used therapeutically and PTHrP is a major cause of hypercalcemia.

Major Hormonal Regulators of Calcium Balance

PTH

$1,25(OH)_2D$

Calcitonin

PTHrP

PARATHYROID HORMONE

PTH is an 84–amino acid polypeptide produced by the parathyroid glands in response to low extracellular calcium. PTH secretion and production are exquisitely responsive to any decrease in the concentration of plasma ionic calcium, which is recognized by the calcium-sensing receptor on parathyroid cells. PTH secretion is suppressed when the extracellular calcium level is high. PTH interacts with cell surface receptors on bone and renal tubules. PTH-occupied receptors interact with membrane G-proteins, resulting in activation of adenyl cyclase and increased formation of cyclic adenosine monophosphate (cAMP). cAMP initiates a cascade of cellular phosphorylations that result in cellular action:

> PTH + receptor → altered G-protein → increased cAMP
> and other messengers → increased calcium

PTH increases plasma calcium by increasing the number and activity of osteoclasts (bone-resorbing cells), but PTH does not interact with osteoclasts directly. Instead, PTH interacts with receptors on osteoblasts (bone-forming cells) and elicits responses that cause osteoclast precursors to become mature osteoclasts.

Major Actions of PTH

Increases release of calcium and phosphorous from bone

Increases renal tubular reabsorption of calcium (and magnesium)

Increases renal phosphate excretion

Increases renal conversion of $25(OH)D$ to active $1,25(OH)_2D$

Net result: increased plasma calcium and decreased plasma phosphorous

---

Osteoclast precursor cells are found in the monocyte-macrophage fraction of blood. Differentiation into osteoclasts is controlled by two proteins made by osteoblasts: (1) receptor activator of nuclear factor kappa B ligand (RANKL), which remains on the osteoblast surface, and (2) macrophage-colony stimulating factor (M-CSF). When these proteins combine with their receptors on osteoclast precursor cells, these precursors are committed to become mature osteoclasts (Fig. 7-2). PTH increases synthesis of RANKL and M-CSF.

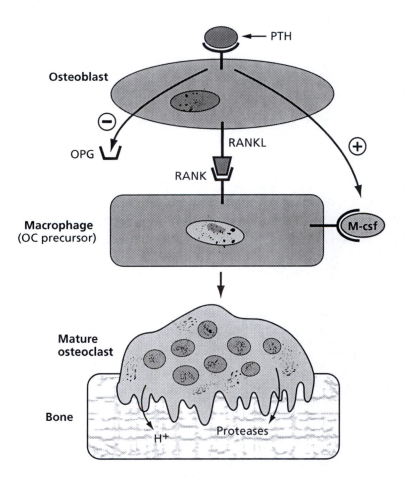

Fig. 7-2. Effect of PTH on Osteoclast Maturation and Bone Resorption

PTH interaction with its receptors on osteoblasts stimulates osteoblast production of M-CSF and RANKL. Interaction of these proteins with their receptors on monocyte/macrophage osteoclast precursors induces these cells to become mature osteoclasts with multiple nuclei and ruffled borders. Osteoclasts secrete acid (H^+) and proteases that dissolve bone and release calcium. RANKL is attached to the osteoblast surface. Interaction of RANKL with RANK, its receptor on macrophage osteoclast precursors, allows the osteoblasts and the osteoclast precursors to make the necessary contact. PTH suppresses osteoblast production of OPG, a soluble decoy receptor protein that competes with RANK for RANKL. Thus, when PTH increases, RANKL–RANK interaction and osteoclast maturation proceed relatively unopposed. M-CSF = macrophage colony–stimulating factor; RANKL = receptor for activation of nuclear factor kappa B ligand; RANK = receptor for activation of nuclear factor kappa B; OPG = osteoprotegerin; OC = osteoclast.

Many other factors affect RANKL. For example, RANKL interaction with its receptor, receptor activator of nuclear factor kappa B (RANK), is blocked by osteoprotegerin (OPG), another osteoblast protein. OPG is a soluble "decoy" receptor that competes with RANK for RANKL. The amount of bone resorption by osteoclasts depends on the balance of RANKL and OPG. PTH inhibits OPG synthesis, leaving RANKL interaction with RANK unopposed (Fig. 7-2). RANKL also stimulates activity of mature osteoclasts.

In the kidney, PTH stimulates calcium reabsorption at the distal tubule and strongly inhibits phosphorous reabsorption proximally and distally. This salvages calcium, prevents hyperphosphatemia, and reduces the risk of calcium phosphate deposition in tissues. PTH increases the activity of the renal enzyme 1α-hydroxylase, which converts inactive 25(OH)D to active $1,25(OH)_2D$. $1,25(OH)_2D$ acts on the intestinal mucosa cells to increase calcium and phosphorous absorption from the intestine. PTH also inhibits bicarbonate reabsorption. The resulting tendency to acidosis inhibits calcium binding to albumin and increases ionized calcium availability.

PTH regulation by extracellular calcium involves feedback loops (Fig. 7-3). Hypocalcemia stimulates PTH synthesis and release. Hypercalcemia suppresses PTH. Both PTH secretion and action are impaired if the magnesium concentration is very low, but magnesium is a much less important regulator of PTH than calcium.

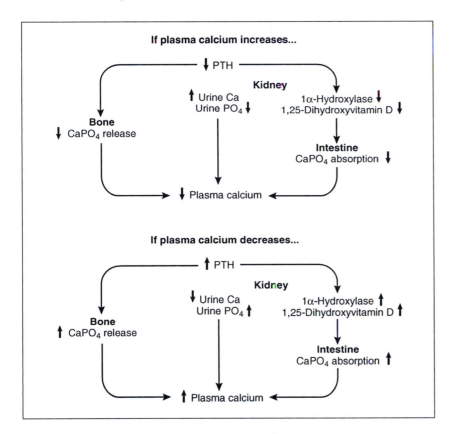

Fig. 7-3. Feedback Loops Regulating the Plasma Calcium Concentration

Calcium-Regulating Hormones and Metabolic Bone Disease   131

Major Regulators of PTH

Stimulators

Low plasma ionized calcium

Inhibitors

High plasma ionized calcium

Very low plasma magnesium

PARATHYROID HORMONE-RELATED PROTEIN (PTHRP)

PTHrP is a 141–amino acid peptide, which is similar to PTH at the N-terminal (8 of the first 13 amino acids are the same). Circulating levels of PTHrP are usually low, but some solid malignancies secrete PTHrP. PTHrP binds to the PTH receptor as well as PTH and causes similar effects. In bone, PTHrP increases osteoclast activity with release of calcium and phosphorous. In the kidney, PTHrP stimulates an increase in urinary cAMP levels and causes increased calcium retention and increased phosphorous excretion. Patients with high PTHrP have much lower levels of $1,25(OH)_2D$ than patients with high PTH. The reason for this is unknown. Overall, PTHrP action results in increased plasma calcium and decreased plasma phosphorous.

The PTHrP concentration is high at some time in many fetal tissues, where it is believed to affect cartilage development and mineralization. PTHrP is high in amniotic fluid, where it may be involved in placental calcium transport, and in breast milk, where it is presumed to affect calcium transport from the mother to the fetus.

CALCITONIN

Calcitonin is a 32–amino acid peptide, which is secreted primarily by parafollicular C cells of the thyroid gland in response to an increase in extracellular calcium. The main action of calcitonin is to suppress osteoclasts, the bone-resorbing cells. After a meal, plasma calcium increases, calcitonin is secreted, bone resorption is suppressed, and calcium and phosphorous are retained in bone. Calcitonin action opposes action of PTH (Table 7-5).

Calcitonin and PTH should check and balance each other to maintain calcium homeostasis. However, it is unclear whether calcitonin has

Table 7-5. Parathyroid Hormone (PTH) vs. Calcitonin

HORMONE	SOURCE	RECEPTORS	EFFECTS
PTH	Parathyroid glands	Osteoblasts	Increased osteoclast action Increased bone resorption Increased plasma calcium
Calcitonin	Thyroid parafollicular cells	Osteoclasts	Decreased osteoclast action Decreased bone resorption Decreased plasma calcium (transiently)

a significant effect on plasma calcium in adult humans. Thyroid C cells secrete calcitonin in response to acute changes in plasma calcium, but changes in calcitonin secretion in response to chronic hypercalcemia and hypocalcemia are uncertain. People who undergo total thyroidectomy with loss of their thyroid C cells do not develop hypercalcemia and patients with medullary carcinoma of the thyroid have enormous plasma calcitonin levels but do not have hypocalcemia. Calcitonin levels are higher in men than in women and decrease with age, but whether this contributes to bone loss with aging in not known. Calcitonin is found in many other tissues, especially the pituitary and the central nervous system where it may have paracrine actions. Calcitonin is used pharmacologically for treatment of hypercalcemia and osteoporosis (see below).

VITAMIN D

Vitamin D is not a true vitamin, since it can be made by the action of sunlight on the skin. It is a fat-soluble hormone that increases the absorption of calcium from the intestine. When exposed to solar energy in the ultraviolet B (UVB) range, 7-dehydrocholesterol (7-DHC) in the epidermis is transformed to previtamin D_3, which isomerizes over the course of several hours to vitamin D_3 (Fig. 7-4). Vitamin D_3 is also

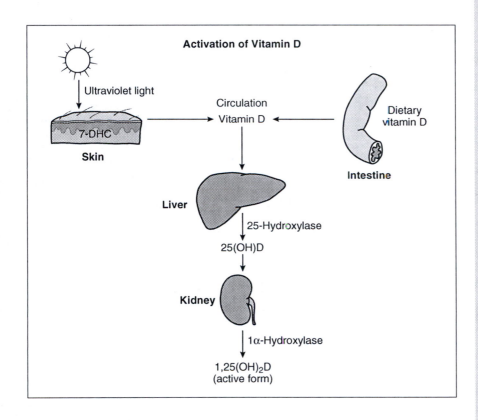

Fig. 7-4. Activation of Vitamin D Obtained from the Diet or Via the Action of Sunlight on Skin

7-DHC = 7-dehydrocholesterol.

Table 7-6. Dietary Sources of Vitamin D

SOURCE	AMOUNT (µG/100 G)	SOURCE	AMOUNT (µG/100 G)
Cod liver oil	125–625	Liver	0.75
Herring	22.5	Egg yolk	1.75
Mackerel	17.7	Cow milk*	0.01–0.10
Salmon, canned	12.5	Butter	0.76
Sardines, canned	7.5	Cheese	0.25
Tuna	5.8	Human milk	0.01–0.25

Note. 1 µg = 25 IU vitamin D. Vitamin D recommended daily allowances (RDAs): 400 IU/day for children, adolescents, pregnant or lactating women; 200 IU/day for adults; RDAs are higher if exposure to sunlight is low.
*In the United States, cow milk is supplemented with vitamin D (400 IU/qt).

available in the diet, mostly from animal sources such as fatty fish, liver, egg yolk, and vitamin D–fortified milk (Table 7-6). Severe nutritional vitamin D deficiency has decreased markedly since fortified milk was introduced. Vitamin D_2 is a similar product found in plants and yeast.

The recommended daily allowance (RDA) of vitamin D (see Table 7-6) is higher for children, adolescents, and pregnant and lactating women. The RDA is based on the assumption that much of the daily requirement will come from exposure to sunlight. This can be a major problem for those who are housebound and those who live in northern latitudes. The amount of UVB available from sunlight diminishes markedly as summer progresses into fall, and at the latitudes of Boston/Minneapolis/Seattle, for example, very little skin production of vitamin D occurs between November and March. Clothing and sunblock prevent vitamin D formation even when more sunlight is available.

Obtaining more vitamin D from sunlight becomes more difficult with age as skin becomes thinner and the content of 7-DHC decreases. Individuals over the age of 70 produce only 30% as much vitamin D as young adults do from the same amount of sunlight. Individuals with high melanin levels in the skin require longer sun exposure for the synthesis of vitamin D_3 because melanin competes with 7-dehydrocholesterol for UVB.

Vitamin D supplements (Table 7-7) are available for those who are unable to obtain adequate vitamin D from their diet and sunlight. Some multivitamin tablets and oral calcium supplements contain vitamin D. It is important for most patients to avoid pharmacologic doses of vitamin D because excess vitamin D and its metabolites can be stored in body fat for a long time and cause prolonged hypercalciuria and hypercalcemia.

Vitamins D_3 and D_2 enter the circulation from the skin or intestine and are carried to the liver bound to vitamin D–binding protein. In the liver they are hydroxylated to 25(OH)D (see Fig. 7-4). This step is poorly regulated so any amount of vitamin D can be converted to

Table 7-7. Vitamin D Supplements

SUPPLEMENT	GENERIC NAME	DAILY DOSE
Vitamin D_3	Cholecalciferol	400–1000 units
Vitamin D_2	Ergocalciferol	400–1000 units
Reduced D_2 (DHT)	Dihydrotachysterol	200 µg
25(OH)Vitamin D_3	Calcifediol	≤20–50 µg
1,25(OH)$_2$Vitamin D_3	Calcitriol	0.25–1.0 µg

25(OH)D, the major storage form of the hormone. The best measurement of vitamin D stores is the 25(OH)D level.

Eventually, 25(OH)D is transported to the kidney where it is hydrolyzed to the active form, 1,25(OH)$_2$D, by the enzyme 1α-hydroxylase. The conversion of 25(OH)$_2$D is highly regulated by feedback loops. A decrease in ionized calcium elicits an increase in PTH, which stimulates renal 1α-hydroxylase activity. PTH also stimulates renal excretion of phosphorous, and lower plasma phosphorous stimulates 1,25(OH)$_2$D production. 1,25(OH)$_2$D also regulates its own production. A low level of 1,25(OH)$_2$D stimulates its synthesis.

Major Actions of 1,25(OH)$_2$D

Increases calcium absorption from the small intestine

Increases phosphorous absorption from the small intestine

When plasma ionized calcium is increased, the pathways operate in reverse. High calcium suppresses PTH, 1α-hydroxylase activity decreases, and activation of 25(OH)D decreases. High plasma phosphorous and a high 1,25(OH)$_2$D level also suppress 1α-hydroxylase activity. These feedback loops normally insure an adequate supply of 1,25(OH)$_2$D while preventing hypercalcemia due to overproduction of the active hormone (see Fig. 7-4).

1,25(OH)$_2$D acts like a steroid hormone. Its target tissues contain a 1,25(OH) receptor, which is similar to other steroid hormone receptors. When 1,25(OH)$_2$D binds to its receptor, and the 1,25 (OH)$_2$D-receptor complex binds to the appropriate response element in the nucleus, altered gene transcription results in protein synthesis. 1,25(OH)$_2$D increases calcium absorption by increasing synthesis of calcium-binding protein, which increases calcium transport across the intestine. 1,25(OH)$_2$D also increases intestinal absorption of phosphorous.

The increased availability of both calcium and phosphorous promotes bone mineralization. 1,25(OH)$_2$D also stimulates synthesis of several proteins in osteoblasts. However, the actions of 1,25(OH)$_2$D on bone are complex. If the plasma calcium level cannot be maintained by calcium from the diet, 1,25(OH)$_2$D stimulates the differentiation of precursor cells into osteoclasts.

Notes

Major Regulators of 1,25(OH)$_2$D

Stimulators

Low plasma ionized calcium → high PTH

Low plasma phosphorous

Low 1,25(OH)$_2$D

Inhibitors

High plasma ionized calcium → low PTH

High plasma phosphorous

High 1,25(OH)$_2$D

Many non–calcium-regulating cells also contain 1α-hydroxylase and 1,25(OH)$_2$D receptors. They produce 1,25(OH)$_2$D, which acts locally to suppress cell proliferation and to increase cell differentiation. These mechanisms are not well understood.

Failure of Calcium Homeostasis

The elegant, interlocking control mechanisms that maintain calcium within the normal range occasionally fail, resulting in hypercalcemia, hypocalcemia, or failure to maintain normal bone. The nomenclature of some of the disorders can be confusing. For example, hyperparathyroidism indicates overproduction of PTH, but this is not always associated with hypercalcemia. The term *primary hyperparathyroidism* is used when the primary problem is excess parathyroid tissue secretion of PTH that is not suppressed by high calcium. *Secondary hyperparathyroidism* refers to parathyroid hyperplasia and high circulating PTH levels that are an appropriate response to prolonged hypocalcemia. Prolonged secondary hypoparathyroidism can lead to *tertiary hyperparathyroidism*, in which excess PTH continues to be secreted even after the hypocalcemia has been corrected. Tertiary hyperparathyroidism results from a combination of excess parathyroid tissue and acquired defects in the parathyroid tissue response to calcium.

HYPERCALCEMIA

Hypercalcemia results from excessive resorption of bone or increased calcium absorption from the intestine with inadequate renal excretion of the excess calcium. In the past, when measuring the serum calcium level was impossible or uncommon, hypercalcemia went undiagnosed until the symptoms or signs were severe. Now hypercalcemia presents most often as an abnormal laboratory measurement in patients who are asymptomatic or who have symptoms (e.g., weakness, fatigue) that might be due to other causes. It is important to be sure that the calcium level is not falsely elevated due to dehydration or hemoconcentration during blood drawing, which may result in high albumin and total calcium levels, but a normal ionized calcium level. If this is suspected, subtracting 0.8 mg/dL per each gram of albumin over a level of 4.0 g/dL will provide a rough estimate of the true total calcium level.

Symptoms and Signs of Hypercalcemia

Hypercalcemia has been described as the disease of the "-ones" (rhymes with "stones"):

- Stones: kidney stones, nephrocalcinosis, thirst, polyuria, and metabolic acidosis
- Bones: bone pain and fractures
- Groans: anorexia, dyspepsia, and constipation
- Moans: fatigue, myalgia, proximal muscle weakness, and joint pain
- Overtones: depression, memory loss, confusion, lethargy, and coma

Obviously hypercalcemia affects many organ systems. Impaired renal concentrating ability causes the polyuria and thirst. The resulting dehydration makes the hypercalcemia worse. Bone pain and fractures occur only with severe or prolonged bone resorption. Gastrointestinal symptoms occur more frequently. Hypercalcemia makes nerve and muscle hypoexcitable and results in the neuromuscular abnormalities listed above. The rate of cardiac repolarization is increased, and the electrocardiogram may show a short Q-T interval. Joint pain is due to calcium deposition in joints and tendons and to chondrocalcinosis. Patients with hypercalcemia have excess hypertension, but the mechanism is not known.

Causes of Hypercalcemia

Primary hyperparathyroidism and hypercalcemia associated with malignancy account for 90% of hypercalcemia. Other major causes include an abnormal calcium sensor protein, vitamin D excess, drugs, and prolonged immobilization.

Major Causes of Hypercalcemia

Too much PTH
Primary hyperparathyroidism
Multiple endocrine neoplasia (MEN) syndromes
Too much PTHrP
Hypercalcemia of malignancy
Abnormal calcium sensor protein
Familial hypocalciuric hypercalcemia
Too much vitamin D
Exogenous: excess ingestion
Endogenous: granulomatous diseases, malignancy
Tumor cytokines, which stimulate osteoclasts
Drugs
Prolonged immobilization

Hypercalcemia Due to Primary Hyperparathyroidism (excess PTH). Eighty percent of primary hyperparathyroidism is due to hypersecretion from a single parathyroid adenoma. The remainder is due to parathyroid hyperplasia (all parathyroid glands are enlarged and overactive). Parathyroid carcinoma is rare.

Hypercalcemia due to a parathyroid adenoma is common (incidence is 1 in 500–1000), especially in middle-aged women. Most patients have mild hypercalcemia and are asymptomatic or have only vague, nonspecific complaints. Classic renal manifestations include hypercalciuria (24-hr calcium excretion >240 mg in women and >300 mg in men), increased urine phosphorus, and reduced creatinine clearance. Twenty percent of patients have kidney stones. Cortical bone mineral density may be low due to excess bone resorption, Surprisingly, trabecular bone is often spared. Complications of severe disease include subperiosteal bone resorption and erosion of the distal tufts of the fingers, which can be seen on industrial grade x-ray film (Fig. 7-5). Bone cysts (osteitis fibrosa cystica) occur in less than 2% of cases. The diagnosis is confirmed by the classic laboratory findings shown in Table 7-8. No treatment except maintaining good hydration is necessary for patients with mild disease. Surgery is recommended for patients with symptoms or plasma calcium ≥1 mg/dL above the upper limit of normal, 24-hour urine calcium >400 mg, kidney stones, or bone mineral density ≤2.5 standard deviations (SD) below the young adult mean.

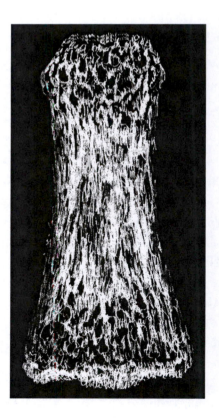

Fig. 7-5. Phalanx in a Patient with Severe Hyperparathyroidism

Note the subperiosteal and intracortical bone resorption.

Table 7-8. Abnormal Calcium States: Circulating Concentrations

DISORDER	CALCIUM	PHOSPHOROUS	1,25(OH)$_2$D	PTH*
Hypercalcemia				
Hyperparathyroidism	High	Low	High	High
PTH-related peptide (PTHrP)	High	Low	Normal	Low
Vitamin D excess	High	High	High	Low
Hypocalcemia				
Hypoparathyroidism	Low	High	Low	Low
Pseudohypoparathyroidism	Low	High	Low	High
Vitamin D deficiency	Low	Low	Low	High
Resistance to 1,25(OH)$_2$D	Low	Low	High	High
Renal failure	Low	High	Low	High

*PTH = parathyroid hormone

Hypercalcemia due to parathyroid hyperplasia occurs as part of two familial, autosomal dominant multiple endocrine neoplasia (MEN) syndromes. MEN-1 is the association of parathyroid hyperplasia with pituitary and pancreatic islet cell tumors. Mutations in the MEN-1 gene, a tumor suppressor gene that codes for the protein menin, have been mapped to chromosome 11. MEN-2A is the association of parathyroid hyperplasia with pheochromocytoma and medullary carcinoma of the thyroid (MTC). The MEN-2A gene, a RET oncogene, is located on chromosome 10. Parathyroid involvement is unusual in MEN-2B, which is associated with MTC, pheochromocytoma, and mucosal neuromas. The clinical and laboratory manifestations of MEN-associated hypercalcemia are the same as for a parathyroid adenoma. Hypercalcemia treatment involves surgical removal of most parathyroid tissue.

Hypercalcemia Due to Malignancy. Tumors usually cause hypercalcemia by producing circulating factors that affect bone resorption. Tumor production of circulating PTHrP is the most common cause of hypercalcemia associated with malignancy. This occurs most often with squamous cell cancers, usually late in the course, when the disease is severe. Patients have hypercalcemia, hypophosphatemia, high urine calcium and phosphorous, and high PTHrP. The PTH level is low because it is suppressed by the hypercalcemia (see Table 7-8). Although PTHrP stimulates renal 1α-hydroxylase, the 1,25(OH)$_2$D level is usually within normal limits, and absorption of calcium from the intestine is not increased. The reason for this is not known.

Causes of Malignancy-Induced Hypercalcemia

Tumor PTHrP
Tumor 1,25(OH)$_2$D
Tumor cytokines

Notes

Some lymphomas produce enough $1,25(OH)_2D$ to cause hypercalcemia. This is thought to be due to excessive conversion of $25(OH)D$ to $1,25(OH)_2D$ by tumor cells. Laboratory values are similar to those expected for vitamin D excess (see Table 7-8). PTH is suppressed by the hypercalcemia.

Some tumors like multiple myeloma produce cytokines, which strongly stimulate osteoclasts. Release of both calcium and phosphorus from bone causes hypercalcemia and hyperphosphatemia, especially if the tumor-associated kidney disease impairs calcium and phosphorus excretion. PTH is suppressed in response to the hypercalcemia, and $1,25(OH)_2D$ is low due to low PTH, high phosphorus, and renal disease.

Hypercalcemia due to bone destruction by invasive tumor metastases is likely to be due to local tumor production of cytokines or PTHrP. This is thought to be the mechanism causing hypercalcemia in patients with breast cancer.

Hypercalcemia Due to Excess Vitamin D. The amount of vitamin D in most over-the-counter multivitamin tablets is too small to cause hypercalcemia if taken as recommended. High doses can cause hypercalciuria and hypercalcemia, especially in patients taking calcium supplements or patients with another problem with calcium regulation. Since vitamin D is fat soluble, depletion of accumulated body stores can take some time.

Hypercalcemia can be due to excessive endogenous $1,25(OH)_2D$ production. Conversion of $25(OH)D$ to $1,25(OH)_2D$ by some lymphomas has been described. This also occurs with granulomatous diseases, including sarcoidosis, tuberculosis, leprosy, and silicone-induced granulomatosis. Levels of calcium, phosphorous, and $1,25(OH)_2D$ are high (see Table 7-8), despite PTH suppression by hypercalcemia. Macrophage 1α-hydroxylase does not respond to PTH and is not down-regulated by high $1,25(OH)_2D$. Patients with granulomas sometimes have worse hypercalcemia and hypercalciuria in the summer, when sun exposure increases their $25(OH)D$ stores.

Hypercalcemia Due to Calcium Receptor Mutations. Familial hypocalciuric hypercalcemia (FHH) is an autosomal dominant disorder caused by mutations in the calcium receptor gene located on chromosome 3. Under normal conditions, if plasma ionized calcium increases, more calcium occupies the calcium receptor on parathyroid cells, less PTH is released, and calcium decreases to normal. Families with FHH have defective receptors, so a higher level of calcium is required to lower PTH.

Patients with FHH have lifelong hypercalcemia, which is usually asymptomatic. They have relatively low urine calcium, considering the hypercalcemia (renal calcium clearance/creatinine clearance <0.01) and borderline high serum magnesium. Serum phosphorous is mildly depressed. Their PTH levels are slightly high or normal (not suppressed by the high calcium as would be expected). They usually require no treatment. Hypercalcemia persists even after subtotal parathyroidectomy. Hypocalciuria also persists due to the abnormal calcium receptor on renal tubule cells. Total parathyroidectomy causes hypocalcemia.

Family screening should be done to prevent unnecessary surgery in other affected members. Occasionally newborns who are homozygous for the abnormal receptor gene develop severe hypercalcemia.

Other Causes of Hypercalcemia. Hydrochlorothiazide (HCTZ) increases calcium reabsorption by the kidney. This can cause hypercalcemia, particularly in the setting of very mild (often previously undiagnosed) hyperparathyroidism. Lithium can cause hypercalcemia by raising the set point for suppression of PTH by calcium. Vitamin A intoxication causes excessive osteoclast activation. Vitamin D intoxication is described above. High acute or chronic calcium ingestion can cause hypercalcemia, usually in the setting of renal impairment. The milk-alkali syndrome is the association of hypercalcemia, metabolic alkalosis, and renal impairment after ingestion of calcium plus an absorbable alkali such as calcium carbonate.

Immobilization, prolonged bed rest, and weightlessness in space flight are associated with marked bone resorption. Growing children and adults with an underlying disorder causing high bone turnover, such as hyperparathyroidism or hyperthyroidism, are particularly vulnerable to developing hypercalcemia in this setting.

Evaluation of Hypercalcemia

- Review symptoms, signs, and duration (a long course is more likely to be benign)
- Check family history to rule out MEN or FHH
- Physical examination
- Laboratory values: serum calcium, albumin, phosphorous, PTH, 25(OH)D, creatinine, magnesium; urine calcium and creatinine
- X-rays: abdomen for kidney stones and any site of bone pain
- Bone densitometry

All of these are not necessary in every case. It is usually not necessary to measure PTHrP. A low PTH level rules out hyperparathyroidism. Most of the time an underlying malignancy is obvious because hypercalcemia is a late manifestation.

Treatment of Hypercalcemia

Patients should keep themselves hydrated, discontinue any medications contributing to hypercalcemia, and avoid immobilization as much as possible. No other treatment may be necessary for patients with mild hypercalcemia who are asymptomatic.

When hypercalcemia is severe enough to require immediate treatment, volume depletion should be corrected with hydration, which reduces plasma calcium by increasing renal excretion. Intravenous bisphosphonates such as pamidronate and zoledronic acid are strong inhibitors of osteoclastic bone resorption. Calcitonin also suppresses osteoclast activity, but the effect is transient, perhaps due to down-regulation of receptors. Glucocorticoids inhibit tumor cytokine release. They also inhibit intestinal calcium absorption, which is useful in cases of vitamin D excess. Oral phosphate binds ingested calcium but may cause diarrhea and hyperphosphatemia. The combination of hypercalcemia and hyperphosphatemia increases the risk of soft tissue calcification. Dialysis may be required if severe hypercalcemia is accompanied by renal failure.

Parathyroidectomy is the treatment of choice when a parathyroid adenoma or parathyroid hyperplasia causes symptomatic or severe hypercalcemia.

HYPOCALCEMIA

Symptoms and Signs of Hypocalcemia

Most symptoms of hypocalcemia are due to increased neuromuscular irritability. Numbness and tingling occur around the mouth and in the fingertips and toes. More severe or rapidly developing hypocalcemia elicits muscle cramps and pain, irritability, impaired mentation, and seizures. Severe hypocalcemia causes congestive heart failure, a prolonged Q-T interval on the ECG, laryngospasm, bronchospasm, and tetany (spontaneous spasms of the muscles of the face and extremities). Panicky patients may hyperventilate and become hypocapnic and alkalotic, which makes the problem worse. Alkalosis causes increased binding of calcium to albumin, decreasing ionized calcium even further. Prolonged hypocalcemia causes intestinal malabsorption, posterior cataracts, basal ganglia calcifications, and extrapyramidal neurologic symptoms. Defective dentition occurs if hypocalcemia begins in childhood.

Latent tetany can be elicited by tapping over the facial nerve in front of the ear lobe (facial spasm = Chvostek's sign) or by inflating a blood pressure cuff above the systolic pressure for 2 minutes (carpal spasm = Trousseau's sign).

If hypocalcemia presents as an unexpected laboratory abnormality, it is important to be sure that ionized calcium really is low and that hypocalcemia is not just the result of low protein-bound calcium. A rough correction for low albumin can be made by adding 0.8 mg/dL to the total serum calcium for every 1.0 g/dL of albumin level lower than 4.0 g/dL.

Causes of Hypocalcemia

The most common causes of hypocalcemia are PTH and vitamin D deficiency. Hypocalcemia due to PTH or vitamin D resistance or an abnormal calcium receptor protein does not occur often, but these disorders and hypocalcemia due to renal failure, severe hyperphosphatemia, or both illustrate major mechanisms of hormone action on calcium homeostasis.

CASE STUDY: *CONTINUED*

Ms. R. presented with asymptomatic primary hyperparathyroidism. The differential diagnosis included the MEN syndromes because her father had kidney stones and hypertension. However, these are common disorders in the general population. Neither of Ms. R.'s daughters nor her sisters had hypercalcemia, and Ms. R. presented no evidence for another endocrine disorder. The high urine calcium ruled out FHH. There was no evidence of malignancy, and the high PTH level ruled out either PTHrP or vitamin D toxicity as the primary cause of the hypercalcemia. The small amount of vitamin D in her multivitamin tablets was not enough to cause hypercalcemia, but it could exacerbate hypercalcemia as a result of another condition. When her hypercalcemia worsened, Ms. R. underwent surgery, which confirmed the presence of a parathyroid adenoma.

After her accident, Ms. R. spent 3 years undergoing rehabilitation before she was able to resume modest activity at home. Two years later she noted increasing weakness and pain in her arms and legs and occasional tingling in her fingers and toes and around her mouth. Her only medication was an anticonvulsant to prevent seizures. Her physical examination revealed a tender sternum and tibiae, proximal muscle weakness, positive Chvostek's sign, and slight hyperreflexia. Her electrocardiogram (ECG) showed a normal Q-T interval. Laboratory tests revealed: calcium 5.8 mg/dL (low); PTH high; albumin normal; phosphorous 2.1 mg/dL (low); 25(OH)D and 1,25(OH)$_2$D low; and urine calcium and phosphorous low.

Causes of Hypocalcemia

PTH deficiency: surgical, hypomagnesemia, autoimmune, congenital
PTH resistance
Vitamin D deficiency
Vitamin D resistance
Abnormal calcium receptor protein
Renal failure (secondary hyperparathyroidism)
Severe hyperphosphatemia
Other: drugs, pancreatitis, transfusion of citrated blood

Hypocalcemia Due to PTH Deficiency. The most common cause of PTH deficiency is surgical damage or removal of the parathyroid glands during thyroid surgery, radical neck dissection, or extensive parathyroid surgery. Transient hypocalcemia for the first few days after removal of a parathyroid adenoma can occur due to edema, hemorrhage, low magnesium, or the "hungry bones" syndrome (patients with very active PTH-induced bone resorption rapidly redeposit calcium and phosphorous in bone when the PTH-producing adenoma is removed). Prolonged postsurgical hypocalcemia indicates permanent damage.

Hypomagnesemia causes hypocalcemia because adequate magnesium is needed for both PTH synthesis and secretion.

Autoimmune hypoparathyroidism can be familial or sporadic and occur alone or as part of a polyglandular deficiency syndrome. The most common association is hypoparathyroidism + adrenal insufficiency (Addison disease) + mucocutaneous candidiasis (moniliasis), or HAM syndrome. The moniliasis usually occurs first, then the hypoparathyroidism, and then the adrenal insufficiency. Polyglandular autoimmune hypoparathyroidism can also be associated with any of the following: vitiligo, alopecia, pernicious anemia, coeliac disease, hypothyroidism, hypogonadism, or type 1 diabetes mellitus.

Hypoparathyroidism in newborns due to congenital absence of the parathyroid glands is associated with other congenital anomalies in several syndromes. Isolated absence of the parathyroid glands is inherited as an X-linked or autosomal recessive disorder.

PTH deficiency is characterized by low PTH, low calcium, high phosphorous, and low $1,25(OH)_2D$ despite normal renal function (see Table 7-8). Urine calcium is low. Treatment involves giving enough calcium and vitamin D supplements to keep plasma calcium in the low-normal range. Higher calcium levels are not desirable because without PTH to help retain urine calcium patients are at risk for hypercalciuria and kidney stones. Calcium supplements are preferred to a diet high in dairy products because the latter also contain phosphorous.

Hypocalcemia Due to PTH resistance (pseudohypoparathyroidism [PHP]). Hypocalcemia occurs despite normal parathyroid activity if bone and kidney are resistant to PTH as a result of a defect in the PTH receptor, an abnormal G-protein associated with the receptor, defective generation of cAMP, or failure anywhere in the subsequent cascade of phosphorylations. Calcium is low, but the PTH level is high because the parathyroid glands oversecrete PTH in an attempt to compensate. This situation, referred to as PHP, is one of the causes of *secondary hyperparathyroidism*, so called because the high PTH level is secondary to the hypocalcemia. Resistance to PTH results in high plasma phosphorous and low $1,25(OH)_2D$ (see Table 7-8). The classic test for PHP is the PTH infusion test. Patients with PHP do not have a normal increase in urinary cAMP and renal phosphorous excretion in response to PTH.

There are several variants of PHP depending on the site of the defect. Patients with PHP type Ia have only 50% of the normal level of the $G_{S\alpha}$ subunit of the G-protein that responds to PTH receptor occupancy. They can have the same $G_{S\alpha}$ defect in other glands, resulting in a diminished response to thyroid-stimulating hormone (TSH), follicle-stimulating hormone (FSH), and luteinizing hormone (LH). Patients with PHP Ia have a distinct phenotype that includes obesity, short stature, round facies, brachydactyly (short 4th and 5th metacarpals giving a knuckle-knuckle-dimple-dimple appearance to the hand), subcutaneous ossification, and mental retardation. This phenotype was first described by Fuller Albright, so PHP Ia is also called Albright hereditary osteodystrophy (AHO).

Genetic disorders of $G_{S\alpha}$ demonstrate imprinting, the transcription of genes from only one parental allele. PHP Ia is inherited only from an affected mother. When the abnormal gene is inherited from an affected father, patients have the skeletal and developmental defects, but they do not have PTH resistance. Calcium and PTH levels and urine cAMP responses to PTH infusion are normal. This variation is called *pseudopseudohypoparathyroidism (PPHP)*. Patients with PHP Ib have PTH resistance but not the skeletal and developmental abnormalities. The treatment of PHP is similar to the treatment for primary hypoparathyroidism.

Hypocalcemia Due to Vitamin D Deficiency. Vitamin D deficiency occurs because of defective supply or defective processing. Problems with obtaining enough vitamin D from the diet and adequate sunlight exposure have been discussed. Malabsorption syndromes exacerbate any dietary deficiency. With severe liver and kidney disease, vitamin D cannot be hydroxylated to 25(OH)D and 1,25(OH)$_2$D. Catabolism of vitamin D is accelerated by drugs such as anticonvulsants, which increase activity of the liver P450 enzyme system. Phenytoin also inhibits calcium absorption in the intestine.

Major Causes of Vitamin D deficiency

Diet low in vitamin D
Malabsorption of vitamin D
Little sun exposure
Severe liver disease
Renal failure
Increased catabolism

Vitamin D deficiency in childhood results in *rickets*, which is characterized by formation of disordered excess cartilage, poor bone formation at the epiphyseal growth plate, and poor mineralization of osteoid in cortical and trabecular bone (Fig. 7-6). Infants with rapidly growing bones develop widened cranial sutures, a soft calvarium prone to deformity, bulging costochondral junctions (rachitic rosary on the anterior chest), wrist enlargement, and delayed eruption of teeth. Older children develop deformities due to pressure on weakened growth plates in weight-bearing bones, resulting in bowed legs (genu varum) or knock knees (genu valgum).

In adults the epiphyseal growth plates have fused. Severe vitamin D deficiency results in defective bone mineralization *(osteomalacia)*.

Bone biopsies show increased osteoid (unmineralized bone). The major clinical finding is diffuse bone pain. X-rays of the long bones may show thin radiolucent lines (Looser's lines) perpendicular to the cortex; these are not fractures. Both children and adults develop muscle weakness.

Laboratory findings (see Table 7-8) include a low calcium level and a high PTH level in response to the hypocalcemia (another example of secondary hyperparathyroidism). Calcium may be low-normal if the high PTH causes enough bone resorption and renal calcium retention to compensate for the poor calcium absorption from the intestine. Phosphorous levels are low, partly due to decreased absorption from the intestine and partly due to the action of PTH on the kidneys. Serum 25(OH)D levels are low. Conversion of 25(OH)D to $1,25(OH)_2D$ is increased in response to the high level of PTH, and $1,25(OH)_2D$ can remain in the normal range until the vitamin D deficiency is severe.

Treatment of vitamin D deficiency involves improving the diet; increasing sunlight exposure, when possible; and supplementing with some form of vitamin D. Overtreatment results in hypercalciuria and hypercalcemia.

Hypocalcemia Due to Vitamin D Resistance. Rare genetic defects in vitamin D metabolism result in ineffective vitamin D action even though the supply of vitamin D is normal. Patients with severe defects present with childhood rickets; milder defects may result in osteomalacia later.

Vitamin D–dependent rickets type I (VDDR-I) is an autosomal recessive disorder caused by a mutation in the gene for renal 1α-hydroxylase.

> Defective 1α-hydroxylase → low $1,25(OH)_2D$ → low calcium → high PTH

Phosphorous is low due to decreased absorption from the intestine and PTH-induced renal excretion. In the past, patients were treated with very large doses of vitamin D—hence the name "vitamin D–dependent" rickets—resulting in very high levels of 25(OH)D or some other metabolite, which has some activity. Now patients are treated with $1,25(OH)_2D$.

Vitamin D–dependent rickets type II (resistance to $1,25(OH)_2D$) is an autosomal recessive disorder caused by a mutation in the $1,25(OH)_2D$ receptor or to a postreceptor defect, so there is no response to $1,25(OH)_2D$.

> Resistance to $1,25(OH)_2D$ → low calcium → high PTH → high $1,25(OH)_2D$

The resulting hypocalcemia elicits a high level of PTH, which stimulates conversion of 25(OH)D to $1,25(OH)_2D$. Phosphorous is low as in VDDR-I. These patients also develop alopecia, indicating that $1,25(OH)_2D$ has some action on hair follicles. If the defect is mild, patients sometimes respond to vitamin D supplements. However, half the patients do not respond even to very high doses. These patients are treated with very high doses of calcium.

Hypocalcemia Due to Renal Failure. Patients with kidney disease often develop hypocalcemia that leads to high PTH levels (secondary hyperparathyroidism). Loss of renal function results in loss of renal 1α-hydroxylase and inability to convert $25(OH)D$ to $1,25(OH)_2D$. Calcium absorption from the intestine is severely compromised. Patients with kidney failure are unable to excrete phosphorous, so phosphorous levels are high. Hyperphosphatemia lowers calcium levels directly (calcium + phosphorous $\rightarrow CaPO_4$). Hyperphosphatemia also suppresses 1α-hydroxylase.

Renal failure $\rightarrow$ low $1,25(OH)_2D$ and high phosphorous $\rightarrow$ low calcium $\rightarrow$ high PTH

Prolonged renal failure results in significant, even severe, parathyroid hyperplasia. The high PTH increases osteoclast bone resorption, which releases both calcium and phosphorous. Since the phosphorous cannot be excreted, the hyperphosphatemia becomes even worse. Bone resorption results in bone pain and fractures.

Treatment includes $1,25(OH)_2D$, calcium supplements, and phosphorous binders. If treatment of hypocalcemia is successful, parathyroid hyperplasia regresses. Prolonged hypocalcemia can cause progressive parathyroid hyperplasia to the point where the parathyroid tissue appears autonomous. PTH production remains higher than normal, even if the underlying renal disease is corrected by renal transplant. If hypercalcemia also develops, the patients have developed tertiary hyperparathyroidism.

Hypocalcemia Due to an Abnormal Calcium Sensor (hypercalciuric hypocalcemia). Mutations in the calcium receptor protein on parathyroid and renal tubule cells can cause a gain in receptor function. These patients have low or low-normal PTH because the calcium receptor is oversensitive to extracellular calcium, and PTH secretion is suppressed. They have hypocalcemia, hypercalciuria, and hypomagnesemia. These abnormalities are the opposite of those in families with FHH (see above) who have a decrease in calcium receptor function. Symptomatic patients should be given just enough vitamin D to raise the calcium enough to suppress their symptoms. Asymptomatic patients should not be treated.

Hypocalcemia Due to Severe Hyperphosphatemia. Normally, the product of the calcium times phosphorous concentrations is less than 60. If $[Ca] \times [P]$ is ≥ 70 after an oral or intravenous phosphorous load, $CaPO_4$ tends to precipitate in soft tissues. High phosphorous also suppresses renal 1α-hydroxylase, and the decrease in $1,25(OH)_2D$ also contributes to hypocalcemia. Hyperphosphatemia severe enough to cause hypocalcemia occurs in renal failure, after chemotherapy, or in rhabdomyolysis, which causes massive cellular lysis with release of intracellular phosphorous.

Other Causes of Hypocalcemia. Drugs that effectively suppress osteoclasts and decrease calcium release from bone (e.g., the bisphosphonates) can cause hypocalcemia. Transfusion with citrated blood or administration of contrast dyes, which contain the calcium chelator EDTA, can cause hypocalcemia.

Patients with pancreatitis can develop profound hypocalcemia, but the mechanisms are uncertain. Release of pancreatic lipase results in excessive release of free fatty acids, which bind calcium. These patients also have hypomagnesemia, which impairs PTH secretion and action.

Metabolic Bone Diseases

Metabolic bone diseases involve abnormal activity of packets of bone known as bone-forming units (BFUs). The normal balance between bone formation and bone resorption is upset, resulting in either loss of bone mass or formation of abnormal bone. The major metabolic bone diseases are osteoporosis, osteomalacia, and Paget disease of bone.

Major Metabolic Bone Diseases

Osteoporosis—a disorder of excessive bone resorption
Osteomalacia—a disorder of bone formation
Paget disease—a disorder of bone remodeling

BONE BALANCE AND BONE MASS

In young people the main bone processes are modeling and growth. Growth factors, hormones and exercise stimulate osteoblasts directly, and bone mass increases. Acquisition of bone mass is nearly complete by the end of adolescence, but another 5% to 10% of bone mass accumulates in the third decade of life when it reaches its peak. Peak bone mass is largely genetically determined, although it is affected by many other factors, including nutrition, activity, and illness. It is higher in men than in women and is higher in blacks than in whites or Asians.

CASE STUDY: *CONTINUED*

Ms. R. developed classic symptoms and signs of hypocalcemia (perioral and peripheral tingling and Chvoste's sign) as a result of vitamin D deficiency. The high PTH level ruled out damage to her parathyroid glands during her earlier surgery as the cause. Her low vitamin D level was due to prolonged lack of exposure to sunlight plus anticonvulsant-induced catabolism of vitamin D from her diet. Ms. R.'s bone and muscle pain and weakness suggested that she had developed osteomalacia.

After bone mass has reached its peak, the main process in adult BFUs is remodeling or repair of damaged bone. A hormonal or physical activation stimulus removes lining cells and exposes the bone surface (activation phase). This attracts osteoclasts that dig a resorption cavity (resorption phase). Eventually this process ceases, and a cement line is formed to cement together the old and new bone. Osteoblasts fill in the cavity with new matrix (osteoid), which is mineralized over a period of months (formation phase). Osteoblasts left behind become osteocytes, which receive signals via a wide network of canaliculi and help maintain bone health. The whole cycle takes 3 to 6 months or more. In adults, bone resorption and bone formation are linked or coupled, and bone formation occurs only after bone resorption.

The extent of bone turnover depends on the *rate* of activation of BFUs and the *number* of BFUs activated. After age 30 or so, bone formation cannot keep up with bone resorption and a small amount of

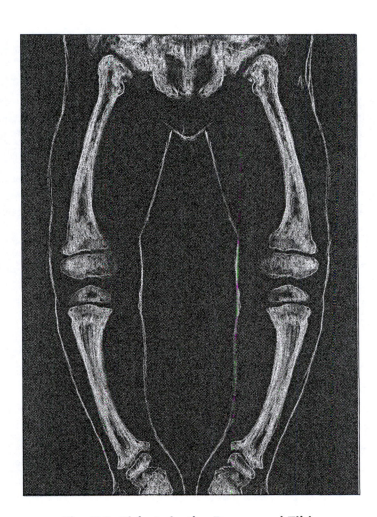

Fig. 7-6. Rickets in the Femur and Tibia

The metaphyses are widened, irregular, and cupped. The bones, in general, are demineralized.

bone can be lost with each cycle. Therefore, anything that activates BFUs and increases bone turnover is likely to contribute to bone loss. Both PTH and thyroid hormone increase the rate of bone turnover. Trabecular bone, which turns over more rapidly than cortical bone, is more vulnerable.

In premenopausal women, estrogen acts as a brake on bone turnover. Estrogen is believed to inhibit release of cytokines that activate osteoclasts. After menopause the suppressive action of estrogen is gone, sensitivity to PTH increases, and osteoclast activity increases. This results in a high bone turnover state, with deeper resorption cavities than usual. Osteoblast activity cannot keep up, bone trabeculae become eroded through, and trabecular connections are lost. Bone density and bone strength are decreased. Although sensitivity to PTH is increased during this period, the excess calcium and phosphorous released from bone actually keep PTH somewhat suppressed, resulting in more calcium loss in urine and less activation of vitamin D. Less calcium is absorbed from the GI tract, increasing total body calcium loss even more. Women lose up to 25% of their trabecular bone and 10% of their cortical bone during the decade after menopause.

Healthy men continue to produce testosterone, although the free testosterone level decreases with age. If testosterone decreases significantly, the increase in bone turnover is comparable to that in postmenopausal women. Young adult men who lack functional estrogen receptors or aromatase, the enzyme that converts testosterone to estrogen, have unclosed epiphyses and osteoporosis. Men clearly need estrogen for normal bone maturation and repair.

After the first postmenopausal decade, the effects of estrogen deprivation diminish and aging changes become dominant. Vitamin D activation and calcium absorption decrease with age. Plasma calcium decreases slightly and PTH increases slightly (but still remains in the normal range). Bone resorption increases to maintain plasma calcium. Osteoblasts become less and less active and fail to fill the resorption cavities. This may be due to failure of local growth factors. Slow loss of 25% of cortical and trabecular bone occurs with aging over a lifetime in both sexes.

Major Regulators of Bone Mass

Genes	Weight
Hormones	Habits (alcohol, smoking)
Calcium	Drugs
Exercise	

Normal changes in bone mass with age are shown in Fig. 7-7. Low bone mass is the major predictor of future fractures, and adults who start with a high peak bone mass at age 30 are better protected. Bone quality also matters, but this is difficult to measure.

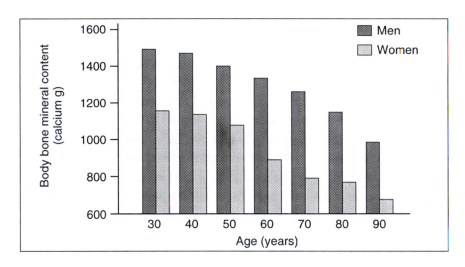

Fig. 7-7. Changes in Bone Mass with Age

Changes in bone mass are indicated by changes in total body calcium content.

Additional Determinants of Bone Mass

Although genes and age are major determinants of bone mass, many other factors also contribute. Major hormone effects on bone are summarized in Table 7-9. Hormone actions at the cellular level are complex. PTH increases osteoclast activity, but under some conditions PTH stimulates bone formation by osteoblasts. Osteoblasts have three possible fates: (1) osteoblasts remaining as new bone is formed can become part of a network of osteocytes that support bone; (2) osteoblasts remaining on the surface when bone matrix production stops can become bone lining cells; and (3) osteoblasts can undergo programmed cell death (apoptosis). When given intermittently, PTH increases osteocyte and lining-cell formation and decreases osteoblast apoptosis, especially in trabecular bone.

1,25(OH)$_2$D contributes to bone formation by stimulating absorption of calcium and phosphorous, but large doses stimulate osteoclasts. Glucocorticoids suppress bone formation and also suppress calcium

Table 7-9. Major Hormone Effects on Bone

INCREASED BONE RESORPTION	DECREASED BONE RESORPTION
Parathyroid hormone	Estrogen
Parathyroid hormone–related peptide	Calcitonin
DECREASED BONE FORMATION	**INCREASED BONE FORMATION**
Glucocorticoids	Testosterone
	Growth hormone
INCREASED BONE TURNOVER	Insulin-like growth factor-1
Hyperparathyroidism	
Hyperthyroidism	

Note. Under selected conditions, parathyroid hormone stimulates bone formation.

absorption from the intestine. Insulin-like growth factor-1 exerts local effects.

More factors that affect bone mass are listed in Table 7-10. High calcium intake during childhood and adolescence increases peak bone mass. In adults a good calcium intake helps overcome the decrease in efficiency of calcium absorption with aging.

Bone mass decreases or increases in response to unloading or loading. Bone is lost rapidly with immobilization, bed rest, and weightlessness (as in space station residence). Increased bone mass with habitual activity has been shown in children, adolescents, and young women. Trained athletes have higher bone mass. However, women whose training leads to weight loss and amenorrhea have low bone mass due to loss of estrogen. The increased exercise does not completely compensate for this loss. In nonathletes, controlled exercise trials have shown gains in bone mass of 1% to 3%. Exercise also increases strength and coordination, which provide protection against falls.

Obese people have higher bone mass, partly due to the increased musculoskeletal effort of moving a heavier load. Also, adipose tissue contains aromatase, the enzyme that converts androgens to estrogens that are stored in fat. Obese postmenopausal women have higher estrogen stores.

Alcohol inhibits osteoblast activity. Smoking is associated with smaller bone mass. The mechanism is not certain, but smokers tend to be thinner. Drugs can cause loss of bone by acting on bone directly (heparin, glucocorticoids) or indirectly by increasing vitamin D catabolism (anticonvulsants) or decreasing calcium absorption (glucocorticoids).

Table 7-10. Major Risk Factors for Osteoporotic Fractures

Aging	**Drugs**
Genetic	Glucocorticoids
White or Asian woman	Heparin
Small peak bone mass	Anticonvulsants
Low body mass index (kg/m^2)	
Family history of osteoporosis	**Habits**
	Smoking
Nutritional	Excessive alcohol intake
Malnutrition	Low activity or immobilization
Malabsorption	
Low calcium intake	**Other**
Low vitamin D	Increased propensity to fall
	Poor vision
Diseases	Poor coordination
Neoplasms affecting bone	Medications decreasing alertness
Rheumatic diseases causing local bone loss	Poor quality bone
	Previous osteoporotic fracture
Hormonal	
Hypogonadism	
Glucocorticoid excess	
Hyperthyroidism	
Hyperparathyroidism	

OSTEOPOROSIS

Osteoporosis is defined as loss of bone mass *plus* accumulated microarchitectural damage resulting in enough bone fragility that fracture is likely with minimal trauma. Minimal trauma is defined as less trauma than that from a fall from a standing height. For women, the World Health Organization also defines osteoporosis as a bone mineral density (BMD) more than 2.5 SD below the young adult mean. Osteopenia is defined as BMD from 1.0 to 2.4 standard deviations below the young adult mean. These are working definitions based on the increase in fractures in studies in white women. These definitions are now used for other groups of women and men, although the fracture studies have not been done.

Osteoporosis is loss of bone mass plus accumulated microarchitechtural damage resulting in enough bone fragility that fracture is likely with minimal trauma.

Osteoporotic bone is characterized by low bone mass, loss of horizontal trabeculae, and areas of microdamage (Fig. 7-8), but composition of the remaining bone is normal. Patients with osteoporosis due to menopause and aging losses have normal calcium and phosphorous levels unless another illness prevents the feedback control loops from operating normally.

Most fractures occur at sites containing trabecular bone, which turns over more rapidly and contains less calcium than cortical bone.

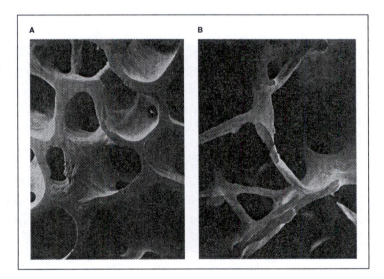

Fig. 7-8. Scanning Electron Micrograph of Trabecular Bone in a Healthy Young Woman (A) and a Postmenopausal Woman with Osteoporosis (B)

In B note the thinner trabeculae and loss of horizontal trabecular connections. (*Source:* Reprinted with permission from Dempster DW, et al. A simple method for correlative light and scanning electron microscopy of human iliac crest bone biopsies. *J Bone Min Res* 1:19, 1986).

Table 7-11. Lifetime Osteoporotic Fracture Risk*

FRACTURE SITE	USUAL AGE	PREVALENCE (BY AGE 80+)
Wrist	50+	24%
Spine	60+	33%
Hip	70+	15%

*Caucasian women in the United States.

The major sites of osteoporotic fractures, time of occurrence, and the lifetime risk for white women are shown in Table 7-11. Black women usually have a higher bone mass than white women and have far fewer fractures. Men have a larger peak bone mass, the diameters of their wrists and vertebral end plates are larger, and they have more cortical bone, which is more highly mineralized and turns over slowly. Men rarely have wrist fractures. They have fewer vertebral fractures than women, and the fractures occur approximately 10 years later. Men have approximately half as many hip fractures as women.

Hip fractures are the most devastating in terms of pain, acute morbidity, long-term disability, mortality, and cost. Less than one-third of those who have a hip fracture return to their prefracture level of function 1 year later. Women at highest risk for a hip fracture are women who are thin or frail or at high risk for falling, women who have already had a vertebral fracture, and women whose mothers had a hip fracture.

Osteoporosis Evaluation

Risk factors for low bone mass (see Table 7-10) predict risk for fractures in populations better than in individuals. Biochemical markers of osteoclast activity (urine pyridinolines or cross-linked N- and C-telopeptides) measure breakdown products of type 1 collagen, the major protein of bone. Markers of osteoblast activity (propeptides of type 1 collagen, osteocalcin, and bone-specific alkaline phosphatase) are osteoblast proteins. These are used primarily for research studies at this time, since there is little longitudinal information in individual patients and day-to-day variation is large. Levels of osteoclast products change several months before levels of osteoblast products. Low levels of both formation and resorption markers indicate that bone turnover has been suppressed.

Osteoporosis Evaluation

Risk factor assessment
Tests (if contributing conditions suspected)
    Hyperparathyroidism—calcium and PTH levels
    Hyperthyroidism—TSH level
    Vitamin D deficiency—25(OH)D level
Bone mineral density measurement
X-rays (if fractures suspected)

Bone mineral density (bone calcium/unit area) measured by dual energy x-ray absorptiometry (DEXA) of the hip or spine is currently the best predictor of future fracture risk. Other sites, including the wrist and forearm, can also be measured by DEXA. Usually it takes at least 1 year to measure significant changes. A DEXA scan should be obtained if the information will influence treatment. X-rays are less sensitive and do not show changes in bone density until one-third of the bone has been lost. X-rays are helpful for sites not measured by DEXA (e.g., the thoracic spine) and when fractures are suspected.

Patients with osteoporosis should be evaluated for hyperparathyroidism, hyperthyroidism, hypogonadism, and vitamin D deficiency, depending on the level of suspicion.

Osteoporosis Prevention and Treatment

Prevention of bone loss is ideal because restoration of major bone loss often is not possible. Pharmacological treatments either suppress bone resorption by osteoclasts (calcium, bisphosphonates, estrogen or an estrogen analog, calcitonin), increase bone formation by osteoblasts (low-dose PTH, testosterone), or improve the calcium supply (calcium supplements, vitamin D).

Osteoporosis Prevention and Treatment

Increase calcium supply
- Calcium
- Vitamin D

Exercise

Prevent falls

Decrease osteoclast action
- Calcium
- Bisphosphonates
- Estrogen
- Selective estrogen receptor modulators
- Calcitonin

Increase osteoblast action
- PTH
- Testosterone

Bisphosphonates are potent osteoclast inhibitors containing phosphate groups that allow them to bind tightly to hydroxyapatite. They prevent vertebral and hip fractures. Estrogen also prevents vertebral and hip fractures, but the risks of estrogen must be weighed against the benefits (see Chapter 12). A progestin must be added to prevent hyperstimulation of the endometrium, unless the woman has had a hysterectomy. Concern about the effect of estrogen on breast cancer risk and withdrawal bleeding limits patient acceptance of hormone replacement therapy. Selective estrogen receptor modulators (SERMs) interact with estrogen receptors and function as estrogen agonists in some tissues and antagonists in others, depending on their interaction with DNA and transcription factors. One of these compounds is raloxifene, which stabilizes bone density and has been shown to reduce vertebral fractures, but not hip fractures, without stimulating the uterus or breast. The long-term effects of SERMs are not known. Calcitonin, which can be given as a nasal spray, has been shown to reduce vertebral fractures but not hip fractures.

Testosterone is used to treat bone loss in hypogonadal men (see Chapter 11). It is not clear whether testosterone effects result from conversion of testosterone to estrogen, or whether testosterone has an independent anabolic effect on bone.

Suppression of osteoclast activity can result in hypocalcemia and secondary hyperparathyroidism. Patients treated with osteoclast inhibitors often need a calcium supplement unless dietary calcium intake exceeds 1000 mg/day. They may need a vitamin D supplement also. Since $1,25(OH)_2D$ has complex actions on bone and often results in hypercalciuria, a physiologic dose of vitamin D such as 400 to 800 IU/d, which can be converted to active vitamin D as needed, is usually recommended when a supplement is required.

Since bone formation is coupled to bone resorption, any intervention that suppresses osteoclast activity eventually results in lower osteoblast activity, and bone mass reaches a plateau. For patients who already have low bone density or osteoporotic fractures, a stimulator of bone formation could be ideal.

PTH can stimulate osteoblast activity and increase bone mass as discussed above. When a synthetic fragment composed of the first 34 amino acids (hPTH[1-34]) is given daily as a small, subcutaneous dose, cortical bone width and trabecular thickness are increased, trabecular architecture is preserved, and vertebral and nonvertebral fractures are reduced. The long-term safety of hPTH is not known, so using it longer than 2 years is not recommended.

Whatever the level of bone mass, it is important to decrease the risk of falling and to encourage exercise when possible.

OSTEOMALACIA

Osteomalacia is a disorder of bone mineralization resulting in accumulation of unmineralized osteoid, bone and muscle pain, weakness, and sometimes fractures. Osteomalacia and rickets caused by vitamin D deficiency have been described. Osteomalacia accompanied by calcium deficiency also may be accompanied by bone loss, because hypocalcemia elicits increased PTH, which increases bone resorption.

Osteomalacia is a disorder of bone mineralization resulting in accumulation of unmineralized osteoid, bone and muscle pain, and weakness.

Osteomalacia can also be due to phosphorous deficiency. The inherited forms are due to a genetic defect in phosphorous transport in the renal tubule or to a humoral factor that stimulates renal phosphorous secretion. They are associated with a defect in synthesis of $1,25(OH)_2D$. X-linked hypophosphatemia is also associated with defective osteoblast function. Patients are treated with oral phosphorous with $1,25(OH)_2D$ to increase calcium absorption.

Major Causes of Osteomalacia

Vitamin D deficiency
Calcium deficiency
Phosphorous deficiency

Acquired hypophosphatemia can be due to very low phosphorous intake (unusual) or excessive binding of ingested phosphate by aluminum-containing antacids. More often, hypophosphatemia results from excessive renal phosphorous loss. Fanconi syndrome and other forms of renal tubular acidosis are associated with renal phosphorous wasting. Tumor-induced or oncogenic osteomalacia is characterized by phosphaturia, hypophosphatemia, and low $1,25(OH)_2D$. The tumors produce a humoral factor that affects phosphate reabsorption at the proximal renal tubule. The tumors are often small and very difficult to find, but bone healing occurs if the tumor can be removed.

Major features of osteoporosis and osteomalacia are compared in Table 7-12.

Table 7-12. Manifestations of Osteoporosis and Osteomalacia

SYMPTOMS AND SIGNS	OSTEOPOROSIS	OSTEOMALACIA
Bone pain	Yes (with fractures)	Yes
Increased bone resorption	Yes	No
Decreased bone formation	Yes	Yes
Decreased bone mass	Yes	Yes
Bone composition normal	Yes	No (increased osteoid)
Muscle weakness	No	Yes
Serum calcium and phosphorous	Usually normal	Often low

CASE STUDY: *CONTINUED*

Ms. R. was treated for osteomalacia with high doses of calcium and vitamin D, and her bone and muscle pain and weakness resolved. Her calcium and vitamin D doses were decreased to more physiologic levels. Two years later, at the age of 67, Ms. R. developed sudden back pain while making her bed. Physical examination revealed loss of 1.5 inches in height from 2 years before and new tenderness over her mid-thoracic spine. Her calcium, albumin, phosphorous, 25(OH)D, and creatinine levels were normal. Spine x-rays revealed two thoracic vertebral fractures. A DEXA scan of her left hip showed low bone density.

PAGET DISEASE OF BONE

Paget disease is a disorder of bone remodeling. Giant multinucleated osteoclasts resorb bone, which is followed by compensatory but disorderly formation of woven bone by osteoblasts. Bone turnover is high, but resorption and formation are coupled and plasma calcium and phosphorous are usually normal. Mineralization is normal. The result: local areas of enlarged, abnormally vascular, easily deformed bone that feel warm due to the increased blood flow. Paget disease may affect one bone or several. The most common sites are the pelvis, femur, skull, tibia, and spine, but other bones may also be involved. X-rays show mixed areas of sclerosis and lucency.

Many patients are asymptomatic and are diagnosed when either an elevated alkaline phosphatase (reflecting increased bone formation) or an abnormal x-ray is obtained during the workup for an unrelated problem. Pain can be due to the increased blood flow, deformity, nearby nerve impingement, and abnormal stresses and degeneration of nearby joints if posture and gait are affected. Skull involvement can result in increased head size and deafness. Neoplastic degeneration occurs but is unusual (<1%).

The cause is unknown, though a virus is suspected, and there is a genetic component. Paget disease is common in Northern Europe, North America, Australia, and New Zealand. Treatment involves suppressing the osteoclasts, mostly with bisphosphonates, the same agents used to treat osteoporosis but at higher doses because the rate of bone turnover in Paget disease is higher. It is unclear whether patients with mild disease (no symptoms and alkaline phosphatase <1.5–2 × normal) should be treated to prevent progression.

Ms. R. now has osteoporosis. She has had two vertebral fractures with minimal trauma. She no longer has symptoms and signs of osteomalacia, and her x-rays did not show Paget disease. Her risk factors for osteoporosis include being a postmenopausal white woman with a family history of osteoporosis; previous high bone turnover due to hyperparathyroidism, low vitamin D, and modest calcium intake in the past; and a period of prolonged immobilization. It is unfortunate that no preventive therapy was instituted after her accident.

Ms. R. was urged to continue her calcium and vitamin D supplements. She will increase her exercise, if possible when her back pain lessens, and will take extra precautions against falling. She will also begin taking a bisphosphonate.

REVIEW QUESTIONS

Directions: For each of the following questions, choose the *one best* answer.

Questions 1 and 2

1 Ms. R. is a 60-year-old woman who consults her physician because her mother has osteoporosis and just fractured two vertebrae. Ms. R. has a history of exercise-induced asthma. She does not smoke and drinks an occasional glass of wine. She dislikes dairy products but drinks a glass of calcium-supplemented orange juice daily. She takes no medications and refuses estrogen and progesterone because her sister has breast cancer. The physical examination reveals a thin, healthy appearing woman. When her bone mass is measured, it is found to be low. The physician would be most likely to recommend

A thyroxine to suppress bone turnover
B calcium to stimulate bone resorption
C a bisphosphonate to suppress osteoclasts
D vitamin D to suppress osteoblast activity
E calcitonin to stimulate osteoclasts

2 Two years later Ms. R.'s asthma worsens, and she is started on chronic glucocorticoid therapy. The physician should be aware that glucocorticoids cause bone loss by

A suppressing vitamin D activation
B suppressing bone resorption

C inhibiting bone formation

D increasing calcium absorption from the intestine

E increasing osteoblast proliferation

3 James T. is a 65-year-old man whose laboratory studies before knee replacement surgery reveal the following: calcium, 11.0 (normal: 8.5–10.5 mg/dL); phosphorous, 2.2 (normal: 2.3–4.5 mg/dL); and albumin and creatinine, normal. The urine calcium-to-creatinine ratio is low. Parathyroid hormone (PTH) is mildly increased. Mr. T. is unconcerned because he feels well except for knee pain, and both his son and granddaughter have high plasma calcium. They have no symptoms. The most likely cause of this man's hypercalcemia is

A parathyroid hormone–related protein (PTHrP)

B primary hyperparathyroidism

C secondary hyperparathyroidism

D abnormal calcium sensor protein

E vitamin D toxicity

4 An elderly man with a long smoking history is admitted to the hospital with complaints of weakness, fatigue, constipation, lethargy, and weight loss. Chest x-ray reveals a mass, which proves to be a squamous cell carcinoma. He also has high calcium and low phosphorous levels that are most likely due to excess

A endogenous $1,25(OH)_2D$

B calcium-binding protein

C parathyroid hormone (PTH)

D calcitonin

E parathyroid hormone–related peptide (PTHrP)

5 In clinic one afternoon a physician sees four patients with elevated PTH levels, but only one has hypercalcemia. Which patient is it most likely to be?

A A 66-year-old man complaining of weakness, lethargy, and constipation; x-rays reveal osteoporosis and a kidney stone

B A 74-year-old woman who has a very limited diet and has been housebound because of a stroke; she complains of bone pain, and a bone biopsy reveals osteomalacia

C A 32-year-old man who has renal failure; he has not been treated with any medications

D A 27-year-old woman who is short, with a round face and hand deformities; she is resistant to PTH and several other hormones

Directions: The group of questions below consists of lettered choices followed by several numbered items. For each numbered item, select the appropriate lettered option with which it is most closely associated. Each lettered option may be used once, more than once, or not at all.

Questions 6-9

For each clinical scenario presented below, select the most likely laboratory test results. Assume that the albumin level is normal.

A High calcium, high phosphorous (PO_4), low parathyroid hormone (PTH), high $1,25(OH)_2$ vitamin D

B High calcium, low PO_4, high PTH, high $1,25(OH)_2D$

C High calcium, low PO_4, low PTH, normal $1,25(OH)_2D$

D Low calcium, high PO_4, high PTH, low $1,25 OH)_2D$

E Low calcium, high PO_4, low PTH, low $1,25(OH)_2D$

F Low calcium, low PO_4, high PTH, low $1,25(OH)_2D$

6 An 82-year-old malnourished woman from a nursing home has bone pain and tenderness, muscle weakness, and tingling around her mouth. An iliac crest biopsy shows poorly mineralized osteoid (bone matrix).

7 A 45-year-old man recently underwent a near-total thyroidectomy for thyroid cancer. He complains of muscle spasms. His Chvostek and Trousseau signs are positive.

8 A lethargic 65-year-old woman has complained of fatigue, depression, weakness, and constipation for 15 years. She has been taking several over-the-counter vitamin preparations for years. Abdominal x-rays reveal three kidney stones, and her urine calcium is high. Her PTH level is low.

9 A 3-year-old girl has been confined indoors and is poorly nourished. She is weak, her legs are bowed, and during the physical examination she cries when palpation exerts pressure on her bones.

References

Brown EM: Familial hypocalciuric hypercalcemia and other disorders with resistance to extracellular calcium. *Endocrinol Metab Clin North Am* 29: 503–522, 2000.

Crandall C: Parathyroid hormone treatment for osteoporosis. *Arch Int Med* 162: 2297–2309, 2002.

Krall EA, Wehler C, Garcia RI, et al: Calcium and vitamin D supplements reduce tooth loss in the elderly. *Am J Med* 111: 452–456, 2001.

Manolagas SC: Birth and death of bone cells: basic regulatory mechanisms and implications for the pathogenesis and treatment of osteoporosis. *Endocr Rev* 21: 115–137, 2000.

Marx SJ: Hyperparathyroid and hypoparathyroid disorders. *N Engl J Med* 343: 1863–1875, 2000.

NIH Consensus Development Panel: Osteoporosis prevention, diagnosis and therapy. *JAMA* 285: 785–795, 2001.

Notes

Peacock M: Primary hyperparathyroidism and the kidney: biochemical and clinical spectrum. *J Bone Miner Res* 17: N87–N94, 2002.

Thomas MK, Demay MB: Vitamin D deficiency and disorders of vitamin D metabolism. *Endocrinol Metab Clin North Am* 29: 611–628, 2000.

Writing Group for the Women's Health Initiative Investigators: Risks and benefits of estrogen plus progestin in healthy postmenopausal women. *JAMA* 288: 321–333, 2002.

8

Pancreatic Islet Hormones, Diabetes Mellitus, and Hypoglycemia

Elizabeth R. Seaquist, M.D.

■ CHAPTER OUTLINE ■

■ LEARNING OBJECTIVES ■

At the completion of this chapter, the student will:

1. understand how insulin and glucagon maintain normal blood glucose concentrations.
2. understand the pathogenesis of type 1 diabetes and type 2 diabetes.
3. be able to distinguish type 1 diabetes from type 2 diabetes based on clinical and laboratory information.
4. be able to identify the acute and chronic complications of diabetes and strategies to prevent them.
5. understand the approaches to treatment of type 1 and type 2 diabetes.
6. understand the causes and consequences of hypoglycemia.

163

CASE STUDY: *INTRODUCTION*

Ms. Anderson is a 21-year-old college student who presented to the college health service because of frequent urination during the previous week. She had been drinking more fluids and feeling more hungry than usual. Despite her good appetite, she had lost about 10 pounds over the semester. She had always been healthy and was taking no medication. Her grandmother was recently diagnosed with diabetes.

On physical exam, she appeared well. Her height was 5'5" and weight was 120 lb. Her blood pressure was 110/75 mm Hg, her pulse was 76 beats/minute, and neither changed when she moved from a supine to standing position. Her general examination was unremarkable.

Laboratory data revealed the following: glucose, 320 mg/dL (normal: 70–110 mg/dL); sodium, 135 mEq/L (normal); potassium, 3.9 mEq/L (normal); bicarbonate, 22 mEq/L (normal: 23–29 mEq/L); creatinine, 0.8 mg/dL (normal); urinalysis, 4+ glucose (normal: 0 glucose). Blood for an insulin level was sent to an outside laboratory. The level was less than 2 µU/mL (low).

Regulation of Blood Glucose Concentration

Normal blood glucose concentrations are maintained by a balance between glucose coming into and exiting the blood space (Figure 8-1).

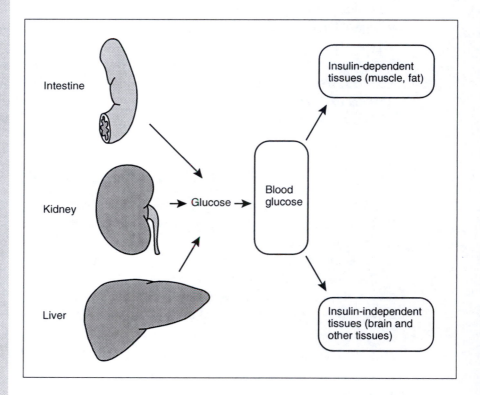

Fig. 8-1. Regulation of Blood Glucose Concentration

Hormones from the pancreatic islet are of primary importance in maintaining this balance.

Pancreatic Islet Structure and Hormones

The endocrine pancreas consists of the islets that are dispersed throughout the exocrine pancreas. Four different hormones are secreted from four different cell types in the islet, as shown in Fig. 8-2.

Major Islet Cell Hormones

Insulin
Glucagon
Somatostatin

Insulin is generated from its precursor proinsulin. In the secretory granule, proinsulin is cleaved into the 51–amino acid insulin peptide and the 31–amino acid C-peptide (for connecting peptide). They are cosecreted in an equimolar ratio. C-peptide can be used as an indicator of endogenous insulin secretion (Fig. 8-3).

The regulation of islet hormone secretion is complex. Glucose is the most important stimulator of insulin release. The metabolism of glucose alters the ATP to ADP ratio in the islet beta cell, thereby favoring the closure of ATP-dependent potassium channels on the cell membrane. With closure of these channels, the membrane depolarizes and calcium enters through voltage-dependent calcium channels. This increase in intracellular calcium concentrations somehow facilitates the release of insulin from secretory granules.

Because of the order in which islet cells are perfused, the upstream hormone modulates the function of the downstream cell. Perfusion goes from the core to the mantle of the islet such that the beta cell has a paracrine effect on the alpha and the delta cells, and the alpha cell has a paracrine effect on the delta cell.

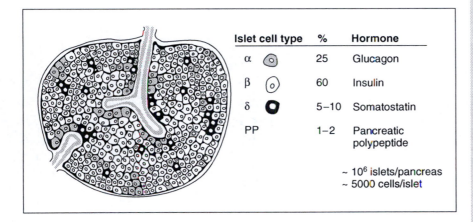

Islet cell type		%	Hormone
α	⊚	25	Glucagon
β	⊙	60	Insulin
δ	●	5–10	Somatostatin
PP		1–2	Pancreatic polypeptide

~ 10^6 islets/pancreas
~ 5000 cells/islet

Fig. 8-2. Structure of Pancreatic Islet

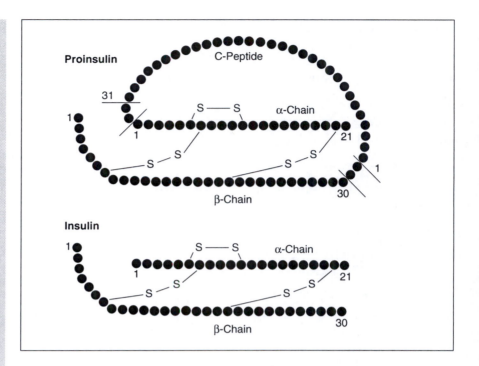

Fig. 8-3. Structure of Proinsulin and Insulin

Proinsulin is cleaved into insulin and C-peptide in the secretory granule. Insulin is composed of α- and β-chains that are joined by two sulfhydryl bridges. Each *dot* represents an amino acid. *Slashes* indicate points of cleavage. *Numbers* refer to the position of the amino acid on the α- and β-chains and C-peptide. The final α- and β-chains contain 21 and 30 amino acids, respectively.

Pancreatic islets are richly innervated. Parasympathetic nerves travel via the vagus nerve and may play a role in the cephalic phase of insulin release that occurs at the sight and smell of food. The sympathetic nerves have a role in the acute response to stress in which insulin secretion is inhibited and glucagon secretion is stimulated (Table 8-1). In addition, many neuropeptides, including vasoactive intestinal peptide (VIP), cholecystokinin (CCK), galanin, and neuropeptide Y (NPY), are found within islet nerve terminals.

Table 8-1. Modulators of Insulin and Glucagon Secretion

INSULIN SECRETION (BETA CELL)		GLUCAGON SECRETION (ALPHA CELL)	
Stimulators	**Inhibitors**	**Stimulators**	**Inhibitors**
Glucose	Somatostatin	Arginine	Somatostatin
Arginine	Epinephrine	Hypoglycemia	Glucose
Leucine			Insulin
Secretin and other intestinal hormones			
Acetylcholine			
Glucagon			
Glucagon-like peptide-1			

INSULIN AND GLUCAGON ACTIONS

Insulin and glucagon oppose each other in regulating glucose metabolism (Table 8-2). Insulin acts to move glucose into insulin-sensitive tissues such as muscle and fat and enhances the storage of fuels. Insulin promotes the storage of glucose as glycogen by increasing the rate of glycogen synthesis and decreasing the rate of glycogenolysis in both liver and skeletal muscle. Through its inhibitory effects on both lipolysis and proteolysis, insulin also promotes the storage of fats and proteins. Glucagon opposes all of these actions of insulin. Glucagon increases blood glucose concentrations by increasing gluconeogenesis and by increasing glycogenolysis in the liver. Somatostatin inhibits the secretion of both insulin and glucagon and reduces the effects of these hormones.

Under healthy conditions, the pancreatic islet secretes a small amount of insulin throughout the day in order to maintain normal plasma glucose concentration. This basal level of insulin secretion is particularly important in regulating the rates of gluconeogenesis and glycogenolysis in the liver and kidney. In response to eating, insulin secretion is increased to prevent excessive postprandial glucose excursions. The rise in blood glucose and amino acid concentrations after a meal stimulates insulin release directly. Insulin secretion is also stimulated by glucagon-like peptide 1 (GLP-1), which is released from the intestine after a meal. Compounds like GLP-1, which augment insulin secretion in response to a rise in glucose, are called *incretins*.

The amount of insulin secreted by the endocrine pancreas to maintain normal glucose tolerance is tightly regulated by the arterial glucose concentration; thus, in healthy individuals the range of glycemia is not large.

The actions of both insulin and glucagon on target cells are mediated by cell surface receptors that bind each hormone specifically. The insulin receptor is a tetrameric structure consisting of two α-subunits (M_r = 135,000) and two β-subunits (M_r = 95,000) joined together by disulfide bonds. The α-subunits are extracellular in location and contain the insulin-binding site, which is rich in cysteine residues. The β-subunits span the plasma membrane and serve to anchor the receptor to the cell. Single cysteine residues are believed to be important in the formation of the α_2–β_2 complex (Fig. 8-4).

Table 8-2. Metabolic Actions of Insulin and Glucagon

	INSULIN	GLUCAGON
Lipolysis	↓	↑
Ketogenesis	↓	↑
Gluconeogenesis	↓	↑
Glycogenesis	↑	↓
Glycogenolysis	↓	↑
Glycemia	↓	↑

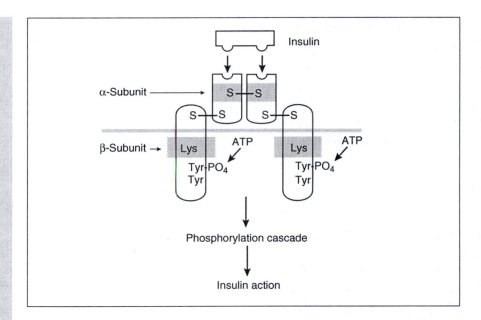

Fig. 8-4. Insulin Interaction with Insulin Receptor

Insulin interaction with its receptor results in phosphorylation of the receptor. This initiates a series of phosphorylations, which results in insulin action. Lys = lysine; Tyr = tyrosine; ATP = adenosine triphosphate; $TyrPO_4$ = tyrosine phosphate.

When insulin binds to the extracellular α-subunits, a signal is transmitted across the plasma membrane that activates the intracellular tyrosine kinase domain of the β-subunits. A series of intramolecular transphosphorylation reactions in which one β-subunit phosphorylates its adjacent partner on a specific tyrosine residue then commences. Once activated, the insulin receptor phosphorylates a number of other proteins on tyrosine residues, such as members of the insulin receptor substrate family (IRS 1–4) and signaling molecules such as Shc. Once these proteins are phosphorylated, they alter the activity of other downstream effectors of insulin action. Signals transmitted through the IRS proteins mediate the metabolic effects of insulin on glucose transport and glycogen synthesis. Signals transmitted through the Shc pathways mediate the effects of insulin on mitogenesis and growth (Fig. 8-4).

The glucagon receptor is a G-protein–linked receptor. Like other receptors in this family, the glucagon receptor has seven transmembrane-spanning domains that couple glucagon binding to adenylate cyclase through G-protein effectors.

GLUCOSE TRANSPORTERS

Glucose movement from the blood into tissue requires the action of a glucose transporter (GLUT). GLUTs are membrane-associated glycoproteins with 12 transmembrane domains, a cytoplasmic NH_2 terminus and a COOH terminus, and a large extracellular loop. Five glucose transporters have been identified (Table 8-3). Insulin regulates the

Table 8-3. Location of Glucose Transporters (GLUT)

GLUT	LOCATION
GLUT-1	Ubiquitous, also in placenta
GLUT-2	Beta cell, liver, kidney, and intestine
GLUT-3	Ubiquitous
GLUT-4	Muscle and fat
GLUT-5	Jejunum

action of GLUT-4. Following insulin binding to its receptor, GLUT-4 is translocated to the cell membrane to facilitate glucose transport.

Pathogenesis of Diabetes: Abnormal Insulin Secretion and Insulin Resistance

To maintain normal glucose tolerance, an individual must have both normal insulin secretion and normal sensitivity to insulin. Absolute insulin deficiency or abnormalities in both insulin secretion and insulin action can lead to diabetes. Diabetes can be either primary or secondary to other diseases such as exocrine pancreatic disease, drugs, hormonal disorders like acromegaly or glucagonoma, or genetic syndromes. Primary diabetes is classified as type 1 or type 2 diabetes mellitus, depending on the pathogenesis.

> **Diabetes mellitus** is a disorder of glucose metabolism resulting in hyperglycemia as a result of absolute insulin deficiency or abnormalities in insulin secretion and insulin action.

TYPE 1 DIABETES MELLITUS (TYPE 1 DM)

This form of diabetes was formerly known as juvenile onset diabetes, ketosis-prone diabetes, or insulin-dependent diabetes mellitus (IDDM).

Pathophysiology

Type 1 DM is caused by an absolute deficiency of insulin. It occurs because of autoimmune destruction of the pancreatic beta cells. It is believed to arise in genetically susceptible individuals who are exposed to an environmental factor that initiates the autoimmune response. The nature of this environmental factor is unknown, but it is hypothesized to be a viral infection, an environmental toxin, or dietary component. Once the triggering event occurs, beta-cell destruction ensues, and there is progressive loss of the beta cells over years. The rate at which this destruction occurs is variable, but beta-cell attrition is believed to be more rapid in persons who are diagnosed in childhood. Overt diabetes does not appear until approximately 90% of the beta cells are destroyed.

Major Classes of Diabetes

Primary diabetes

Type 1 DM

Type 2 DM

Secondary diabetes

Due to pancreatic destruction

Due to other hormonal diseases

Due to genetic syndromes

Autoimmune destruction of pancreatic beta cells can sometimes be detected in children by measurement of circulating islet-cell antibodies. Between 50% to 85% of children with type 1 DM have antibodies to islet cells (ICA, islet-cell antibodies) present in their serum at the time of diagnosis, and some children also have antibodies to insulin. These are not antibodies directed against the antigen that incites the autoimmune process, but are antibodies generated in response to the destruction of the beta cell. Adults do not usually have detectable concentrations of these antibodies in the serum at the time of diabetes diagnosis, perhaps because the onset of the autoimmune destruction of their beta cells occurred years earlier and their rate of beta-cell destruction was so slow that antibody production disappeared.

In contrast to ICA, antibodies to the enzyme glutamic acid decarboxylase (GAD) are thought to be important in the autoimmune destruction of beta cells. Anti-GAD antibodies are often detected in children and adults at the time diabetes is diagnosed.

Prevalence

In the United States, approximately 0.3% of the population develop type 1 DM by 20 years of age. The worldwide prevalence varies significantly. The highest prevalence is found in Finland, where two to three times as many people develop type 1 DM as in the United States. Japan has a rate that is about one-tenth that of the rate in the United States. Type 1 DM is rare in African Americans, Hispanics, and Native Americans.

Clinical Features

The peak age of onset of type 1 DM occurs between the ages of 10 and 16 and coincides with puberty. A second peak of onset occurs in the late 30s and early 40s. Patients with type 1 DM are usually lean. Presenting symptoms include the following:

- Excessive urination (*polyuria*), which occurs because of glucosuria (osmotic diuresis)
- Excessive thirst (*polydipsia*), which occurs in response to dehydration

- Excessive hunger (*polyphagia*), which occurs because of persistent loss of calories as a result of glucosuria and the possible effects of diabetes on satiety signals in the brain
- Unexplained weight loss, which occurs because of the inability to eat enough calories to compensate for loss of glucose in the urine

---

Symptoms and Signs of Hyperglycemia

Excessive urination (polyuria)

Excessive thirst (polydipsia)

Excessive eating (polyphagia)

Weight loss

Additional clinical features are shown in Table 8-4.

TYPE 2 DIABETES MELLITUS (TYPE 2 DM)

This form of diabetes was formerly known as adult onset diabetes or non–insulin-dependent diabetes mellitus (NIDDM).

Pathophysiology

Type 2 DM occurs because of abnormalities in *both* insulin secretion and insulin action, as shown in Fig. 8-5. Which defect comes first has long been the subject of debate, but current research suggests that different populations may start with different primary defects. Some populations may have a primary defect in insulin secretion, which can lead to hyperglycemia when coupled with the insulin resistance. Others may have the primary defect in insulin resistance but will not develop

Table 8-4. Comparison: Type 1 Diabetes Mellitus (type 1 DM) and Type 2 Diabetes Mellitus (type 2 DM)

	TYPE 1 DM	TYPE 2 DM
Synonyms	IDDM, juvenile-onset diabetes	NIDDM, adult-onset diabetes
Age of onset	Usually <30 years	Usually >40 years
Ketosis	Common	Rare
Body weight	Nonobese	Obese (80%)
Prevalence	0.5%	6%–10%
Genetics	HLA-associated, 40%–50% concordance rate in twins	Non–HLA-associated, 95%–100% concordance rate in twins
Circulating islet cell antibodies	50%–85%	<10%
Treatment with insulin	Necessary for survival	Not necessary for survival
Complications	Frequent	Frequent

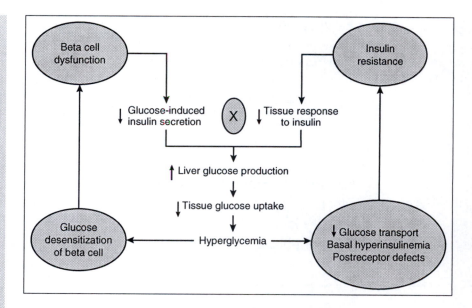

Fig. 8-5. Multiplier Hypothesis

Both defective glucose-induced insulin secretion and defective tissue response to circulating insulin are required for type 2 DM to manifest. These two defects in concert lead to increased liver glucose production, decreased cellular glucose uptake, and hyperglycemia. Hyperglycemia then leads to glucose desensitization of the beta cell. This leads to further impairment of beta-cell function. Hyperglycemia is also associated with decreased glucose transport, basal hyperinsulinemia, decreased insulin binding, and postreceptor defects—all of which promote insulin resistance. Progressive impairment in insulin secretion and insulin sensitivity ultimately produce the syndrome of type 2 DM.

hyperglycemia until their beta cells become unable to secrete enough insulin to maintain normal blood glucose concentrations. In either case, the result is that glucose production from the liver increases and glucose uptake into tissues decreases. The hyperglycemia that ensues exacerbates the problem by leading to further impairment of beta-cell function and insulin action.

Abnormal insulin secretion in type 2 DM is specific to glucose-stimulated insulin secretion. Insulin secretion in response to other stimuli shown in Table 8-1 is normal. Causes of abnormal insulin secretion include the following:

- *Mutations in the gene for glucokinase.* Some families have an unusual autosomal dominant form of type 2 DM called maturity onset diabetes of the young (MODY), which is due to a mutation in glucokinase. This leads to abnormal glucose sensing in the beta-cell and impaired insulin secretion.
- *Mutations in transcription factors.* Other forms of MODY have been linked to mutations in transcription factors that regulate transcription of genes involved in beta cell metabolism.
- *Abnormalities in insulin action.* These may also contribute to abnormal insulin secretion.

Environmental factors such as obesity and lack of exercise increase insulin resistance and contribute to the development of type 2 DM. Insulin resistance can also arise because of a defect in one or more areas of insulin action. Causes of insulin resistance include the following:

- *Prereceptor defects.* These are rare problems due to either an abnormal insulin molecule or antibodies to insulin that prevent it from binding to its receptor.
- *Receptor defects.* These rare abnormalities include syndromes of severe insulin resistance in which the available number of receptors is decreased; unusual autoimmune disorders in which antibodies directed against the insulin receptor prevents hormone binding and subsequent action; or mutations in the receptor that alter the affinity for insulin.
- *Postreceptor defects.* These include mutations in the insulin-receptor gene that prevent the receptor from participating in normal insulin signal transduction; abnormalities of the intracellular messengers mediating the effect of insulin; and increased activity of protein tyrosine phosphatases, which dephosphorylate the phosphorylated tyrosines needed for normal insulin-receptor activation. Insulin-receptor function is also attenuated by increased serine-threonine phosphorylation of the β-subunit. Chronic elevations in insulin levels and counter-regulatory hormones like glucagon, cortisol, and catecholamines, and cytokines like TNF-α are believed to increase insulin resistance through this mechanism.

Causes of Insulin Resistance

Prereceptor defects
Abnormal insulin
Anti-insulin antibodies
Insulin-receptor defects
Decreased receptor number
Abnormal receptors
Antibodies to receptor
Postreceptor defects

Prevalence

In the United States, 6% to 10% of the population develops type 2 DM. The prevalence rate is higher in African Americans, Hispanics, and Native Americans.

Clinical Features

Most patients with type 2 DM present over the age of 40 years, although MODY presents in childhood. Most patients with type 2 diabetes are obese and have a strong family history of the disease. There is a growing concern about the increase of type 2 DM in children related to an increase in the prevalence of childhood obesity.

Approximately 50% of Americans with type 2 diabetes do not know they have the disease, because either their hyperglycemia is not severe enough to cause symptoms or they do not recognize the symptoms of hyperglycemia. The diagnosis is often made in asymptomatic individuals when they are being evaluated for another problem. Patients with type 2 DM can present with the same symptoms and signs as patients with type 1 DM if they are sufficiently hyperglycemic.

Prevention

People at increased risk for developing type 2 DM can be identified by a family history of the disease, obesity, or a history of diabetes during pregnancy. Randomized prospective studies have shown that the risk of developing type 2 DM can be reduced over the short term by intensive efforts to reduce weight and increase exercise. Use of the medication metformin to reduce insulin resistance also reduces the risk of developing type 2 DM.

Laboratory Evaluation of Diabetes Mellitus

The hallmark of diabetes is hyperglycemia. The Expert Committee on the Diagnosis and Classification of Diabetes Mellitus of the American Diabetes Association has formulated the diagnostic criteria for diabetes mellitus listed in Table 8-5. Symptomatic patients who present with blood glucose concentrations greater than 200 mg/dL or patients who display ketonuria and clearly have type 1 diabetes usually require no further evaluation to make the diagnosis of diabetes.

Asymptomatic patients with blood glucose concentrations greater than 200 mg/dL or symptomatic patients with random blood glucose concentrations less than 200 mg/dL (11.1 mM) should have their glucose concentrations measured in the fasting state. If the fasting plasma glucose concentration is greater than or equal to 126 mg/dL (7.0 mM) on two or more occasions, the diagnosis of diabetes is made. However, if they have fasting glucose concentrations less than 126 mg/dL (7.0 mM), they may have diabetes or impaired glucose tolerance, or may be normal. Such patients may not need to undergo additional diagnostic testing if the initial recommendations of weight loss and increased exercise would be the same whether or not they meet the

Table 8-5. Diagnostic Criteria for Diabetes

TEST	DIABETES MELLITUS	IMPAIRED GLUCOSE TOLERANCE
Fasting glucose (on 2 or more occasions)	≥126 mg/dL (7.0 mM)	110–125 mg/dL (6.1–6.9 mM)
OGTT* (2-hr plasma glucose)	≥200 mg/dL (11.1 mM)	140–199 mg/dL (7.8–11.0 mM)

* OGTT = oral glucose tolerance test

official diagnostic criteria for diabetes. When an official diagnosis must be made, an oral glucose tolerance test is done in which 75 grams of glucose is ingested at time zero, and a blood sample for measurement of plasma glucose is obtained at 2 hours. Table 8-5 lists the blood glucose responses to this test required for the designation of diabetes or impaired glucose tolerance. Persons with impaired glucose tolerance do not always go on to develop diabetes, but many do so, especially if they are obese.

In clinical practice, laboratory evaluation is often enhanced by the measurement of glycosylated hemoglobin. Glucose contains a carbonyl group that can react with an N-terminal amino acid of a protein such as hemoglobin. This reaction is called glycation or glycosylation. The amount of hemoglobin glycosylated is directly related to the degree of hyperglycemia. Hemoglobin A_{1c} (HbA_{1c}) is the largest subfraction of hemoglobin, and glycosylation of this subfraction is measured most frequently. Since the life span of a red blood cell is approximately 90 days, the percentage of glycosylated hemoglobin (or glycosylated HbA_{1c}) provides information about the level of glycemia for the past 2-3 months. Glycosylated hemoglobin measurements are not part of the official diagnostic criteria for diabetes, but these values correlate well with fasting glucose values, and high glycosylated hemoglobin is used as a marker for diabetes and an indicator of glucose control.

Treatment of Diabetes

The goal of diabetes therapy is twofold: (1) to correct the symptoms of diabetes and (2) to normalize plasma glucose concentration as much as possible in order to prevent the long-term complications of diabetes. When designing a treatment program, it is useful to consider therapies that will correct the underlying pathophysiologic defect that led to the diabetes in the first place. Since type 1 DM develops because of insulin deficiency that results from beta-cell destruction, the appropriate therapy for type 1 DM patients is insulin replacement. Patients with type 2 DM have defects in both insulin secretion and insulin action.

CASE STUDY: *CONTINUED*

Ms. Anderson presented at the college health service with classic symptoms of hyperglycemia. Her laboratory data confirmed that she was hyperglycemic without any other electrolyte abnormalities. Her serum insulin level was inappropriately low for her plasma glucose level, indicating an insulin-deficiency state. This, her young age, lean weight, and lack of a strong family history for type 2 DM, all support the diagnosis of type 1 DM. Ms. Anderson was placed on insulin therapy and encouraged to receive ongoing care with her diabetes care team. For the next 2 years she managed her diabetes very well.

Therapy for these individuals should be directed to overcome these metabolic abnormalities. The specific strategies used to meet the goals of therapy depend on the type of diabetes present.

MANAGEMENT OF TYPE 1 DM

Type 1 DM requires that patients take insulin to sustain life. Patients with this disorder have an absolute insulin deficiency, and therapies are designed to replace insulin in as physiologic a way as possible. To replicate the normal pattern of insulin secretion in a person with type 1 DM, insulin must be present throughout the day at a level sufficient to maintain normal glycemia and must be increased after meals to prevent hyperglycemia. Ideally, the person administering exogenous insulin should know the insulin dose that maintains normal plasma glucose concentrations under a variety of circumstances. Unfortunately, determining the correct dose of insulin necessary to meet the metabolic needs of the moment and estimating the actual pharmacokinetics of the available insulin preparations are very difficult. Many patients with type 1 DM find it impossible to achieve consistent normoglycemia.

The insulin preparations commonly used for the treatment of diabetes include the short-acting lyspro, aspart, and regular insulins and the intermediate-acting neutral protamine Hagedorn (NPH), glargine, Lente, and Ultralente insulins. As shown in Table 8-6, all of these insulins, except lyspro and aspart, have a lag time between the time of injection and the time they begin to affect blood glucose concentrations. They have different times of peak effect and predicted duration of action. Depending on the schedule and preferences of a given patient, these insulins can be used alone or in combination, as shown in Fig. 8-6.

In designing treatment strategies for patients with type 1 DM, it is essential to remember that each blood glucose concentration is the result of three variables: the food eaten and absorbed, the exercise performed (exercise increases sensitivity to insulin), and the insulin taken in the hours before measurement. To achieve normoglycemia in type 1 DM, many patients find a schedule with consistent times for insulin injection, meals, and exercise—in which meal and exercise content also remain stable—allows them to reach their treatment goals more

Table 8-6. Pharmacokinetics of Insulin Action

INSULIN	ONSET OF ACTION (HR)	PEAK ACTION (HR)	AVERAGE DURATION OF ACTION (HR)	MAXIMUM DURATION (HR)
Regular	0.5–1.0	2–3	3–6	4–6
Lyspro	Immediate	1–2	2–4	4
Aspart	Immediate	1–3	3–5	5
Lente	3–4	4–12	12–18	16–20
Ultralente	6–10	None	18–20	20–30
NPH	1–4	4–10	10–16	14–18
Glargine	1–2	None	22–24	24

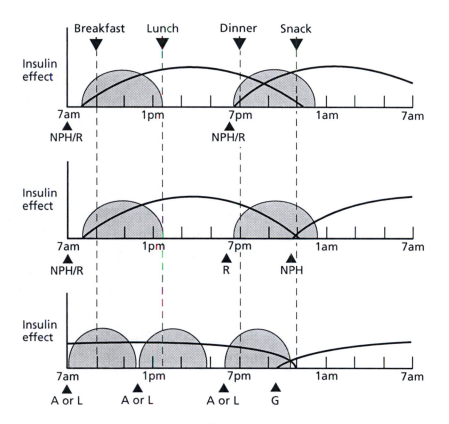

Fig. 8-6. Insulin-Dosing Regimen

Three insulin-dosing regimens are shown. *Top*, the expected insulin effect derived from a twice daily injection schedule, *middle*, a schedule with three injections daily, *bottom*, a more vigorous four-injection daily regimen. The short-acting regular (R), lyspro (L), or aspart (A) insulins are used to prevent postprandial hyperglycemia. The intermediate-acting insulin neutral protamine Hagedorn (NPH) and the long-acting insulin glargine (G) provide basal coverage. Shaded areas indicate action times of regular and aspart or lispro insulin. NPH/R = a mixture of NPH and regular insulin.

easily. If one of these three variables changes, the other two must be adjusted if normoglycemia is to be maintained.

MANAGEMENT OF TYPE 2 DM

Type 2 DM results from defects in both insulin secretion and insulin action. Therefore, treatments are designed to improve insulin secretion and to overcome insulin resistance. Most clinicians follow a stepped approach to treating type 2 DM. Diet and exercise are generally the first line of therapy unless the patients are very symptomatic or hyperglycemic. If the patient is obese, as most persons with type 2 DM are, the primary goal of diet therapy should be calorie reduction to achieve weight loss. Weight loss, however it is achieved, decreases insulin resistance.

If adequate glycemic control cannot be obtained through changes in diet and exercise, pharmacologic therapy is added. Blood-glucose lowering drugs act by increasing insulin secretion, lowering hepatic glucose output, slowing the rate of starch digestion, or increasing the efficiency of glucose uptake by muscle. Oral hypoglycemic agents are usually tried first, but insulin can also be given.

The biguanide metformin is often the first choice for obese patients because it lowers hepatic glucose production and reduces hepatic insulin resistance and is not associated with weight gain. Sulfonylureas work by increasing insulin secretion. These drugs bind to specific receptors on pancreatic beta cells, which cause ATP-dependent potassium channels to close, calcium channels to open, and insulin secretion to occur. Thiazolidenediones are insulin-sensitizing agents that work by altering the transcription rates of insulin-regulated genes. These drugs are believed to serve as agonists for the peroxisome proliferator activated γ nuclear receptor (PPARγ). The mechanisms of action of the oral hypoglycemic agents, their expected effects on blood glucose, and their side effects are summarized in Table 8-7.

Locations for Control of Hyperglycemia

Control glucose entry from intestine

Control liver glucose output

Control muscle glucose uptake

Augment pancreatic insulin secretion

Over the course of time, most patients with type 2 DM find that the original oral medication used to treat their diabetes is no longer

---

CASE STUDY: CONTINUED

Two years after her diagnosis of diabetes, Ms. Anderson developed a severe gastroenteritis that resulted in nausea and vomiting. She was unable to eat and her fluid intake was decreased. She reduced her insulin doses substantially because she thought this would help her avoid hypoglycemia during her illness-imposed fast. However, her blood glucose became very high, and she presented to the emergency room feeling lightheaded and weak. In the emergency room, she was found to have orthostatic changes in blood pressure and pulse, but the rest of her examination was normal. Laboratory data included the following: sodium, 129 mEq/L (normal: 138–147 mEq/L); potassium, 4.0 mEq/L (normal); bicarbonate, 15 mEq/L (normal: 23–29 mEq/L); glucose, 540 mg/dL (normal: 70–110 mg/dL); blood urea nitrogen (BUN), 30 mg/dL (normal: 10–20 mg/dL); creatinine, 2.2 mg/dL (normal: 0.6–1.2 mg/dL); and pH, 7.2 (normal 7.4). Serum ketones were high and ketonuria was present.

Table 8-7. Major Drugs for the Treatment of Type 2 DM

DRUGS	SITES OF ACTION	EFFECTS ON GLYCEMIA		SIDE EFFECTS
		FPG (MG/DL)	HBA₁C (%)	
Sulfonylureas	**Pancreas**			
Glyburide	Increase insulin secretion	$\downarrow$50–60	$\downarrow$1.0–1.5	Hypoglycemia, weight gain
Glipizide				
Glimiperide				
Tolazamide				
Biguanides	**Liver**			
Metformin	Decrease hepatic glucose production	$\downarrow$50–60	$\downarrow$1.0–1.5	Anorexia, diarrhea, lactic acidosis in susceptible individuals
Inhibitors of starch digestion	**Small intestine**			
Acarbose	Delay starch and sucrose digestion	$\downarrow$PP–PG	$\downarrow$0.5–1.0	Flatulence, diarrhea and abdominal pan
Miglitol	Delay glucose absorption			
Thiazolidenediones	**Muscle, liver, and fat**			
Pioglitazone,	Increase muscle glucose uptake	$\downarrow$20–50	$\downarrow$0.6–1.0	Weight gain, edema, increased plasma volume
Rosiglitazone	Decrease liver glucose output			

Note. FPG = fasting plasma glucose; PP-PG = postprandial plasma glucose; HbA1c = hemoglobin A1c; $\downarrow$ = decreased.

adequate. To prevent hyperglycemia, oral medications with different mechanisms of action can be combined or insulin can be added. Eventually it may be necessary to give combinations of insulins or to give insulin several times daily. Patients with type 2 DM do not require insulin to maintain life, but they may need insulin therapy to control hyperglycemia.

Complications of Diabetes

ACUTE COMPLICATIONS

The acute complications of diabetes involve the immediate effects of hyperglycemia on fluid and electrolyte balance. Because of the osmotic diuresis that ensues during hyperglycemia, dehydration occurs in patients who are unable to maintain sufficient water intake. Excessive and prolonged hyperglycemia can lead to a life-threatening illness in patients with both type 1 DM and type 2 DM. However, the pathophysiology depends on the type of diabetes present.

Acute Complications of Diabetes
Dehydration
Diabetic ketoacidosis
Hyperosmolar coma

Type 1 DM

Hyperglycemia in a patient with type 1 DM indicates insulin deficiency and carries the risk of developing ketoacidosis. Diabetic ketoacidosis (DKA) is characterized by extreme hyperglycemia (generally >300 mg/dL), an increased anion gap, metabolic acidosis (usually pH < 7.3) and an increase in the concentrations of total blood ketones (usually > 5 mM). In the setting of absolute insulin deficiency, glucagon action on adipose tissue and the liver are unopposed. Consequently, lipolysis is unrestrained and free fatty acids accumulate in the blood. These free fatty acids are transported to the liver where they provide energy for gluconeogenesis. Excess free fatty acids, which cannot be completely oxidized, are converted by the liver to ketones: acetate, acetoacetate, and β-hydroxybutyrate. These appear in the blood as organic acids and are excreted in the urine, producing ketonuria. Proteolysis is increased in the absence of insulin, and the amino acids provide substrate for gluconeogenesis. Hepatic glucose output increases, since glucagon stimulates both gluconeogenesis and glycogenolysis. Glucose utilization decreases, because without insulin glucose uptake by muscle is decreased. Persistent hyperglycemia causes an osmotic diuresis, which leads to extreme dehydration, inadequate renal function, and growing acidosis. These relationships are outlined in Fig. 8-7.

The presence of acetone may impart a fruity odor to the patient's breath. In addition to hyperglycemia, glucosuria, ketonemia, and ketonuria, patients present with low bicarbonate as a result of the acidosis and elevated blood urea nitrogen and creatinine as a result of dehydration. Total body potassium and phosphorous are depleted by gastrointestinal loss because DKA is frequently accompanied by nausea and vomiting and by diuresis and acidosis. However, serum levels may be normal because of shifts to the extracellular space in the presence of acidosis. Serum sodium may be low because plasma volume is expanded by the excess glucose.

The treatment of DKA requires that insulin be administered to correct the insulin-deficient state and to overcome the excess glucagon effect. Insulin decreases lipolysis and ketone-body formation and increases glucose uptake into fat and muscle. The dehydration and electrolyte abnormalities associated with DKA must be corrected by the administration of intravenous fluids. It is essential to determine and treat whatever caused the severe metabolic decompensation. Illness, with its attendant rise in the insulin-opposing hormones cortisol and epinephrine, is a common cause of DKA. Undetected myocardial ischemia, pregnancy, or poor compliance with the diabetes care regimen may also be responsible.

Type 2 DM

Hyperglycemia in a patient with type 2 DM can lead to hyperosmolar coma. Insulin deficiency is not absolute, so significant ketosis and severe acidosis (DKA) usually do not occur. However, these patients can develop hyperglycemia and dehydration, which are much more severe

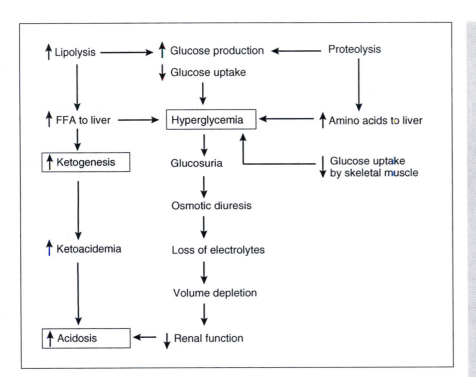

Fig. 8-7. Metabolic Consequences of Severe Insulin Deficiency (Diabetic Ketoacidosis)

In the setting of severe insulin deficiency, the ratio of glucagon to insulin is shifted in favor of glucagon, resulting in lipolysis and ketogenesis. Lipolysis contributes fuel (free fatty acids) for gluconeogenesis. Insulin deficiency results in increased proteolysis, which contributes amino acids for gluconeogenesis. Glucagon stimulates both gluconeogenesis and glycogenolysis. Liver glucose production increases. Glucose uptake by muscle is markedly decreased. Acidosis and renal insufficiency occur in response to the rising blood concentrations of ketones and glucose. If insulin deficiency is left untreated, diabetic ketoacidosis occurs.

than that seen in patients with DKA. Hyperosmolar coma is characterized by an increase in blood glucose to greater than 600 mg/dL, profound dehydration due to the hyperglycemia, and increased serum

---

CASE STUDY: CONTINUED

Two years after her diagnosis, Ms. Anderson presented with diabetic ketoacidosis, which developed as a result of inadequate insulin dosing in the setting of an acute illness. This illustrates the importance of educating patients in how to adjust their diabetes therapy under a variety of circumstances. When she presented with DKA, Ms. Anderson was significantly dehydrated, as demonstrated by her orthostatic hypotension and elevated BUN and creatinine levels. She was treated with intravenous fluids and insulin and was taught appropriate sick-day management techniques. She made a quick and complete recovery.

osmolality to greater than 320 mOsm/kg. Bicarbonate remains greater than 15 mEq/L (normal: 23–29 mEq/L), pH remains greater than 7.3 (normal: 7.4), and severe ketosis is absent. This syndrome usually occurs in elderly patients and may be precipitated by illness or drugs. Therapy depends on detection and treatment of the underlying cause of the disorder, aggressive hydration, and replacement of electrolyte deficiencies. Hyperglycemia improves with hydration alone, since increased plasma volume increases renal blood flow and allows excess glucose to be excreted in the urine. However, insulin is usually included in the treatment program.

CHRONIC COMPLICATIONS

Chronic complications of diabetes arise when tissues that are freely permeable to glucose are exposed to chronic hyperglycemia. These complications of diabetes mellitus can be categorized as microvascular and macrovascular, as shown in Fig. 8-8.

CASE STUDY: CONTINUED

Fifteen years later, Ms. Anderson returned to her physician's office seeking help in managing her diabetes. During the previous week, she had experienced a severe hypoglycemic reaction while working at home alone in the afternoon. When her family came home for dinner, they found her unconscious on the floor. The paramedics were called and found her blood glucose to be 20 mg/dL (normal fasting glucose: 70–110 mg/dL). After receiving an intravenous injection of glucose, she regained consciousness. Although this was the first time she had ever needed paramedics to treat an insulin reaction, she had recently experienced difficulty in detecting low blood sugars. On several occasions over the last few months, she had been unaware that she was hypoglycemic until a family member noted that she was confused. With some difficulty, they persuaded her to drink a glass of juice to help restore her blood sugar to normal. Ms. Anderson also said that she was often surprised to find her fasting blood sugars were around 40 mg/dL because she had no symptoms of hypoglycemia.

On physical examination, her blood pressure was 150/95 mm Hg with a heart rate of 96 beats/minute. Her fundoscopic exam was significant for dot hemorrhages and hard exudates in both eyes. Her neurologic exam revealed absent deep tendon reflexes in her legs and markedly decreased sensation in a stocking distribution to mid-calf bilaterally. Examination of her feet revealed normal pulses and mild edema. The rest of her examination was unremarkable.

Her laboratory data were significant: glycosylated hemoglobin of 7.8% (normal: 4.5–6.0%); glucose level, 240 mg/dL (normal: 70–110 mg/dL); creatinine, 2.5 mg/dL (normal: 0.6–1.2 mg/dL); and urinalysis, 4+ protein (normal: 0 protein).

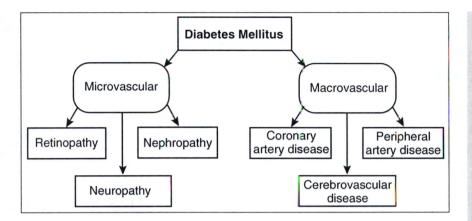

Fig. 8-8. Chronic Complications of Diabetes Mellitus

The chronic complications of diabetes are classified according to the size of the blood vessels affected by the disease. In microvascular complications, small arterioles and capillaries are affected by hyperglycemia, whereas in macrovascular complications, the affected vessels are large arteries. Microvascular complications are unique to diabetes, but macrovascular complications also occur in the nondiabetic population.

All these complications can occur in patients with both type 1 and type 2 diabetes, but all patients with diabetes do not develop complications. Other factors, such as genetic susceptibility, are also believed to play a role. Nonetheless, reduction of hyperglycemia is effective in preventing the development and progression of the long-term complications of diabetes. In the Diabetes Control and Complications Trial, a prospective randomized study in which patients with type 1 DM were randomized to receive either standard therapy or intensive therapy for more than 5 years, the group that received intensive therapy significantly reduced their risk of developing all the microvascular complications of diabetes.

The reason that chronic hyperglycemia results in long-term complications is uncertain. Current evidence supports four hypotheses:

- formation of advanced glycation end products (AGEs)
- increased flux through the polyol pathway
- activation of protein kinase C
- increased flux through the hexosamine pathway

Tissue proteins are nonenzymatically *glycated* or *glycosylated* by glucose in direct proportion to the ambient glycemia. The products are ultimately converted into highly reactive carbonyl compounds and reactive oxidative species that can cause proteins to become abnormally cross-linked to each other. This alters both protein structure and function. Because these advanced glycation end products (AGEs) can be very long-lived, and because they can continue to react with proteins even after blood glucose concentrations are normalized, hyperglycemia may have lasting effects on the integrity of tissue proteins (Fig. 8-9). This may be particularly true in the extracellular matrix,

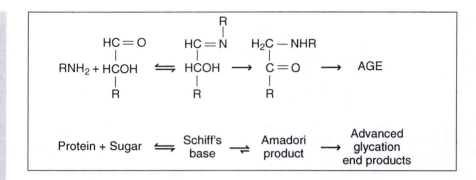

Fig. 8-9. Formation of Advanced Glycation End Prpoducts (AGEs)

Formation of AGEs begins with reversible interactions between a protein amino group (RNH_2) and a sugar molecule containing a reactive aldehyde group (HC=O) to form a glycated protein (Schiff's base). Further rearrangement of the glycated protein leads to the irreversible production of AGEs.

where AGE-modified proteins alter both matrix-matrix and matrix-cell interactions. Increased cross-linking of lens proteins leads to lens opacities (cataracts). Intracellular proteins such as basic fibroblast growth factor can also be AGE-modified, leading to changes in cellular mitogenic activity. AGEs can also interact with specific receptors on many cell types, including endothelial cells, glomerular mesangial cells, and macrophages. Binding of AGEs to these receptors can result in altered gene expression.

Chronic Complications of Diabetes
Microvascular complications (affect arterioles and capillaries)
Nephropathy
Neuropathy
Retinopathy
Macrovascular complications (affect larger vessels)
Myocardial infarctions
Strokes
Ischemic ulcers
Amputations

Chronic hyperglycemia increases flux through the polyol pathway. This results in increased accumulation of intracellular sorbitol, a sugar alcohol made from glucose by the enzyme aldose reductase (Fig. 8-10). Sorbitol accumulation increases intracellular osmotic pressure and causes fluid retention. When sorbitol accumulation occurs in the lens, fluid accumulation can cause blurred vision. This resolves after a period of improved glucose control. Sorbitol accumulation has also been shown to impair sodium-potassium-adenosine-triphosphatase

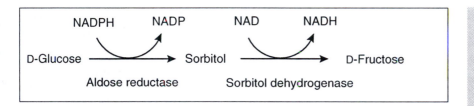

Fig. 8-10. Flux Through the Polyol Pathway

Aldose reductase converts D-glucose into sorbitol. The rate of this reaction is dependent on the cellular concentration of glucose. NAD = nicotinamide adenine dinucleotide; NADH = the reduced form of NAD; NADP = nicotinamide adenine dinucleotide phosphate; NADPH = the reduced form of NADP.

$(Na^+\text{-}K^+\text{-}ATPase)$ activity, leading to decreased adenosine triphosphate (ATP) concentrations and cell death.

Chronic hyperglycemia induces increased protein kinase C activity. Activation of this enzyme in retinal and renal tissue has been associated with abnormalities in blood flow, vascular permeability, angiogenesis, and proinflammatory gene expression. Hyperglycemia also increases flux through the hexosamine pathway. During hyperglycemia, fructose-6-phosphate is diverted from glycolysis to pathways that require UDP-N-acetylglucosamine. This, in turn, results in changes in gene expression and protein function.

These mechanisms for the development of diabetes complications can ultimately be linked by overproduction of superoxide by the mitochondrial electron transport chain in the setting of hyperglycemia. These mechanisms also can be linked to the vascular endothelium dysfunction, platelet abnormalities, and defects in supporting cells such as retina pericytes or glomerular mesangial cells that are associated with development of long-term complications of diabetes.

Diabetic Nephropathy

Diabetic nephropathy occurs in 20% to 40% of patients after 5 to 10 years of diabetes. Thickening of capillary basement membranes and the mesangium of the glomeruli results in glomerular sclerosis and renal insufficiency. The onset of nephropathy is heralded by the appearance of albumin in the urine. Because early treatment of diabetic nephropathy slows the rate of progression to renal failure, all patients with diabetes should be screened for the presence of albumin in their urine. Patients can be categorized as having either normal renal function, microalbuminuria (30–300 mg albumin/day) or macroalbuminuria-proteinuria (>300 mg albumin/day). Once the stage of proteinuria is reached, the glomerular filtration rate begins to fall. Patients with type 1 DM develop hypertension at this time. Progression of hypertension and worsening renal function results in end-stage renal disease after 15 to 25 years of diabetes in 20% to 30% of patients.

Progression of diabetic nephropathy is strongly associated with acceleration of and earlier death from atherosclerosis. The mechanisms other than hypertension are uncertain.

Pathogenesis of nephropathy is the same in patients with type 2 DM, but these patients are often older and the course may be complicated by hypertension and atherosclerosis that were already present when the diagnosis of diabetes was made.

Development and progression of microalbuminuria and proteinuria can be prevented or delayed by good control of glycemia and hypertension. Treatment with an angiotensin-converting enzyme inhibitor has been shown to slow the rate of progression toward end-stage renal disease. Angiotensin receptor antagonists also reduce albuminuria.

Diabetic Neuropathy

The manifestations of diabetic neuropathy are protean. Patients can develop neurologic complications at any time after diagnosis, and more than one type of neuropathy may appear in the same patient. The number of diabetic patients who develop neuropathy is difficult to determine, since abnormalities on testing are not always associated with symptoms. However, most diabetic patients experience some symptoms related to neurologic complications at some point in their lives. The major types of neuropathy are listed in Table 8-8.

Table 8-8. Diabetic Neuropathies

NEUROPATHY	SYMPTOMS	PHYSICAL SIGNS	TREATMENT
Distal symmetric sensori-motor neuropathy	Paresthesias or pain in stocking/glove distribution	Decreased reflexes, decreased sensation, muscle wasting	Foot care education, pain management
Autonomic neuropathy			
Cardiac	Lightheadedness	Orthostatic hypotension and resting tachycardia	Fludrocortisone, compression stockings
Gastrointestinal	Early satiety, nausea, vomiting, constipation, diarrhea		Prokinetic agents such as metoclopramide
Genitourinary	Impotence, retrograde ejaculation		Phosphodiesterase type 5 inhibitors; penile or urethral injections with papaverine, phento-lamine, prostaglandin E_2; vacuum or implantable device
Amyotrophy	Severe pain, weakness, weight loss	Muscle weakness, cachexia	Supportive care or gluco-corticoid, self-limited
Mononeuritis multiplex	Weakness or loss of sensation in distribution of single nerve—often one of cranial nerves III-VI	Muscle weakness or decreased sensation in the distribution of a single nerve	Self-limited

Diabetic Retinopathy

Some degree of retinopathy occurs in more than 90% of patients with diabetes, but vision-threatening complications occur in less than 30%. Patients have usually had diabetes for 5 years before the first signs of retinopathy become apparent, but new eye problems can develop at any time. Retinopathy occurs in predictable stages, as listed below.

- Background or nonproliferative retinopathy
    —Development of microaneurysms in weakened retinal capillary walls
    —Dot and blot hemorrhages as a result of the escape of erythrocytes from microaneurysms
    —Hard exudates as a result of extravasation of serous fluid from capillaries into the retina
- Preproliferative retinopathy
    —Cotton wool spots as a result of retina ischemia and infarction in the nerve layer
- Proliferative retinopathy
    —Neovascularization: fragile new vessels develop in response to ischemia

Vision loss from diabetic retinopathy occurs because of hemorrhage of the fragile new blood vessels into the vitreal cavity. The accumulation of blood can obscure vision, but it is the subsequent fibroproliferative changes in the clot that result in retinal detachment and permanent vision loss. Early detection of preproliferative and proliferative retinopathy allows treatment with photocoagulation. This eliminates the neovascularization and decreases the stimulus to additional proliferation. Because patients are asymptomatic until serious vision loss occurs, they must be screened for the development of retinopathy each year.

Macrovascular Complications

Patients with diabetes experience cardiovascular disease more frequently and at an earlier age than do people without diabetes, and the outcome is more severe. All the major blood vessels are affected, and atherosclerosis extends to the blood vessels in the feet. Women with diabetes are not protected from developing coronary heart disease before menopause as are women without diabetes. Diabetes synergizes with other risk factors for coronary heart disease. For example, both diabetes and smoking increase the risk for a myocardial infarction threefold, but in women with diabetes the combination of diabetes and smoking increases the risk *13-fold*. A thromboembolic stroke is 2 to 3 times more likely to occur in patients with diabetes, the incidence of peripheral vascular disease is 4 times greater, gangrene is 15 times more common, and the amputation rate is 2 to 4 times greater.

The reason for the increased severity of atherosclerosis is not known, but several abnormalities contributing to atherosclerosis and thrombosis have been implicated. These include endothelial dysfunction; increased fibrinogen; increased platelet aggregation; small dense lipoproteins, which are readily taken up into vessel walls; increased glycosylated and oxidized low density lipoproteins (LDLs); and increased stiffness of blood vessels resulting from abnormal cross-linking of glycated proteins.

Increased atherosclerosis is found even in patients with only mild impairment in glucose metabolism. Their glucose levels may be in the normal or impaired glucose tolerance range, but they have hyperinsulinemia, indicating that they are insulin resistant. These patients are also likely to have central obesity, hypertension, hypertriglyceridemia, and low HDL cholesterol. This constellation of abnormalities is known as the *metabolic syndrome* (previously called insulin resistance syndrome or syndrome x). The metabolic syndrome is strongly associated with the development of coronary heart disease.

Macrovascular disease is the most common cause of death in all patients with diabetes mellitus. For this reason, management of cardiovascular risk factors is of particular importance in the diabetic patient, and hypertension and hyperlipidemia warrant particularly aggressive treatment.

Some complications of diabetes can be attributed to the presence of both microvascular and macrovascular disease. Foot ulcers that fail to heal and ultimately lead to amputation are usually due to neuropathy and insufficient blood flow to the feet because of atherosclerosis. In patients with peripheral neuropathy, injury to the feet is common because they do not detect pain with foot trauma. These injuries are often left untreated because the patient is unaware of their presence. Infection sets in and the wound increases in size. To heal such an injury, sufficient tissue oxygenation must be present. When atherosclerosis is present in the arteries of the affected leg, sufficient oxygen is not available, and the ulcer heals slowly, if at all.

Impotence is another complication that is usually due to a combination of microvascular and macrovascular disease. To achieve and sustain an erection, a man must have normal neural function and sufficient delivery of arterial blood to the corpora cavernosa to develop tumescence. Men with diabetic neuropathy and diffuse atherosclerosis in the pelvic arteries can become impotent because of neurologic dysfunction and inadequate blood flow.

Hypoglycemia

Hypoglycemia refers to a lower than normal blood glucose level. Hypoglycemia is dangerous because glucose is the primary fuel of the brain. During periods of insufficient glucose delivery, cerebral activity is impaired. To maintain normoglycemia, counterregulatory mechanisms are activated in response to a fall in blood glucose (Table 8-9).

Table 8.9. Hypoglycemia Counter Regulation

PLASMA GLUCOSE	HORMONE RESPONSE TO HYPOGLYCEMIA
80–85 mg/dL (4.4–4.7 mM)	Insulin ↓
65–70 mg/dL (3.6–3.9 mM)	Glucagon ↑
65–70 mg/dL (3.6–3.9 mM)	Epinephrine ↑
65–70 mg/dL (3.6–3.9 mM)	Growth hormone ↑
55–60 mg/dL (3.1–3.3 mM)	Cortisol ↑

Note: In patients with long-standing diabetes, the glucagon response is absent. The epinephrine response may be absent, or the glucose threshold may be decreased.

The increases in glucagon and epinephrine stimulate glycogenolysis and gluconeogenesis to restore normoglycemia acutely. The increases in cortisol and growth hormone are important in recovery from prolonged hypoglycemia, but they contribute little to restoring normoglycemia in the acute setting.

Symptoms of hypoglycemia usually begin when the plasma glucose concentration falls to 45–50 mg/dL (normal: 70–110 mg/dL) and can be divided into two categories:

1. Adrenergic symptoms are due to excessive secretion of epinephrine in response to hypoglycemia. These symptoms include sweating, tremor, tachycardia, anxiety, and hunger.
2. Neuroglycopenic symptoms are due to dysfunction of the central nervous system (CNS) when glucose delivery to the brain is impaired. These symptoms include dizziness, headache, clouding of vision, blunted mental activity, loss of fine-motor skill, confusion, abnormal behavior, convulsions, and loss of consciousness.

Hypoglycemia occurs most frequently in patients with type 1 DM and is usually due to difficulty in matching exogenous insulin injections with anticipated blood glucose levels. Hypoglycemia is a particularly serious problem for patients attempting to normalize their blood glucose concentrations using intensive insulin regimens. In fact, the intensively treated group in the Diabetes Complications and Control Trial had a 2 to 3 times greater risk of developing hypoglycemia than the control group receiving standard treatment. The risk of hypoglycemia often limits how successfully blood glucose concentrations can be normalized in patients with diabetes.

Notes

Hormones Counter-Regulating Hypoglycemia
Glucagon
Epinephrine
Growth hormone
Cortisol

HYPOGLYCEMIA UNAWARENESS

Patients with long-standing diabetes are at particular risk for developing *hypoglycemia unawareness*, which occurs when they no longer experience the warning symptoms of hypoglycemia that prompt them to eat when their blood glucose concentration is very low. Patients who have had type 1 DM for 5 or more years lose their ability to release glucagon secretion in response to hypoglycemia and become dependent on the release of epinephrine. Unfortunately, their epinephrine response is attenuated. Therefore, they may not have a rise in catecholamine before their blood glucose decreases to a level too low to sustain cerebral function.

The cause of hypoglycemia unawareness is uncertain, but may relate to alterations in the delivery of glucose to the brain in well-controlled diabetic patients. In patients with hypoglycemia unawareness, the symptomatic response to hypoglycemia often can be restored if they allow their blood glucose concentrations to be somewhat higher for several weeks.

HYPOGLYCEMIA UNRELATED TO DIABETES

Hypoglycemia can also occur in people who do not have diabetes. Determining whether the insulin concentration is high or low can help to diagnose the cause of hypoglycemia. High insulin concentrations occur because of excessive release of insulin from the pancreas or

---

CLINICAL CASE: *RESOLUTION*

Fifteen years after her diagnosis of diabetes, Ms. Anderson presented with hypoglycemia unawareness. Her clinical course suggested that she no longer had hypoglycemia-induced glucagon or catecholamine secretion. She was instructed on how to avoid hypoglycemia by more consistent timing of her medications, snacks, and exercise and by adjusting her insulin doses. Family members were taught how to give glucagon in an emergency situation.

Ms. Anderson also displayed physical findings consistent with diabetic retinopathy and peripheral diabetic neuropathy. The presence of edema, proteinuria, and an elevated creatinine indicated that she also had diabetic nephropathy. She was referred to an ophthalmologist for careful evaluation. She was given intensive instruction in appropriate foot-care techniques and asked to examine her feet daily. She was given antihypertensive therapy with an ACE inhibitor, which has been shown to retard progression of diabetic nephropathy.

Because patients with proteinuria are at increased risk for atherosclerosis, blood pressure control is particularly important. She should also have her fasting lipid profile measured (see Chapter 9) and treatment for hyperlipidemia instituted, if necessary.

because of surreptitious administration of exogenous insulin. Measurement of the serum C-peptide concentration differentiates between endogenous or exogenous hyperinsulinemia because C-peptide is secreted in equimolar amounts with endogenous insulin. When insulin secretion is excessive, C-peptide levels are elevated in proportion to the insulin concentration. In the presence of exogenous insulin, C-peptide concentrations are low because secretion of both C-peptide and endogenous insulin is suppressed.

Causes of hypoglycemia associated with excessive insulin secretion include insulin-producing tumors and the use of drugs like sulfonylureas, pentamidine, quinine, and monoamine oxidase inhibitors, which stimulate insulin release. Patients with very rapid gastric emptying following gastric surgery may also develop hypoglycemia with high insulin levels. In these patients with alimentary hypoglycemia, the rapid absorption of food provides a strong stimulus for insulin secretion. Since insulin secretion lags behind absorption, hyperinsulinemia persists after the disappearance of nutrients from the gastrointestinal tract, and hypoglycemia occurs.

Hypoglycemia can also occur in the setting of low insulin concentrations. When gluconeogenesis is decreased, as occurs with alcohol excess, liver failure, severe malnutrition (usually in children or the elderly), and growth hormone or cortisol deficiency, hypoglycemia can occur with fasting. Large mesenchymal tumors that produce insulin-like growth factors can also lead to low insulin hypoglycemia.

REVIEW QUESTIONS

Directions: For each of the following questions, choose the *one best* answer.

Questions 1 and 2

A 58-year-old man comes to the physician's office complaining of recent onset of fatigue, a 20-lb weight loss, and the need to urinate 2 or 3 times each night. He is 6' tall and weighs 275 lbs. His blood pressure is 135/88 mm Hg and does not change with movement from a supine to upright position. He has no other abnormalities. Laboratory data reveal a fasting glucose of 270 mg/dL. Urinalysis reveals high urine glucose but no ketones.

1 What is the most likely cause of this man's symptoms?

   A Type 1 diabetes mellitus (type 1 DM)
   B Type 2 diabetes mellitus (type 2 DM)
   C Diabetes insipidus
   D Urinary tract infection

2 Further evaluation of this patient would be most likely to reveal

A increased insulin resistance
B severe beta-cell depletion
C evidence for other autoimmune disorders
D propensity to develop ketoacidosis

3 A 45-year-old man has had type 2 diabetes for 5 years. He has been following a weight-reduction diet and has increased his exercise. He is interested in minimizing his risk of developing long-term complications of diabetes. Which of the following is most likely to be the best long-term strategy to help him achieve his goal?

A Monitoring his blood pressure annually and examining his fundi every 5 years
B Maintaining his blood glucose as close to normal as possible
C Avoiding all alcohol consumption
D Exercising at least 3 times each week and examining his feet every 6 months
E Increasing his fasting hepatic glucose output to avoid hypoglycemia

4 A 37-year-old man with a 22-year history of type I diabetes mellitus comes to the physician's office with his wife for marital counseling. The wife feels the husband has suffered a personality change. If she offers him something to eat when she thinks he is having an insulin reaction, he becomes belligerent. This behavior is in marked contrast to his former even-tempered manner. He says that he used to become sweaty and shaky during insulin reactions, but during the last year he has had no symptoms when his blood sugar levels are low. What is the most likely cause of his mood swings and personality change?

A After 22 years of diabetes, he is frustrated when others tell him what to do
B He has lost increased cortisol and growth-hormone secretion in response to hypoglycemia
C He has lost his ability to secrete catecholamines in response to hypoglycemia
D He has increased glucagon secretion in response to hypoglycemia

Questions 5-8

For each case history that follows, select the diagnosis that is most appropriate.

A Type 1 diabetes mellitus (type 1 DM)
B Type 2 diabetes mellitus (type 2 DM)
C Diabetic ketoacidosis
D Marked insulin resistance

5 A 30-year-old Native American man is found to have glucose in his urine during a physical examination. He had slightly high blood glucose concentrations 2 years ago but was never told that he had diabetes. He feels well. Both of his parents, his two older brothers, and several aunts and uncles have diabetes. All are taking pills to control their blood sugar. On physical examination he weighs 280 lb and his height is 5′9″. His laboratory data include the following: fasting plasma glucose concentration, 160 mg/dL (normal: 70–110 mg/dL); glycosylated hemoglobin, 10.0% (normal: 4.5%–6.0%); and urinalysis remarkable only for the presence of glucose.

6 A 25-year-old woman comes to the physician's office because of a 2-week history of polyuria and polydipsia. She reports feeling ravenously hungry and asks if she can finish her lunch while she talks to you. In the last month she has eaten more than usual but has lost 10 lb. All of her family members are well. On physical examination she is 5′4″ tall and weighs 120 lb. Her blood glucose concentration is 280 mg/dL. Other laboratory data include C-peptide concentration of 50 pg/mL (normal: 500–2500 pg/mL) and glucosuria.

7 A 12-year-old boy is brought to the emergency room by his parents because he had become increasingly lethargic over the last 4 hours. He stayed home from school because of abdominal pain and lightheadedness. His mother reports that he has been getting up twice at night to urinate for the last few days, and she thinks he has lost weight. On physical examination his supine blood pressure is 100/60 mm Hg, and his supine heart rate is 90 beats/min. His upright blood pressure is 80/45 mm Hg, and his upright heart rate is 130 beats/min. His laboratory data include the following: plasma glucose concentration, 450 mg/dL (normal fasting concentration: 70–110 mg/dL); arterial pH of 7.1 (normal: 7.35–7.45); and urinalysis remarkable for the presence of glucose and ketones.

8 A 65-year-old woman comes to the physician's office because she feels tired all the time. She attributes this to the extra work at home caring for her father who was recently discharged from the hospital following amputation of his foot. On physical examination, she is 5′7″ and weighs 250 lb. Laboratory data reveal the following: plasma glucose concentration, 124 mg/dL (normal fasting concentration: 70–110 mg/dL); glycosylated hemoglobin, 6.5% (normal: 4.2%–6.0%); and a C-peptide concentration of 2500 pg/mL (normal: 500–2500 pg/mL).

Questions 9–13

For each of the patients with diabetes mellitus described below, select the complication that is most likely to be present.

A Diabetic retinopathy
B Peripheral vascular disease
C Diabetic nephropathy
D Diabetic neuropathy

9 A 34-year-old day-care worker has had type I diabetes mellitus for 30 years. She complains of bloating after she eats, intermittent nausea and vomiting. She feels lightheaded if she rises quickly from the floor after reading stories to the children. On physical examination, her supine blood pressure is 180/95 mm Hg with a pulse of 110 beats/minute, and her upright blood pressure is 90/50 mm Hg with a pulse of 110 beats/minute. Her neurologic examination demonstrates absent deep tendon reflexes and loss of light touch sensation in her feet. The remainder of her examination is unremarkable.

10 A 72-year-old retired electrician comes into the clinic complaining that his feet feel like someone is giving him electric shocks at night when he is trying to sleep. He has had type 2 diabetes for 7 years. His examination is significant for absent vibration and pinprick in his feet and lower legs. His dorsalis pedis pulses are palpable.

11 A 23-year-old librarian who developed type 1 diabetes mellitus at age 11 comes to the physician's office for a routine visit. He has no complaints and reports that his blood glucose values measured at home range from 80 to 250 mg/dL. His blood pressure is 140/88 mm Hg. Examination of his fundi reveals several hard exudates, some arterioventricular nicking, and several microaneurysms, although his visual acuity is normal at 20/20. His urinalysis is unremarkable.

12 A 28-year-old medical student who developed type 1 diabetes mellitus at age 9 comes to the physician's office for a routine visit. She has no complaints and reports that the blood glucose values measured at home range from 90 to 230 mg/dL. Her blood pressure is 145/94 mm Hg. Her visual acuity is 20/20. Her 24-hour urinary albumin excretion rate is 300 mg/day.

13 A 58-year-old basketball coach with a 10-year history of type 2 diabetes presents because of a sore on his foot that developed 2 weeks ago. His legs often ache during basketball practice as he runs along with the players. The aching stops when he stops running. There is an ulcer on his second right toe that measures 0.5 × 0.5 cm. His right foot is cooler than the left, and the pulses on the right are weaker. On neurologic examination his deep tendon reflexes are present in all limbs, and his light touch sensation is normal.

References

Atkinson MA, Eisenbarth GS: Type 1 diabetes: new perspectives on disease pathogenesis and treatment. *Lancet* 358: 221, 2001.

Brownlee M: Biochemistry and molecular cell biology of diabetic complications. *Nature* 414: 813–820, 2001.

Cryer PE: Hypoglycemia: the limiting factor in the glycemic management of type 1 and type 2 diabetes. *Diabetologia* 45: 927–948, 2002.

Frank RN: Diabetic retinopathy. *N Engl J Med* 350: 48–58, 2004.

Inzucchi SE: Oral antihyperglycemic therapy for type 2 diabetes. *JAMA* 287: 360–372, 2002.

Nathan DM. Initial management of glycemia in type 2 diabetes mellitus. *New Engl J Med* 347: 1342–1344. 2002.

Pessin J, Saltiel AR: Signaling pathways in insulin action: molecular targets of insulin resistance. *J Clin Invest* 106: 165–169, 2000.

The Expert Committee on the Diagnosis and Classification of Diabetes Mellitus: Report of the expert committee on diagnosis and classification of diabetes mellitus. *Diabetes Care* 20(7): 1183–1197, 1997.

9

Disorders of Lipid Metabolism

Angeliki Georgopoulos, M.D.

■ CHAPTER OUTLINE ■

■ LEARNING OBJECTIVES ■

At the completion of this chapter, the student will:
1. be aware of the structure and function of the lipoprotein classes.
2. be able to describe the pathways of lipoprotein metabolism.
3. understand the mechanisms leading to cholesterol and/or triglyceride elevation.
4. be able to differentiate between primary and secondary lipid disorders.
5. understand the physical and laboratory findings associated with specific hyperlipidemias.
6. understand the approach to treatment for lipid disorders.

CASE STUDY: *INTRODUCTION*

A 47-year-old woman had a heart attack 6 months ago and returned to her physician's office for follow-up. Her history revealed episodes of atypical chest pain for approximately 2 months before her heart attack, but none since the event. Her family history is positive for premature (before age 55 years) coronary artery disease. She recently learned that her father had elevated plasma cholesterol, and her paternal uncle had elevated triglycerides.

She had been feeling tired and the cold weather bothered her more, but she complained of no other health problems. She is still menstruating. She works in a stressful job with frequent deadlines and has been exercising erratically for the past year. A year ago she stopped smoking, and she has been watching her fat and cholesterol intake since the heart attack. She drinks a glass of wine every night and takes aspirin for occasional headache and muscle pain.

Physical examination revealed a 140 lb, 5'7" woman with a blood pressure of 130/85 mm Hg. Her heart rate and rhythm were normal. Examination of her skin revealed bilateral xanthelasmas around her eyelids but no xanthomas. Examination of the neck showed normal carotid pulses and a smooth, enlarged thyroid gland. Her chest was clear, there were no abnormal heart sounds or bruits, and her abdomen was normal. Peripheral pulses were decreased on her right side. The results of her neurologic examination were normal except for slow relaxation of her deep tendon reflexes.

Lipid Function

Cholesterol and fatty acids are the basic lipid molecules. *Cholesterol* is an essential component of cell membranes and a precursor of bile acid and steroid-hormone synthesis. It is synthesized in the liver from two-carbon units (acetyl CoAs) that condense to form 3-hydroxy-3-methylglutaryl CoA, which can be converted to mevalonic acid. This rate-limiting step is catalyzed by the enzyme 3-hydroxyl-3-methylglutaryl CoA reductase (HMGCoA reductase). Conditions that decrease this enzyme activity reduce the amount of cholesterol formed.

Fatty acids are used as fuel and combine with other molecules for the production of complex lipids. They combine with cholesterol to produce cholesterol esters, and with glycerol, phosphate, and choline, serine, or ethanolamine to produce phospholipids. Monoglycerides, diglycerides, and triglycerides (TG) are produced when fatty acids combine with glycerol. Fat (TG) is a source of energy, provides excellent insulation, and cushions the skeleton during falls.

Fat is ingested in the diet or made in the liver. The liver can take up fatty acids from blood or synthesize fatty acids from acetyl CoA derived from glucose or alcohol metabolism and incorporate them into TG. TG are incorporated into larger particles for transport to other tissues.

Lipases are the enzymes that hydrolyze TG to fatty acids and glycerol. The liberated fatty acids can be oxidized by tissues for energy or reconstituted into TG and stored, especially in adipose tissue. Lipoprotein lipase (LpL) is found in capillary endothelial cells in many tissues. LpL removes fatty acids from TG in circulating lipid particles. Hepatic lipase hydrolyzes TG and phospholipid delivered to the liver. Pancreatic lipase hydrolyzes TG in the intestine.

TG stored in adipose tissue is hydrolyzed by hormone-sensitive lipase. Hormone-sensitive lipase is stimulated by epinephrine during fasting, exercise, or stress, and fatty acids are released into the blood. In contrast, insulin suppresses hormone-sensitive lipase and stimulates LpL. After a carbohydrate meal, the rise in glucose stimulates insulin secretion. Hormone-sensitive lipase is suppressed, so lipolysis is decreased and more fatty acids are taken up into adipose tissue for storage as TG.

Lipoproteins

LIPOPROTEIN STRUCTURE

Since lipids are insoluble in water, they are carried in the plasma as lipid–protein structures called *lipoproteins*. Lipoproteins transport lipids between different tissues. Lipoproteins are classified and separated by their density, which is determined by the ratio of lipid to protein (Fig. 9-1).

Classes of Lipoproteins

Chylomicrons
Very low-density lipoprotein (VLDL)
Intermediate density lipoprotein (IDL)
Low-density lipoprotein (LDL)
High-density lipoprotein (HDL)

The protein portion of a lipoprotein is called an *apolipoprotein* and is designated by a capital letter (e.g., apolipoprotein A = apo A). Each apolipoprotein category includes several protein molecules distinguished by roman numerals (e.g., apo A-I) Humans produce all the apolipoprotein A, B, and C subtypes. However, an individual's apo E isoform type is determined by two separate alleles (one from each parent). Homozygotes have only one isoform (e.g., apo E-3/E-3); heterozygotes have two (e.g., apo E-3/E-4). Apo E-3 and apo E-4 are the most common forms. Most apoproteins are produced by the liver,

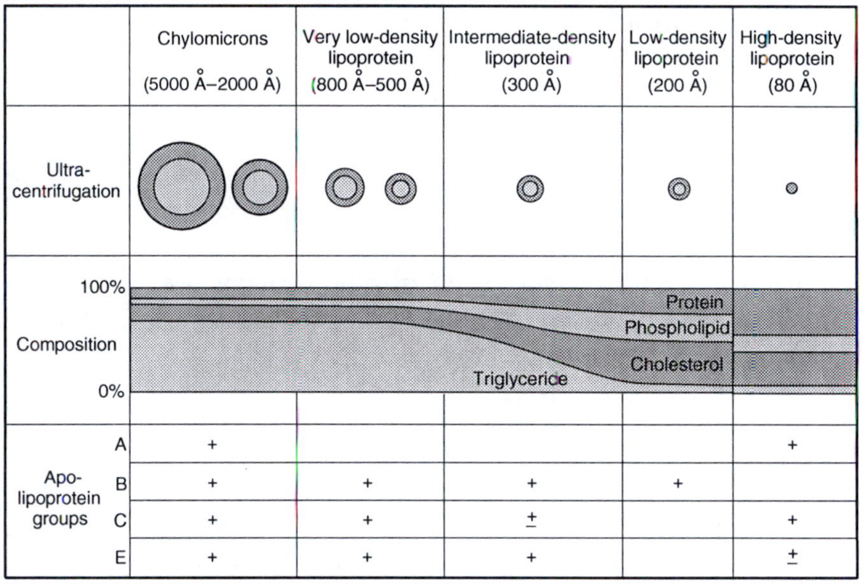

	Chylomicrons (5000 Å–2000 Å)	Very low-density lipoprotein (800 Å–500 Å)	Intermediate-density lipoprotein (300 Å)	Low-density lipoprotein (200 Å)	High-density lipoprotein (80 Å)
Ultra-centrifugation					
Composition (100% to 0%: Protein, Phospholipid, Cholesterol, Triglyceride)					
Apo-lipoprotein groups A	+				+
Apo-lipoprotein groups B	+	+	+	+	
Apo-lipoprotein groups C	+	+	±		+
Apo-lipoprotein groups E	+	+	+		±

Fig. 9-1. Composition of Lipoproteins Classified by Size

(*Source:* Adapted with permission from Bierman EL: Hyperlipoproteinemia, Current Concepts. Kalamazoo. MI: Upjohn, 1984, p 6.)

except for Apo B-48 and A-IV, which are produced by the intestine. Apo E is produced in several tissues, including the central nervous system. ApoE-4 is a risk factor for Alzheimer's disease.

Major Apolipoprotein Types and Subtypes
apolipoprotein A (apo A_I, apo A_{II}, apo A_{IV})
apolipoprotein B (apo B_{100}, apo B_{48})
apolipoprotein C (apo C_I, apo C_{II}, apo C_{III})
apolipoprotein E (apo E_2, apo E_3, apo E_4)

The composition of all lipoproteins is qualitatively similar but quantitatively different. All lipoproteins are spheres. They contain a core of nonpolar (totally insoluble) triglyceride and cholesterol esters. Their surface contains free cholesterol and the detergent-like phospholipids and apolipoproteins that enable them to be soluble in plasma.

The various lipoproteins are distinguished by the proportions of their components (Figure 9-1). Large, light lipoproteins like chylomicrons and very low-density lipoproteins (VLDLs) have cores that are rich in triglycerides. Small, denser lipoproteins such as low-density lipoproteins (LDLs) and high-density lipoproteins (HDLs), which contain more protein, have cores that contain mostly cholesterol esters. Chylomicron remnants and VLDL remnants, including intermediate-density lipoproteins (IDLs), are denser than chylomicrons and

VLDL but lighter than LDL and HDL. Remnants contain approximately equal proportions of cholesterol and triglycerides.

It is important to realize that the composition of circulating lipoprotein particles in the blood is not fixed; it changes through interactions with other lipoproteins, transfer proteins, and enzymes. There is heterogeneity in size and composition even among lipoproteins classified in the same "family" of chylomicrons, VLDLs, remnants, IDLs, LDLs, and HDLs. Besides carrying lipids, the lipoproteins also carry lipid-soluble vitamins (vitamins A, D, and E), lipid-soluble drugs, antioxidant enzymes, and some viruses.

Functions of Apolipoproteins

Solubilize lipids in plasma

Act as ligands for lipoprotein receptors (apo B and apo E)

Act as cofactors for enzymes (apo C-II and apo A-I)

Apolipoproteins are not only solubilizing factors. They play an active role in the metabolism of the lipoproteins. Apo E and apo B act as ligands for lipoprotein receptors in tissues. Apo E has greater affinity for receptors than apo B, so apo E mediates the cellular uptake of the lipoproteins when both are present. When no apo E is present, as in LDL, apo B is the ligand for receptor binding. Ligand-binding by the liver receptors clears the lipoprotein from the circulation. However, ligand-binding to cells in blood vessel walls results in uptake of lipid and formation of foam cells, which initiates atherosclerosis.

Lipoproteins containing apo B can be atherogenic (promote atherosclerosis). There is only one apo B per lipoprotein particle; therefore the blood concentration of apo B reflects the number of potentially atherogenic particles in the circulation. Apo B is found in all lipoproteins except HDL.

HDL, which contains large amounts of apo A-I, is considered antiatherogenic (prevents atherosclerosis). Apo A-I is a ligand for HDL-binding to peripheral tissues.

Some apolipoproteins act as enzyme cofactors. Apo C-II is a cofactor for the enzyme lipoprotein lipase (LPL). Apo A-I and possibly apo D are cofactor(s) for the enzyme lecithin cholesterol acyltransferase (LCAT), which transfers fatty acids to cholesterol to form cholesterol esters.

Apolipoprotein (a) [apo(a)] is a special protein that binds by a disulfide link to the apo B of LDL to form a lipoprotein called Lp(a). Apo(a) is structurally homologous to plasminogen and is considered atherogenic and thrombogenic.

METABOLIC PATHWAYS

Exogenous Pathway

This pathway involves metabolism of ingested fat (Figure 9-2). Dietary triglyceride is partially hydrolyzed in the intestine by

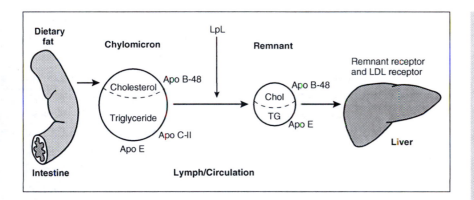

Fig. 9-2. Exogenous Pathway of Lipoprotein Metabolism

LDL = low-density lipoprotein; Apo = apolipoprotein; LpL = lipoprotein lipase; Chol = cholesterol; TG = triglyceride.

pancreatic lipase before being absorbed. Triglycerides are reformed in intestinal cells and are incorporated into *chylomicrons*, which also contain a small amount of dietary cholesterol and apolipoproteins (Table 9-1). They are the biggest and lightest lipoprotein particles, and because they contain 80% to 90% triglyceride, they are lighter than plasma and float to the top when a tube of plasma is refrigerated.

Chylomicrons, normally present in the postprandial state but not in the fasting state, are secreted from the intestine into the lymph and transported to the blood via the thoracic duct. They contain apo B-48

Table 9-1. Lipoprotein Classes: Sources and Constituents

CLASS	SITE OF PRODUCTION	MAJOR LIPIDS*	MAJOR APOLIPOPROTEINS
Chylomicrons	Intestine	80%–90% triglyceride	B-48, A-I, A-IV, E, C-I, C-II, C-III
Chylomicron remnants	Circulation	60%–65% triglyceride, 20% cholesterol	B48, E
VLDL	Liver	50%–60% triglyceride, 20% cholesterol	B100, E, C-I, C-II, C-III
IDL from VLDL	Circulation	35% cholesterol, 25% triglyceride	B100, E
LDL from IDL	Circulation	60% cholesterol, 10% triglyceride	B100
HDL	Liver, intestine	25% phospholipid, 20% cholesterol, 5% triglyceride	A-I, A-II, C-I, C-II, C-III,

Note. VLDL = very low-density lipoprotein; LDL = low-density lipoprotein; IDL = intermediate-density lipoprotein; HDL = high-density lipoprotein
*The remainder of the particle is mostly protein.

and acquire additional apolipoproteins from HDL in the lymph and plasma. Circulating chylomicrons interact with plasma HDL and with lipoprotein lipase (LpL) on the endothelial surface of blood vessel walls. LpL attacks the particles and hydrolyzes the triglyceride to release free fatty acids (FFA) and produce remnant particles. Apo C-II is a cofactor for LpL and is required for lipolysis. Hepatic lipase also contributes to lipolysis of chylomicron triglyceride. Surface material liberated during chylomicron lipolysis (phospholipid, free cholesterol, and apolipoproteins other than apo B-48) is added to newly formed HDL. The liberated FFA are bound to albumin and taken up as fuel by peripheral tissues (muscle, adipose) and by the liver. In the liver, FFA are either oxidized or used for synthesis of triglycerides. FFA provide energy (but not substrate) for gluconeogenesis.

Role of Lipases in Lipid Metabolism

Pancreatic lipase hydrolyzes dietary triglyceride in intestine.

Lipoprotein lipase hydrolyzes triglyceride in chylomicrons and VLDL in circulation.

Hepatic lipase hydrolyzes triglyceride and phospholipid in remnant particles and HDL.

Hormone-sensitive lipase hydrolyzes triglyceride in adipose tissue to release free fatty acids into the blood. It is inhibited by insulin and stimulated by epinephrine.

Chylomicron remnants are quickly cleared by specific receptors in the liver and other tissues through a complex process that involves LpL, hepatic lipase, and two receptors—the remnant receptor and the LDL (apo B/E) receptor. Apo E is the ligand for both of these receptors, and abnormalities in the apo E structure or homozygosity for the E-2 isoform reduce remnant clearance.

Chylomicrons deliver dietary triglycerides to tissues for fuel.

Chylomicron remnants deliver dietary cholesterol to the liver.

Endogenous Pathway

In contrast to the exogenous pathway, which operates only after fat ingestion, the endogenous pathway is always active (Fig. 9-3). It involves VLDL synthesis in the endoplasmic reticulum of the liver. VLDL synthesis is driven by fatty acids, which are used for triglyceride synthesis, and by attachment to apo B-100. Microsomal triglyceride transfer protein (MTP) is critical in this process. Defective MTP causes *abetalipoproteinemia*, a disorder characterized by lack of apo B–containing lipoproteins and very low plasma cholesterol levels. The VLDL particles are secreted by the liver and carry endogenous triglyceride and cholesterol in the blood.

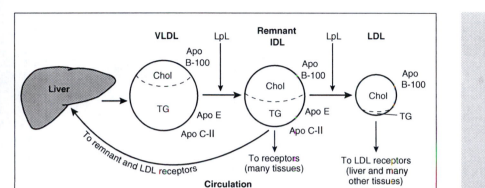

Fig. 9-3. Endogenous Pathway of Lipoprotein Metabolism

CHOL = cholesterol; TG = triglyceride; VLDL = very low-density lipoprotein; LDL = low-density lipoprotein; IDL = intermediate density lipoprotein; Apo = apolipoprotein; LpL = lipoprotein lipase.

The metabolic fate of VLDL in the circulation is similar to that of chylomicrons. VLDL is hydrolyzed by lipoprotein lipase and its cofactor apo C-II. During hydrolysis, surface material is transferred to HDL, and FFA are transferred to peripheral tissues and the liver. This leaves *VLDL remnants*, which have two possible fates: further lipolysis to produce IDL and LDL or removal by the liver via LDL and remnant receptors. Apo E is the main ligand for VLDL remnants and IDL.

If apo E is abnormal, chylomicron remnants and VLDL remnants can remain in the circulation for a long time, where they become cholesterol enriched by ongoing transfer of cholesterol from HDL to the remnants in exchange for transfer of triglycerides to HDL. The transfer is facilitated by cholesterol ester transfer protein (CETP). These cholesterol-rich remnants can be taken up by cells of the blood vessel wall and cause atherosclerosis.

LDL is the final product of VLDL lipolysis. The LDL core contains cholesterol but little triglyceride and only one apolipoprotein per particle: apo B-100, the ligand for LDL removal by liver LDL receptors. Because LDL is the major carrier of cholesterol in the blood, defects in the structure of apo B-100 or the LDL receptor lead to accumulation of LDL and increased blood cholesterol levels.

Circulating LDL delivers cholesterol to cells where it can be used for synthesis of cell membranes, for bile acid production (liver only), and for steroid hormone synthesis (adrenals, ovaries, testes, skin).

Cellular Cholesterol Regulation

Circulating LDL delivers cholesterol to cells where it can be used for synthesis of plasma membranes, bile acid production (liver only), and

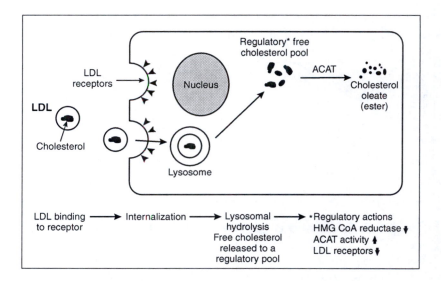

Fig. 9-4. LDL Receptor-Mediated Pathway of Regulation of Intracellular Cholesterol

LDL interacts with receptors, is taken up by the cell, and is degraded in lysosomes to amino acids and cholesterol. The accumulating cholesterol (1) suppresses additional cholesterol synthesis by feedback inhibition of 3-hydroxy-3-methylglutaryl coenzyme A (HMG-CoA) reductase; (2) is converted into cholesterol esters by acylCoA cholesterol acyltransferase (ACAT); and (3) down-regulates LDL receptors so less cholesterol is removed from plasma.

steroid hormone synthesis (adrenals, ovaries, testes, and skin). When LDL is taken up by cells through the LDL receptor (Figure 9-4), it is transferred to lysosomes where free cholesterol is released and used for membrane synthesis. The free cholesterol also enters a regulatory pool. As the size of this regulatory pool increases, further cellular accumulation of free cholesterol is prevented by (1) inhibition of the enzyme HMG-CoA reductase, the rate-limiting step in cholesterol synthesis; (2) a decrease in the number of LDL receptors on the cell membrane, so less cholesterol can enter the cell; and (3) esterification of free cholesterol to cholesterol esters through the enzyme acetyl cholesterol acyltransferase (ACAT).

If the cellular uptake of LDL were to occur only through this pathway, where the amount of intracellular cholesterol is carefully regulated, atherosclerosis would not develop. It is hypothesized that development of atherosclerosis involves lipoprotein uptake by unregulated pathways. Unregulated uptake of oxidized LDL by scavenger receptors is one example of this. Uptake of remnant lipoproteins by macrophages is another.

Reverse Cholesterol Pathway

In contrast to the exogenous and endogenous pathways that deliver cholesterol to the cells and that can lead to the development of

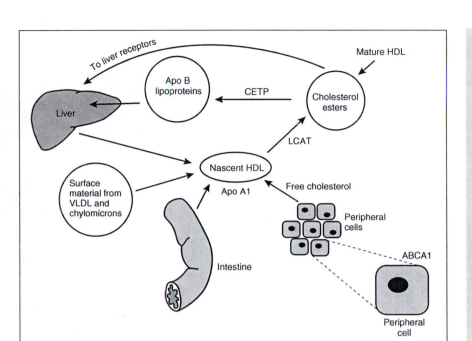

Fig. 9-5. Reverse Cholesterol Pathway Mediated by HDL

ApoA1 on the surface of HDL interacts with the ABCA1 cassette protein (the transporter) on the surface of a cell. This activates movement of cholesterol from the peripheral cell to the nascent HDL particle. ApoA1 also is a cofactor for the enzyme LCAT in the blood. Therefore, ApoA1 facilitates conversion of free cholesterol on the HDL surface to cholesterol esters. The water-insoluble esters go to the HDL core, creating mature, spherical HDL particles. Cholesterol esters can go directly to the liver via HDL binding to liver receptors, or indirectly by being transferred to ApoB-containing lipoproteins through the action of CETP. From the liver, cholesterol can be converted to bile acids and excreted from the body via the intestine. Apo = apolipoprotein; CETP = cholesterol ester transfer protein; LCAT = lecithin-cholesterol acyltransferase; VLDL = very low-density lipoprotein; HDL = high-density lipoprotein.

atherosclerosis, the reverse cholesterol pathway removes cholesterol from the cells and eventually from the body (Fig. 9-5). This process involves nascent HDL, a discoidal form of HDL, which contains apo A-I and phospholipids. Nascent HDL is secreted by the liver and intestine into the blood where it takes up surface components released during lipolysis of triglyceride-rich lipoproteins. Nascent HDL is a good acceptor of cellular cholesterol. Cholesterol is transferred from cells to HDL by either a gradient mechanism or a transport mechanism that seems to involve apo A-I and a cell surface–binding protein (ABCA1), a member of a large family of ATP-binding cassette transporters. Free cholesterol is then converted to cholesterol esters by the enzyme lecithin cholesterol acyltransferase (LCAT). Uptake and esterification of free cholesterol cause the nascent HDL particle to become a mature, spherical HDL_3 particle. As more cholesterol is acquired, the HDL_3 particle becomes a bigger HDL_2 particle.

LCAT (lecithin-cholesterol acyltransferase) is the enzyme in the circulation that esterifies lipoprotein free cholesterol to cholesterol esters by transferring fatty acid from phospholipid. **ACAT** is the enzyme in cells that catalyzes the reaction of free cholesterol with fatty acid to form cholesterol esters.

Cholesterol esters in HDL_2 have three possible fates: (1) They can be exchanged for triglyceride in VLDL, IDL, or chylomicron remnants in the circulation. As mentioned, the transfer is facilitated by CETP. These apo B–containing lipoproteins can be taken up by liver receptors. In the liver, some of the cholesterol is used for synthesis of bile acids, which are then excreted into the intestine and leave the body through the stool. This is the only route by which cholesterol leaves the body. (2) HDL_2 can be further enriched in cholesterol esters and acquire apo E to form HDL_1, which can then be taken up by the liver directly via the apo E receptor. This is not a major pathway in humans who have CETP. (3) HDL cholesterol esters can be taken up by steroid hormone–producing cells in the adrenals and the gonads, in a process facilitated by apo A-I.

Higher levels of HDL cholesterol are associated with decreased risk of atherosclerosis. Disorders associated with low HDL, including some forms of familial low HDL, are associated with premature atherosclerosis. Patients with Tangier's disease have an autosomal recessive disorder resulting in defective ABCA1. This results in defective efflux of cellular cholesterol to nascent HDL, rapid degradation of apo A-I, and low HDL cholesterol levels. Patients who are homozygous for the defective gene accumulate cholesterol esters in macrophages of the reticuloendothelial system and other tissues, including the arterial wall. Patients present with orange tonsils, corneal opacities, hepatosplenomegaly, neuropathy, and premature coronary artery disease.

Cholesterol can only be removed from the body by being delivered to the liver and being excreted as bile acids.

Hyperlipidemias

Hyperlipidemia refers to elevated levels of cholesterol *(hypercholesterolemia)*, triglyceride *(hypertriglyceridemia)*, or both. Hyperlipidemias are due to increased lipoprotein production, decreased clearance of lipoproteins, or a combination of both. The defect can be primary (genetic), secondary (due to diseases or drugs), or a combination of both. Hyperlipidemia is a major risk factor for atherosclerosis and pancreatitis.

Hyperlipidemia is a major risk factor for **pancreatitis,** as a result of high levels of triglyceride from chylomicrons and VLDL, and for **atherosclerosis,** due to high levels of cholesterol (and sometimes triglyceride) from apo B–containing lipoproteins.

CLASSIFICATION: PHENOTYPE VS. GENOTYPE

Hyperlipidemias can be characterized by their phenotype or genotype based on the type of lipid involved (cholesterol, triglyceride, or both). Several primary abnormalities are due to single gene mutations in LpL, apo C-II, apo E, apo B, or the LDL receptor, but primary hypercholesterolemia is usually polygenic in origin. The genes for common disorders such as combined familial hyperlipidemia and familial hypertriglyceridemia are unknown.

The lipoprotein phenotype is like a photograph. It represents the status of lipoprotein metabolism at a specific point in time and gives no information about the dynamics involved (overproduction, decreased clearance, or both). Phenotypes can, however, shift over time. For example, a patient with familial hypertriglyceridemia who develops poorly controlled diabetes could develop chylomicronemia syndrome (see Severe Hypertriglyceridemia) and then revert to modest hypertriglyceridemia when the diabetes is controlled. A genotype can be associated with more than one phenotype (see Familial Combined Hyperlipidemia), especially if a secondary cause is superimposed.

SCREENING

Since chylomicrons and apo B–containing lipoproteins increase the risk of pancreatitis and atherosclerosis, respectively, patients with coronary, peripheral vascular, or cerebrovascular disease and those with pancreatitis should be screened for hyperlipidemia. Patients with a family history of hyperlipidemia or premature (before the age of 55 years in men and 65 years in women) atherosclerosis should also be screened. Since hyperlipidemias are frequently associated with diabetes and renal failure, screening of patients with these diseases is recommended.

These physical findings should also prompt hyperlipidemia screening: xanthomas (cholesterol deposits in skin), xanthelasmas (cholesterol deposits in eyelids), corneal arcus (white ring around the iris) in a young person, lipemia retinalis (cream-colored cast to retinal blood vessels), and turbid fasting plasma (indicates hypertriglyceridemia). Central obesity is associated with insulin resistance, high VLDL, and low HDL. Xanthelasma is also seen in individuals who do not have hyperlipidemia. This is also true of corneal arcus, which is common in the elderly.

Because the prevalence of undesirable lipid levels is so high, and high lipid levels can be treated, the National Cholesterol Education Program III (NCEP-III) guidelines recommend a complete lipid profile every 5 years in everyone, starting at age 20.

Candidates for Hyperlipidemia Screening

Medical history

atherosclerosis (coronary, peripheral, cerebrovascular), pancreatitis, diabetes, renal failure

Family medical history

hyperlipidemia

atherosclerosis in men <age 55

atherosclerosis in women <age 65

Physical findings

xanthomas, xanthelasmas, corneal arcus before age 50, lipemia retinalis, central obesity, turbid fasting plasma

Everyone

at 5-year intervals starting at age 20

Isolated Hypercholesterolemia

Since LDL is the major carrier of cholesterol in the blood, isolated hypercholesterolemia is usually due to decreased clearance or overproduction of LDL. Primary (genetic) causes of decreased LDL clearance include genetic defects in LDL receptors and genetic defects in apo B that prevent interaction with LDL receptors. Secondary causes of decreased LDL clearance include hypothyroidism and a high saturated fat diet. Primary and secondary causes of isolated hypercholesterolemia can coexist. Isolated hypercholesterolemia from any cause is associated with an increased risk of atherosclerosis (Table 9-2).

DECREASED LDL CLEARANCE

Familial Hypercholesterolemia

Familial hypercholesterolemia is a monogenic, autosomal dominant disorder caused by a defect in the LDL receptor. Several defects have been described. The frequency in the United States and other Western populations is 1 in 500 individuals. Homozygotes (frequency 1 in 1 million) have extremely high cholesterol levels (600–1000 mg/dL or 15.5–25.9 mmol/L). Hypercholesterolemia is present in infancy and worsens with age. Severe atherosclerosis develops in childhood, and death usually occurs before the age of 30 years. Heterozygotes usually have cholesterol levels greater than 300 mg/dL or 7.8 mmol/L. They have signs of atherosclerosis by middle age: xanthomas (lipid masses or deposits) over tendons, especially over the Achilles tendon, tendons of the hands, and tendons on plantar surfaces; and xanthelasmas (lipid deposits around the eyes).

Table 9-2. Classification and Clinical Manifestations of Hyperlipidemia

LIPID ELEVATION	LIPOPROTEINS	PANCREATITIS	ATHEROSCLEROSIS	XANTHOMAS[a]
Cholesterol only	LDL	No	Yes	Tendinous Xanthelasmas
Triglyceride only	VLDL	No	Variable	No
Cholesterol and Triglyceride	LDL and VLDL	No	Yes	Xanthelasmas
Cholesterol = Triglyceride	Remnants[b]	No	Yes	Tuberoeruptive Palmar
Triglyceride >>> Cholesterol	Chylomicrons[c]	Yes	No	Eruptive
Triglyceride >> Cholesterol	VLDL and chylomicrons	Yes	Yes	Eruptive

Note. LDL = low-density lipoprotein; VLDL = very low-density lipoprotein
[a] Xanthomas are not always present.
[b] VLDL and chylomicron remnants
[c] Presents in childhood

Major Causes of Isolated Hypercholesterolemia
Decreased LDL clearance

Primary (genetic)
   defective LDL receptors (familial hypercholesterolemia)
   defective apo B
   polygenic causes
Secondary
   hypothyroidism
   high-fat diet

Increased VLDL leading to LDL overproduction

Primary (genetic)
   familial combined hyperlipidemia with increased
   cholesterol *only*
Secondary
   nephrotic syndrome
   glucocorticoids
   anabolic steroids

Familial Defective Apo B

This rare monogenic disorder occurs with a frequency of 1 in 500 to 1 in 1000 in white individuals with hypercholesterolemia. Patients present with the same phenotype as patients with familial hypercholesterolemia, including tendinous xanthomas. It can be differentiated from familial hypercholesterolemia by in vitro studies showing decreased LDL-binding in fibroblasts with normal LDL receptors or by a PCR-based assay of DNA isolated from blood cells.

Polygenic Causes of Hypercholesterolemia

These are more common than monogenic defects. The diagnosis can be made in families with hypercholesterolemia in more than 10% of first-degree relatives after other genetic disorders have been excluded. Patients do not have tendinous xanthomas.

Secondary Causes of Decreased LDL Clearance

Hypothyroidism and a high saturated-fat diet are associated with decreased expression of LDL receptors.

OVERPRODUCTION OF VLDL

LDL is not secreted directly by the liver but is the end product of VLDL metabolism. VLDL particles are better cleared by the liver LDL (B/E) receptor than are LDL particles because VLDL particles contain apo E, which has a higher affinity for the receptor than apo B. Therefore, over-production of VLDL can result in isolated hypercholesterolemia from high LDL, if VLDL particles are cleared effectively but LDL are not.

Familial Combined Hyperlipidemia

Familial combined hyperlipidemia, the most common primary hyper-lipidemia, is an autosomal dominant disorder that occurs with a gene frequency of 1 in 100 to 1 in 200 in the United States. Individuals with this disorder produce large numbers of small apo B–containing particles (Fig. 9-6). Family members can have high VLDL and LDL

CASE STUDY: CONTINUED

Because this woman had atherosclerosis at an early age (less than 65 years) and the physical examination revealed xanthelasmas, she was screened for hyperlipidemia. Her levels were high: total cholesterol, 287 mg/dL (desirable: ≤200 mg/dL) and triglycerides, 295 mg/dL (desirable: ≤150 mg/dL). She does not have isolated hypercholesterolemia.

Her history of cold intolerance and physical findings of an enlarged thyroid and slow reflexes are consistent with the presence of hypothyroidism. A low free thyroxine (FT_4) level and high thyroid-stimulating hormone (TSH) level confirmed the diagnosis of primary hypothyroidism.

A primary (genetic) basis for her hyperlipidemia is indicated by her family history of hyperlipidemia and the early onset of her atherosclerosis. She also has a secondary cause for decreased cholesterol clearance (hypothyroidism).

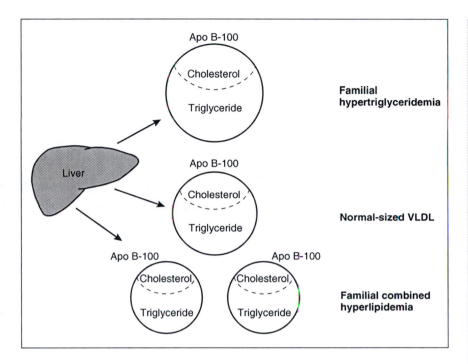

Fig. 9-6. Types of Hypertriglyceridemia

Note the large particle size but normal number of particles in familial hypertriglyceridemia. Note the small size and increased number of particles in familial combined hyperlipidemia. Apo = apolipoprotein; VLDL = very low-density lipoprotein. (*Source:* Adapted with permission from Chait A, Brunzell JD: Endocrine system syllabus, Seattle, WA: Washington University School of Medicine 1994, p 17.)

(combined hyperlipidemia with high triglycerides and high cholesterol) or high VLDL alone (high triglycerides only) or high LDL alone (high cholesterol only), depending on the efficiency of VLDL removal versus the efficiency of LDL removal. The diagnosis of familial combined hyperlipidemia cannot be made in patients who only have high VLDL or LDL, unless the lipid profiles of other family members are known. Patients with this disorder do not have xanthomas but might have xanthelasmas.

Secondary Causes of VLDL Overproduction

Diabetes, nephrotic syndrome, alcohol excess, and drugs such as glucocorticoids and anabolic steroids are associated with VLDL overproduction (see Diabetes, Renal Disease, Drugs).

Isolated Hypertriglyceridemia

Since VLDL is the major carrier of triglyceride in the fasting state, modest isolated fasting hypertriglyceridemia (triglyceride level ≥200–499 mg/) is mostly due to VLDL elevation. Increased VLDL production, decreased VLDL clearance (decreased lipolysis), or both are responsible. There are no xanthomas and no increased risk of pancreatitis associated with triglyceride levels less than 500 mg/dL. However, the combination of a primary (genetic) disorder and a super-imposed secondary disorder can result in severe triglyceride elevation, which changes the clinical picture. The risk for atherosclerosis depends on the cause of the hypertriglyceridemia (see Table 9-2).

Two genetic disorders can result in isolated modest hypertriglyceridemia: familial combined hyperlipidemia and familial hypertriglyceridemia (see Fig. 9-6).

Major Causes of Isolated Mild to Moderate Hypertriglyceridemia

Increased VLDL production, decreased catabolism, or both

Primary (genetic)
  familial hypertriglyceridemia
  familial combined hyperlipidemia

Secondary
  diabetes
  renal failure
  drugs: alcohol, glucocorticoids, estrogen, beta blockers, diuretics

---

OVERPRODUCTION OF VLDL

Familial Hypertriglyceridemia

In patients with this autosomal dominant disorder (gene frequency 1:500), the hypertriglyceridemia is due to production of a *normal number* of very large VLDL particles with extra triglyceride at the core. Since there is only one apo B per particle, no matter how large, apo B is not increased. These particles are poorly lipolyzed by LpL. They are too large to be taken up easily into blood vessels, so this disorder is not considered atherogenic unless patients also have low HDL levels.

Familial Combined Hyperlipidemia

This disorder is described in the section under Isolated Hypercholes-terolemia. Patients can develop isolated hypertriglyceridemia if VLDL particle clearance is less effective than LDL particle clearance. The triglyceride elevation is due to production of an *increased number* of small, dense apo B–containing VLDL particles and remnants that are easily taken up by blood vessels. This disorder is atherogenic.

SECONDARY CAUSES OF VLDL OVERPRODUCTION

Disorders that can lead to VLDL overproduction are common and should be ruled out in all patients with hypertriglyceridemia.

Diabetes

Insulin deficiency or insulin resistance results in activation of hormone-sensitive lipase, which increases lipolysis within adipose tissue. The excess free fatty acids are released into the circulation and are delivered to the liver, which incorporates them into triglyceride packaged in VLDL. Insulin deficiency or insulin resistance also impairs action of LpL, resulting in decreased clearance of VLDL from the circulation. Hypertriglyceridemia improves with better diabetes control.

Renal Disease

Nephrotic syndrome is associated with increased VLDL production. Impaired VLDL lipolysis by LpL and decreased clearance of VLDL and VLDL remnants can contribute to the hypertriglyceridemia. Renal failure of any cause is associated with defective clearance of VLDL and remnants.

Drugs

Alcohol is converted to acetate, which serves as a metabolic fuel, and oxidation of FFA is decreased; instead, the free fatty acids are converted to triglyceride and incorporated into VLDL. Increased glucocorticoids cause insulin resistance, which increases VLDL production. Estrogen increases VLDL production and VLDL clearance; if VLDL clearance is impaired, VLDL and triglyceride levels increase. Diuretics and beta blockers are also associated with increased triglyceride levels. The mechanisms are not clearly understood.

IMPAIRED CLEARANCE OF VLDL AND CHYLOMICRONS

Because VLDL and chylomicrons are cleared by a common pathway, any defect in clearance can result in accumulation of both. The problem is compounded if impaired clearance coexists with increased VLDL production or a high-fat diet, which increases chylomicron production.

SEVERE HYPERTRIGLYCERIDEMIA (CHYLOMICRONEMIA)

Chylomicronemia in Children

This is a rare autosomal recessive disorder (frequency <1:100,000) resulting in chylomicron accumulation due to absent or defective LpL or its cofactor apo C-II. Since chylomicrons contain mostly triglycerides, the triglyceride elevation is much, much greater than the cholesterol elevation. These patients have hypertriglyceridemia at birth, but this is often unrecognized until they present with abdominal pain due to pancreatitis. Eruptive xanthomas can occur on the trunk and the extremities (see Table 9-2). The retina blood vessels may have a creamy cast on fundoscopic examination due to the refraction of light by the high chylomicron content in the blood (lipemia retinalis). If the patient is eating a typical high-fat Western diet, the triglyceride level can be greater than 2000 mg/dL.

Chylomicronemia in Adults

This is a common disorder characterized by increased cholesterol and triglyceride levels as a result of both VLDL and chylomicron elevations. Occasionally, chylomicronemia occurs in patients who are homozygous for a genetic disorder causing hypertriglyceridemia. Most often, especially if the triglyceride level is over 1000 mg/dL, chylomicronemia syndrome is due to a combination of genetic and secondary causes, such as familial combined hyperlipidemia and diabetes. Diabetes is present in 50% of patients with adult chylomicronemia.

Patients can present with pancreatitis, eruptive orange xanthomas on the trunk and extremities, and lipemia retinalis. The underlying cause or causes of the hypertriglyceridemia determine whether or not the disorder is atherogenic (see Table 9-2).

Combined Cholesterol and Triglyceride Elevation

COMBINED CHOLESTEROL AND TRIGLYCERIDE ELEVATION WITH CHOLESTEROL PREDOMINANCE

This is a common hyperlipidemia that results from increased VLDL production leading to increased LDL production. The primary (genetic) cause is usually *familial combined hyperlipidemia*. Secondary causes of VLDL overproduction include diabetes, drugs, and and renal disease. VLDL and LDL clearance may also be decreased. There is no association with pancreatitis or xanthomas, but the risk for atherosclerosis is increased (see Table 9-2).

REMNANT DISEASE (FAMILIAL DYSBETALIPOPROTEINEMIA)

Remnant disease is a rare disorder resulting from an increased number of remnants of triglyceride-rich lipoproteins (VLDL and chylomicrons) in the circulation. The remnants are enriched in cholesterol, resulting in similar proportions of cholesterol and triglycerides. Levels of 300 to 400 mg/dL are typical. The remnants accumulate due to combined defects of overproduction and decreased clearance. Overproduction is due to either a genetic defect, like familial combined hyperlipidemia, or a secondary cause, such as diabetes. Decreased clearance is due to a genetic defect in apo E, the ligand that mediates binding to liver receptors for clearance. Patients with this disorder are usually homozygous for the apo E_2 isoform or carry an abnormal form of apo E.

Usually a secondary cause of remnant overproduction or decreased clearance is required to unmask this type of hyperlipidemia even in someone who is homozygous for the defective apo E-2. Patients with the disorder can have palmar or tuberoeruptive xanthomas. They are at increased risk for atherosclerosis but usually not for pancreatitis (see Table 9-2).

Diagnosis

The diagnosis of hyperlipidemia requires a fasting lipid profile. The period of fasting should be 12 to 14 hours. Chylomicrons formed after the last meal should be cleared after this time, if chylomicron disposal is normal.

The lipid profile includes plasma triglyceride, total cholesterol, and HDL cholesterol levels. With this information the LDL cholesterol level can be calculated using the Friedwald formula. The formula makes three assumptions: (1) the total cholesterol is the cholesterol present in VLDL, LDL, and HDL (no chylomicrons present); (2) most of the triglyceride is contained in the VLDL; and (3) the ratio of triglyceride to cholesterol in VLDL is approximately 5 to 1. The Friedwald formula used for LDL cholesterol (CH) calculation is as follows:

$$LDL_{CH} = total\ cholesterol - (VLDL_{CH} + HDL_{CH})$$
$$VLDL_{CH} = triglyceride \div 5$$

This LDL calculation includes IDL. If the triglyceride level is greater than 400 mg/dL, chylomicrons are present. The formula cannot be used because chylomicron cholesterol would also have to be taken into account. A plasma refrigeration test can then be done to verify the presence of chylomicrons. If plasma containing chylomicrons is refrigerated overnight, the light chylomicrons will float to the top and form a creamy layer.

In patients with a triglyceride level greater than 200 mg/dL, both cholesterol- and triglyceride-rich particles could be atherogenic if

---

CASE STUDY: *CONTINUED*

A full fasting lipid profile was ordered and the results revealed the following: total cholesterol 287 mg/dL, triglycerides 295 mg/dL, and HDL cholesterol 41 mg/dL.

Using the Friedwald formula, the VLDL level was calculated as $295 \div 5 = 59$ mg/dL (normal <30 mg/dL), and the LDL level as $287 - (59 + 41) = 187$ mg/dL. The LDL and VLDL cholesterol levels are both elevated, making it likely that the patient has an atherogenic disorder. Her non-HDL cholesterol was calculated as $287 - 41 = 246$ mg/dL (optimal ≤ 130 mg/dL). All the patient's values are abnormal.

To rule out other frequent causes of secondary hyperlipidemias (e.g., diabetes, renal disease, liver disease), fasting plasma glucose, creatinine, urinalysis, and liver function tests were obtained. Also, a detailed history of drugs that cause secondary hyperlipidemia (e.g., alcohol, diuretics, beta-blockers, estrogens, progesterone, androgens, corticosteroids, retinoic acid) was taken.

No other cause of secondary hyperlipidemia was found.

(1) the particles are remnants or (2) the triglyceride-containing VLDL particles are small, cholesterol enriched, and easily incorporated into blood vessel walls. In these patients, the NCEP-III guidelines recommend considering the level of non-HDL cholesterol, because total atherogenic cholesterol = all apo B–containing particles.

non-HDL cholesterol = total cholesterol − HDL cholesterol

A desirable value for non-HDL cholesterol is ≤130 mg/dL. Non-HDL cholesterol can be determined even in the nonfasting state and provides useful information about atherosclerosis risk. The level of atherosclerosis risk based upon LDL and non-HDL levels is shown in Table 9-3.

Another measurement of atherosclerosis risk is the total cholesterol/HDL ratio. A ratio of 4.5 or lower is desirable.

Desirable Plasma Lipid Levels

Total cholesterol ≤200 mg/dL (≤5.17 mmol/L)
Triglycerides ≤150 mg/dL (≤1.80 mmol/L)
LDL cholesterol ≤100 mg/dL (≤3.38 mmol/L)
non-HDL cholesterol ≤130 mg/dL (≤4.13 mmol/L)
HDL cholesterol ≥40 mg/dL (≥1.16 mmol/L) in men and ≥50 mg/dL (≥1.3 mmol) in women

---

Evaluation for Hyperlipidemia

Is hyperlipidemia present?
Which lipids and lipoproteins are elevated?
Is there a family history of hyperlipidemia (primary disorder)?
Is there a secondary cause?
Is this a combined primary and secondary hyperlipidemia?

Table 9-3. Atherosclerosis Risk Based on LDL and Non–HDL Cholesterol (mg/dL)

CATEGORY OF RISK	LDL	NON–HDL CHOLESTEROL*
Very high	≥190	≥220
High	≥160	≥190
Desirable (primary prevention)	<130	<160
Optimal (secondary prevention	<100	<130

Note. LDL = low-density lipoprotein; non–HDL cholesterol = non–high-density lipoprotein cholesterol
* non–HDL cholesterol = LDL + VLDL + remnants = total cholesterol − HDL

Goals of Treatment

Treatment of chylomicronemia decreases the risk of pancreatitis. Eruptive xanthomas resolve with lowering the triglyceride levels, and tuberous and tendinous xanthomas regress with decreasing cholesterol levels. Hyperlipidemia treatment can result in some regression of atherosclerotic lesions. Lowering plasma LDL has been shown in clinical trials to reduce the risk of fatal and nonfatal myocardial infarctions.

NCEP Guidelines

The NCEP has developed guidelines for the evaluation and treatment of patients at risk for coronary heart disease as a result of hyperlipidemia. *Primary prevention* refers to treatment of patients with no atherosclerosis. *Secondary prevention* refers to treatment of patients who have atherosclerosis.

PRIMARY PREVENTION

Since atherosclerosis is multifactorial, treatment goals for primary prevention are based on the number of atherosclerosis risk factors present in a given patient. The risk factors to be evaluated before deciding on a treatment plan are shown in Table 9-4. Diabetes counts as two risk factors, because in patients with diabetes atherosclerotic events occur earlier, are more severe, and are more likely to be fatal. High HDL >60 mg/dL is a negative risk factor which can be subtracted from the total number of risk factors.

If a patient has only one risk factor, in addition to high LDL, the risk of coronary heart disease in the next 10 years is low. Life-style changes can be instituted at any time, but the use of drugs to lower LDL is recommended if the LDL level is ≥190 mg/dL.

A patient with two or more risk factors in additions to high LDL, carries a higher risk for coronary heart disease (CHD) in the next 10 years, and a more rigorous treatment plan is suggested. The percent risk of CHD over the next 10 years can be calculated by allocating points for increasing age, total cholesterol, HDL, hypertension (treated or untreated), and smoking. Different scales have been derived for men

---

Table 9-4. Major Risk Factors for Development of Atherosclerosis (in addition to LDL cholesterol)

Male >45 years old Female >55 years old	Cigarette smoking	Low HDL (<40 mg/dL) Diabetes counts as 2 risk factors.
Family history of premature coronary heart disease in men <55 years old in women <65 years old	Hypertension (blood pressure >140/90 mm Hg) or treated hypertension	HDL >60 mg/dL is a negative risk factor.

Note. HDL = high-density lipoprotein

and women based on clinical data from the Framingham study (see NCEP guidelines *JAMA* 285: 2486–2497, 2001).

SECONDARY PREVENTION

If CHD or a CHD equivalent is present (abdominal, peripheral, cerebrovascular or carotid artery disease, or diabetes), the task is secondary prevention and the LDL cholesterol goal is ≤100 mg/dL. NCEP recommendations for initiation of lifestyle changes and drug treatment and goals of therapy are shown in Table 9-5.

LIFESTYLE CHANGES

Diet and exercise changes and smoking cessation improve lipoprotein levels. If patients are overweight, caloric intake should be adjusted to achieve ideal body weight. The NCEP-III guidelines recommend a diet containing approximately 15% of calories as protein and 25% to 35% as fat, consisting of <7% saturated fat, up to 20% monounsaturated fat, and 10% polyunsaturated fat. The rest of the calories should come primarily from complex, higher-fiber carbohydrates. Cholesterol intake should be less than 200 mg per day. Decreasing saturated fat intake results in up-regulation of the LDL receptors and increased clearance of apo B–containing lipoproteins. Decreasing total fat intake reduces production of atherogenic chylomicron remnants. Decreasing simple carbohydrate intake and increasing fiber or legumes reduces postprandial glucose and insulin levels and insulin resistance. Dietary stanols/sterols (2 g/day) and viscous fiber (10–25 g/d) help to lower LDL.

Table 9-5. NCEP Recommendations for Initiation of Treatment

CATEGORY OF RISK	LDL GOAL MG/DL (MMOL/L)	LDL LEVEL FOR LIFESTYLE CHANGES	LDL LEVEL FOR DRUG THERAPIES
CHD or CHD equivalent[a] (10-year risk of CHD ≥20%)	<100 (2.6)	≥100 (3.4)	≥130 (3.4)[b]
2+ risk factors and 10-year risk of CHD 10%–20%[c]	<130 (3.4)	≥130 (3.4)	≥130 (3.4)
2+ risk factors and 10-year risk of CHD <10%[c]	<130 (3.4)	≥130 (3.4)	≥160 (3.4)
0–1 risk factors	<160 (4.1)	≥160 (4.1)	≥190 (4.9)[d]

Note. CHD = coronary heart disease; LDL = low-density lipoprotein
[a] CHD equivalents = abdominal, peripheral vascular, cerebrovascular and carotid artery disease, diabetes, and multiple risk factors conferring a 10-year risk of a CHD event ≥20%, based on the Framingham study point scores.
[b] Optional level 100–129 mg/dL (2.6–3.3 mmol/L)
[c] Risk category where Framingham point scores are used to assess the percent risk of CHD over the next 10 years. See *JAMA* 285: 2486–2497, 2001, for calculation of point scores.
[d] Optional level 160–189 mg/dL (4.1–4.9 mmol/L)

Exercise is associated with increased LpL activity, increased uptake of fatty acids by muscle, and fewer triglyceride-rich apo B–containing lipoproteins. Twenty to 30 minutes of exercise 5 to 7 times per week is recommended, when feasible.

Smoking cessation is associated with an increase in HDL and a decrease in postprandial triglyceride-rich lipoprotein levels.

Drug Therapy for Hyperlipidemias

Drugs available for the treatment of hyperlipidemias and their complications are shown in Table 9-6. The drug chosen depends on the lipoprotein abnormality present.

HYPERCHOLESTEROLEMIA

HMG-CoA reductase inhibitors or "statins." These drugs inhibit the rate-limiting step in cholesterol synthesis. The decrease in intracellular cholesterol leads to an increase in the number of functional LDL (B/E) receptors on the liver cell surface and more efficient clearance of LDL (18%–55%) and, to a lesser extent, VLDL and VLDL remnants (7%–30%). Members of this drug family have been shown to decrease cardiovascular morbidity and mortality and total mortality, and to cause regression of atherosclerosis.

Table 9-6. Drugs Used to Treat Hyperlipidemia

DRUG	ACTION	INDICATION	CONCERNS
Niacin	Decreases VLDL production	Increased VLDL and LDL (increased triglycerides and cholesterol)	Increased blood glucose; increased liver enzymes and uric acid, flushing, and GI effects
Gemfibrozil	Increases VLDL and chylomicron clearance	Increased VLDL and chylomicrons (increased triglycerides)	Increased liver enzymes, rare myositis
Fish oil	Decreases VLDL production	Increased chylomicrons (increased truglycerides)	Rare bleeding if combined with anticoagulants or aspirin
HMG-CoA reductase inhibitors ("statins")*	Decrease cholesterol synthesis	Increased LDL (increased cholesterol)	Increased liver enzymes, rare myopathy
Bile acid sequestrants	Increase cholesterol loss from intestine	Increased LDL (increased cholesterol)	Malabsorption of other drugs, GI side effects
Ezetimibe	Inhibits cholesterol absorption from intestine	Increased LDL (increased cholesterol)	Increased liver enzymes

Note. VLDL = very low-density lipoprotein; LDL = low-density lipoprotein; GI = gastrointestinal; HMG-CoA = 3-hydroxy-3-methylglutaryl CoA
* fluvastatin, lovastatin, pravastatin, simvastatin, atorvastatin, ceruvastatin

Ezetimibe. Ezetimibe inhibits intestinal absorption of cholesterol and related plant sterols. Average reduction of LDL is 18% to 20%; triglyceride is reduced 7% to 11%; and HDL is increased by 1% to 5%. The combination of ezetimibe and a statin has a synergistic effect, resulting in LDL and triglyceride reductions of 51% and 29%, respectively, and increases of HDL up to 9%. This combination is associated with higher rates of elevations in liver function tests. The effect of ezetimibe administration on cardiovascular endpoints is not known.

Bile acid sequestrants. Colestipol and cholestyramine are resins that increase fecal loss of cholesterol by binding bile acids in the intestine. This results in an increase in hepatic bile acid synthesis with a corresponding decrease in liver cell cholesterol. This, in turn, increases LDL receptor expression, which leads to increased LDL clearance. LDL cholesterol decreases 15% to 30%. Triglycerides can increase, so these agents are not used for patients with hypertriglyceridemia. Bile acid sequestrants have been shown to decrease the risk of cardiovascular events, but not mortality. Gastrointestinal side effects limit patient acceptance.

Nicotinic acid (niacin). Nicotinic acid decreases release of fatty acids and decreases VLDL and, to a lesser degree, LDL production. Triglyceride levels are decreased by 20% to 50%, LDL is decreased by 5% to 20%, and HDL is increased by 10% to 20%. Nicotinic acid has been shown to decrease 10-year CHD mortality. Side effects are more common with the immediate release form. Absolute contraindications include severe gout, active peptic ulcer disease, and liver disease. Relative contraindications include poorly controlled diabetes, as nicotinic acid may increase plasma glucose.

Surgery and other treatments. In cases of severe hypercholesterolemia with intolerance or inadequate response drugs, ileal bypass surgery has been shown to decrease LDL by 25% and cause regression of atherosclerosis. Alternative therapies for patients with homozygous familial hypercholesterolemia include plasmapheresis and experimental therapies such as portacaval shunting, liver transplantation, and gene therapy.

HYPERTRIGLYCERIDEMIA

The desired plasma triglyceride level is ≤150 mg/dL. Levels between 150 and 199 mg/dL are considered borderline high; levels between 200 and 500 mg/dL are high; and levels >500 mg/dL are very high. It is very important to treat secondary causes of hypertriglyceridemia and address lifestyle factors. Drug treatment is indicated if hypertriglyceridemia is associated with increased risk for atherosclerosis, as in combined familial hyperlipidemia, diabetes, or the *metabolic syndrome* (a cluster of associated abnormalities including hypertriglyceridemia, low HDL, insulin resistance, abnormal fasting glucose, hypertension, and abdominal obesity).

Clinical Characteristics of the Metabolic Syndrome

Insulin resistance

Abdominal obesity (high waist circumference)
- men: >40 in or 102 cm
- women: >35 in or 88 cm

Hypertension

Hyperglycemia: fasting plasma glucose > 100 mg/dL

Triglycerides ≥150 mg/dL

Low HDL
- men: <40 mg/dL
- women: <50 mg/dL

In patients with the *chylomicronemia syndrome*, the risk for pancreatitis is low if triglycerides are reduced to <1000 mg/dL. In children who lack LpL or its cofactor apo C-II, primary treatment is the restriction of fat intake to 10% to 15% of calories. Drugs for treatment of hypertriglyceridemia include nicotinic acid (see above), fibrates, and fish oil.

Fibrates. Members of this drug family (fenofibrate and gemfibrozil) activate transcription factors associated with the alpha form of the peroxisome proliferator–activating receptor (PPARα) that increase LpL

CLINICAL CASE: *RESOLUTION*

This patient's cholesterol and triglyceride levels were elevated to a similar degree. A combination of increased VLDL and LDL is possible. This phenotype is seen in patients with familial combined hyperlipidemia. Given the positive family history of cholesterol elevation in her father and triglyceride elevation in her uncle, the diagnosis of familial combined hyperlipidemia is very likely. Another possibility is VLDL overproduction due to her familial combined hyperlipidemia coupled with apo E-2 homozygosity, which hampers remnant clearance (remnant disease). Special tests of her apo E isoforms and tests to measure remnants would be required make this diagnosis.

This patient should be treated for her hypothyroidism first. If her triglyceride (VLDL) levels remain elevated as a result of primary hyperlipidemia, nicotinic acid or a fibrate would be the first drugs of choice. If she continues to have elevated LDL cholesterol, treatment choices include an HMG-CoA reductase inhibitor, ezetimibe, or a bile acid sequestrant. Combinations of gemfibrozil or nicotinic and an HMG-CoA reductase inhibitor increase the risk for myopathy.

gene transcription and lipolysis. Fibrates also reduce VLDL production by inducing fatty acid oxidation. Triglyceride levels are decreased 20% to 50%; HDL levels are increased 10% to 20%. Gemfibrozil is effective for primary prevention of CHD in patients with increased LDL plus VLDL/remnants and for secondary prevention in patients with mild elevation of triglycerides and low HDL (dyslipidemia). A decrease in total mortality has not been shown. Fibrates are the drugs of choice for the chylomicronemia syndrome. Gemfibrozil use in patients with renal failure must be monitored closely. Fenofibrate lowers LDL, as well as VLDL/remnants, fibrinogen, and uric acid.

Fish oil. The omega-3 fatty acids in fish oil inhibit VLDL synthesis and decrease platelet aggregation. Patients with high triglyceride levels who cannot tolerate a fibrate may benefit from fish oil, 4 to 12 gm/day. Fish oil increases hyperglycemia in some patients with type 2 diabetes.

COMBINED CHOLESTEROL AND TRIGLYCERIDE ELEVATIONS

The first consideration is to reach the goal for LDL cholesterol. An HMG-CoA reductase inhibitor or nicotinic acid is usually the first choice for drug therapy. To achieve the non-HDL goal, a combination of drugs is usually necessary, but combinations of fibrates with statins or nicotinic acid must be used with caution because they increase the risk of liver and muscle damage. If used, lower doses of statins should be prescribed with close monitoring of liver enzymes. If myalgias occur, creatine kinase should be measured.

LOW HDL LEVELS

Effective treatment for low HDL is limited to addressing the factors that raise HDL, namely increasing exercise, when possible; smoking cessation; estrogen replacement in postmenopausal women, if not contraindicated; and treatment of high triglyceride levels. It is uncertain whether a small amount of alcohol should be recommended for patients with normal triglyceride levels. Nicotinic acid or gemfibrozil can be used for patients with CHD or CHD equivalents. All patients with low HDL should be treated vigorously to achieve LDL and non-HDL goals.

REVIEW QUESTIONS

Directions: For each of the following questions, choose the *one best* answer.

Questions 1 and 2

A 22-year-old student who had an asthma attack was treated with prednisone, a glucocorticosteroid, which was to be tapered over the next month. Ten days after starting the medication, she attended a health fair, where her cholesterol was tested and found to be above the optimal range. She was referred to her physician, who ordered a fasting lipid profile and found a total cholesterol of 255 mg/dL), triglyceride of 210 mg/dL, and HDL of 58 mg/dL. The physician consulted a lipid expert to interpret the results.

1 The lipid expert knows that this patient has

A isolated low-density lipoprotein (LDL) elevation
B combined LDL and very low-density lipoprotein (VLDL) elevation
C chylomicron elevation
D isolated VLDL elevation
E combined VLDL and chylomicron elevation

2 If asked whether this is a primary disorder that needs to be treated with lipid-lowering drugs, the lipid expert most likely would reply that

A it is a primary disorder that should be treated with drugs
B it is a secondary hyperlipidemia, and no drugs are necessary
C it is a combined primary and secondary hyperlipidemia, and no drugs are necessary
D it is not known whether this is a primary or secondary disorder, and no drugs are necessary
E it is not known whether this is a primary or secondary disorder, but drugs should be started

3 A 38-year-old obese man with severe coronary atherosclerosis goes to his physician for evaluation of his hyperlipidemia. He has no tendinous xanthomas or xanthelasmas. His blood glucose, urinalysis, liver, thyroid, and kidney function tests are normal. He is taking no medications other than nitroglycerin as needed. His father, who had high cholesterol and triglycerides, died at age 40 of a massive heart attack. His 45-year-old sister, who had normal cholesterol but high triglycerides, just had coronary bypass surgery. The patient's physician orders a fasting lipid profile, which reveals the following: total cholesterol, 338 mg/dL; triglycerides, 165 mg/dL; and HDL, 41 mg/dL. The most likely diagnosis for this patient is

A familial defective apo B
B familial combined hyperlipidemia
C familial hypertriglyceridemia
D familial dysbetalipoproteinemia (remnant disease)
E combined familial and secondary hyperlipidemia

4 A 5-year-old child is brought to the emergency room with severe abdominal pain after attending a birthday party where he ate a cheeseburger, French fries, and a milk shake. Physical examination reveals midepigastric and left upper quadrant tenderness and a vesicular rash on his buttocks and trunk. The diagnosis is pancreatitis.

Which of the following lipid disorders is this child most likely to have?

A familial hypercholesterolemia

B familial combined hyperlipidemia

C familial lipoprotein lipase deficiency

D familial defective apo B

E familial dysbetalipoproteinemia (remnant disease)

5 A 58-year-old computer analyst recently had a heart attack. His overnight refrigerated plasma had a creamy layer on top. His fasting lipid profile is as follows: total cholesterol, 289 mg/dL; triglycerides, 3325 mg/dL; HDL, 13 mg/dL; and fasting plasma glucose, 250 mg/dL (normal: 70–110 mg/dL). His lipid values can best be explained by

A LDL overproduction and decreased clearance by the liver

B normal VLDL synthesis but decreased lipolysis to LDL

C complete lipolysis and clearance of chylomicrons but not VLDL

D up-regulated LDL receptors and increased LDL clearance

E overproduction and decreased clearance of VLDL and chylomicrons

Questions 6 and 7

6 A healthy 29-year-old woman who is taking no medications asks her physician for a prescription for an oral contraceptive containing estrogen and a progestin. Her mother has hypertriglyceridemia but has not had any consequences. Her physician orders a lipid profile, although she is not fasting. Her total cholesterol is 198 mg/dL, and her HDL cholesterol is 32 mg/dL. Does she need a fasting lipid profile?

A her cholesterol level is good, so she does not need a fasting lipid profile

B a complete lipid profile should have been drawn originally, as she had not eaten for 6 hours

C she needs a fasting lipid profile because of her age and family history

D a fasting lipid level profile is not necessary because her mother has no symptoms

E a lipid profile is not needed because oral contraceptives have no effect on lipids

7 Some time later the patient returns for a fasting lipid profile, which reveals the following: total plasma cholesterol, 180 mg/dL; triglycerides, 355 mg/dL; and HDL cholesterol, 35 mg/dL. Her urinalysis, blood glucose, liver, thyroid, and kidney function tests are normal. The patient is most likely to have which of the following disorders?

A familial hypertriglyceridemia

B defective apo B

C familial dysbetalipoproteinemia

D secondary hypertriglyceridemia

E chylomicronemia syndrome

References

Brooks-Wilson A, Marcil M, Zhang, L-H, et al: Mutations in ABC1 in Tangier disease and familial high-density lipoprotein deficiency. *Nature Genetics* 22: 336–345, 1999.

Bucher HC, Griffith MS, Guyatt GH: Effect of HMGCoA reductase inhibitors on stroke. *Ann Int Med* 128: 89–95, 1998.

Dammerman M, Breslow JL: Genetic basis of lipoprotein disorders. *Circulation* 91: 505–512, 1995.

Fuentes F, Lopez-Miranda J, Sanchez E, et al: Mediterranean and low-fat diets improve endothelial function in hypercholesterolemic men. *Ann Intern Med* 134: 1115–1119, 2001.

Hill SA, McQueen MJ, et al: Reverse cholesterol transport—a review of the process and its clinical implications. *Clin Biochem* 30: 517–525, 1997.

Knopp RH: Drug treatment of lipid disorders. *N Engl J Med* 341: 498–511, 1999.

Kraus WE, Houmard JA, Duscha BD: The effects of the amount of exercise on plasma lipoproteins. *N Engl J Med* 347: 1483–1492, 2002.

Prosser MS, Stinnett AA, Goldman PA, et al: Cost-effectiveness of cholesterol-lowering therapies according to selected patient characteristics. *Ann Int Med* 132: 769–779, 2000.

The National Cholesterol Education Program (NECP) Expert Panel: Executive summary of the third report of the National Cholesterol Education Program (NECP) Expert Panel on detection, evaluation, and treatment of high blood cholesterol in adults (Adult Treatment Panel II). *JAMA* 285: 2486–2497, 2001.

10

Obesity

Charles P. Billington, M.D.

■ CHAPTER OUTLINE ■

■ LEARNING OBJECTIVES ■

At the completion of this chapter, the student will:
1. understand the definition of obesity.
2. understand potential causes of obesity.
3. be aware of the medical risks of obesity.
4. understand approaches to treatment for obesity.
5. understand the risks and benefits of treatment of obesity.

CASE STUDY: *INTRODUCTION*

A 35-year-old man came to the clinic because high blood pressure was detected at a health fair screening program. He felt well and had no complaints. The patient said that he weighed approximately 250 pounds when he played football 15 years ago and has gained weight gradually since that time. He stated that he does not eat excessively. He is employed as a restaurant manager and has been working regularly. His job is sedentary, and his leisure pursuits include television, computers, and talking with friends. His mother, father, and brother are also obese. His maternal grandparents had diabetes, and his mother has type 2 diabetes mellitus. On examination his blood pressure was 150/100 mm Hg, and his pulse was 82 beats/min. His height is 6′2″ and his weight is 320 lb. The remainder of his examination was unremarkable except for trace pedal edema bilaterally. Laboratory examination revealed a fasting plasma glucose of 115 mg/dL (normal: 70–100 mg/dL). An electrocardiogram (ECG) showed mild left ventricular hypertrophy.

Introduction

The recognition that obesity poses a risk to health and life dates back to Hippocrates. Concern is heightened now by the understanding that obesity is linked, through its very substantial contribution to the metabolic syndrome, to the development of diabetes mellitus, hypertension, hyperlipidemia, increased risk of heart disease, and other medical problems. Considering these risks, it is even more alarming that the prevalence of obesity is increasing rapidly throughout the world. In the United States there has been an explosion in the prevalence of obesity during the last 20 years. The most recent National Health and Nutrition Survey (NHANES) data indicate that over 30% of the U.S. population is now obese, and nearly 5% have extreme obesity. U.S. public health authorities have identified obesity as the most important public health problem.

DEFINITIONS

Obesity is defined as excess accumulation of body fat. In normal adult men 15% to 22% of the body is composed of fat; in healthy adult women 18% to 33% of the body is composed of fat. Technically, men with more than 22% body fat and women with more than 33% body fat are obese. However, since total body fat is difficult to measure, obesity is usually defined by a surrogate measure, most commonly the comparison of weight to height in the *body mass index* (BMI).

The BMI is now the standard method of reference for U.S. and international health measures. Since normal body weight is more proportional to height squared than to height, the BMI is calculated

Table 10-1. Obesity Defined by Body Mass Index (BMI)

	BMI (KG/M²)
Underweight	<18.5
Normal weight	18.5–24.9
Overweight	25–29.9
Obesity	30–39.9
Extreme obesity	40–

by dividing weight in kilograms by the height in meters squared (kg/m²). A close estimate of BMI can be made by dividing weight in pounds by height in inches squared, then multiplying the result by 704. The normal range for BMI is 18.5 to 24.9 kg/m². Individuals with BMI less than 18.5 kg/m² are considered underweight; individuals with a BMI between 25 and 29.9 kg/m² are considered overweight. Obesity is defined as a BMI of 30 to 39.9 kg/m², and extreme obesity is defined as a BMI greater than 40 kg/m² (Table 10-1). BMIs corresponding to a range of heights and weights are shown in Fig. 10-1.

Very muscular individuals can have an increased BMI without the expected increase in body fat. For these individuals a more technical measure of body fat estimation is required. This condition can usually be discerned by clinical observation.

Calculation of the Body Mass Index (BMI)

$$BMI = weight/height^2 = kg/m^2$$
$$BMI \simeq (pounds/inches^2) \times 704$$

The distribution of body fat is also important. *Upper body,* or *abdominal, obesity* is associated with more medical problems than lower body obesity. The most accurate measurements of upper body obesity are obtained with computed tomography (CT) scanning or magnetic resonance imaging (MRI) of the abdomen, but these methods are too expensive for routine use.

In clinical practice, upper body obesity is assessed by measuring waist circumference. The waist circumference is measured in upright posture at the level of the iliac crests with minimal respiration. Men are more likely to develop central obesity; women are more likely to develop lower body obesity. Thus, upper body obesity is also called android or apple (shape) obesity, while lower body obesity is also called gynoid, gluteal, or pear (shape) obesity. Women with a waist circumference >35 inches and men with a waist circumference >40 inches have central obesity.

BMI →	25	26	27	28	29	30	31	32	33	34	35	36	37	38	39	40
Height						Weight (in pounds)										
4'10"	119	124	129	134	138	143	148	153	158	162	167	172	177	181	186	191
4'11"	124	128	133	138	143	148	153	158	163	168	173	178	183	188	193	198
5'0"	128	133	138	143	148	153	158	164	169	174	179	184	189	194	199	204
5'1"	132	137	143	148	153	158	164	169	174	180	185	190	195	201	206	211
5'2"	136	142	147	153	158	164	169	175	180	186	191	196	202	207	213	218
5'3"	141	146	152	158	163	169	175	180	186	192	197	203	208	214	220	225
5'4"	145	151	157	163	169	174	180	186	192	198	203	209	215	221	227	233
5'5"	150	156	162	168	174	180	186	192	198	204	210	216	222	228	234	240
5'6"	155	161	167	173	179	185	192	198	204	210	216	223	229	235	241	247
5'7"	159	166	172	178	185	191	198	204	210	217	223	229	236	242	248	255
5'8"	164	171	177	184	190	198	203	210	217	223	230	236	243	249	256	263
5'9"	169	176	182	189	196	203	209	216	223	230	236	243	250	257	264	270
5'10"	174	181	188	195	202	209	216	223	230	236	243	250	257	264	271	278
5'11"	179	186	193	200	207	215	222	229	236	243	250	258	265	272	279	286
6'0"	184	191	199	206	213	221	228	235	242	250	258	265	272	280	287	294
6'1"	189	197	204	212	219	227	234	242	250	257	265	272	280	287	295	303
6'2"	194	202	210	218	225	233	241	249	256	264	272	280	288	295	303	311
6'3"	200	208	216	224	232	240	247	255	263	271	279	287	295	303	311	319
6'4"	205	213	221	230	238	246	254	262	271	279	287	295	303	312	320	328

Fig. 10-1. Body Mass Index (BMI) Calculated for a Range of Heights (Measured in Feet and Inches) and Weights (Measured in Pounds)

To determine the BMI for an individual, find that person's height in the left column. Find the weight closest to that person's weight along the row to the right. Go to the top of the column to find the closest BMI. For example, someone who is 5'6" tall and weighs 198 lb has a BMI of 32. Someone who is 6'0" tall and weighs 210 lb has a BMI of 28.5.

Central obesity (abdominal, apple, or android obesity) is defined as
- waist circumference >35 inches in women, and
- waist circumference >40 inches in men.

Central obesity is responsible for most of the increased medical risk.

MEDICAL RISKS

Obesity is a chronic disease that produces medical problems directly and indirectly by increasing risks for other serious conditions. Strong evidence indicates that excess body weight is associated with increased all-cause mortality in a continuous relationship. The slope of the relationship between BMI and mortality is less acute for overweight people but becomes steeper as BMI increases. Higher BMIs are associated with increased development of diabetes mellitus, coronary artery disease, and cancer. It is likely that reducing excess body weight will reduce the risk for these diseases, but more supporting evidence for the positive effect of weight loss is needed. Significant weight loss can ameliorate type 2 diabetes, and there is substantial evidence that loss of approximately 10% of body weight can improve risk factors for heart disease, including hyperglycemia, hypertension, and dyslipidemia. It is believed that prolonged weight reduction would improve health and decrease mortality.

Obesity increases the likelihood of developing a broad range of conditions, which are listed in Table 10-2. The cluster of closely associated disorders that make up the metabolic syndrome—hyperinsulinemia, hyperglycemia (impaired glucose tolerance or diabetes), hypertension, hypertriglyceridemia, and low HDL cholesterol—is closely associated with central obesity and with atherosclerotic vascular disease.

Although data indicate that the risks associated with obesity rise continuously with weights above "ideal," there is uncertainty about the point at which obesity becomes serious enough to warrant medical

Table 10-2. Conditions for Which Risk Is Increased by Obesity

All-cause mortality	Thromboembolic disease	Sleep apnea
Coronary heart disease	Osteoarthritis and gout	Restrictive lung disease
Stroke	Diabetes mellitus	Colorectal cancer
Sudden death	Hypercholesterolemia	Endometrial and breast cancer
Congestive heart failure	Low HDL cholesterol	
Hypertension	Gallstones	

Note. HDL = high density lipoprotein

intervention. One classification of obesity according to the level of risk for complications is shown in Table 10-3.

Causes of Obesity

Obesity results from excess caloric intake relative to energy expenditure. The scientific basis for this is not fully developed, but it is clear that human obesity results from interaction between genes, behavior, and environment.

Human obesity is a group of heterogeneous disorders resulting from interaction between genes, behavior, and the environment.

GENETIC FACTORS

Animal studies showing that obesity can be produced by a mutation in a single gene confirm that there are biological mechanisms regulating body weight and fat mass. The most compelling evidence for this comes from the identification of the protein hormone leptin, which is made in adipose tissue. Leptin is the product of the ob gene. Adipose tissue normally secretes leptin into the circulation, and blood levels of

Table 10-3. Obesity-Associated Risk of Complications Defined by Body Mass Index (BMI)

BMI (KG/M²)	WAIST CIRCUMFERENCE ≤35 INCHES (F) ≤40 INCHES (M)	WAIST CIRCUMFERENCE >35 INCHES (F) >40 INCHES (M)
25–29.9	Increased risk	High risk
30–34.9	High risk	Very high risk
35–39.9	Very high risk	Very high risk
40–	Extremely high risk	Extremely high risk

Note. Risk is increased when comorbid conditions are present (see Table 10-2). F = female; M = male.

leptin correlate with the total fat mass of the body. Neurons expressing leptin receptors are located in the arcuate nucleus of the hypothalamus. These leptin-sensitive neurons project to the paraventricular nucleus of the hypothalamus and to other brain sites and participate in brain information processing that regulates appetite, energy balance, and body weight.

In the ob/ob mouse, an animal with monogenic obesity, a mutation in the ob gene results in a defective form of leptin. The affected mouse overeats dramatically, has reduced metabolic energy expenditure, and gains considerable weight. If normal leptin is administered to the ob/ob mouse, food intake is suppressed, energy expenditure increases, and the animal loses weight. Obesity with a similar phenotype is seen in animals such as the fatty rat with a mutation in the leptin receptor. These animal models show that maintenance of a healthy weight depends on a critical leptin signal about the sufficiency of body fat stores.

Humans also need leptin. A very small number of people have been found with abnormal genes for leptin or leptin receptors. These people have serious obesity. Appetite and body weight decrease when these individuals are given exogenous leptin.

Both animal and human studies indicate a genetic component of obesity. Studies also indicate a genetic contribution to body fat distribution and metabolic rate.

The role of leptin in individuals with normal weight and most individuals with excess body weight is less clear. Leptin levels generally rise along with body weight and body fat content, and that relationship appears to be normal in most people who are obese. Under experimental conditions in animals, leptin inserted directly into the brain can reduce appetite and body weight, but there is little evidence that leptin usually functions to control appetite and body weight among animals or humans with normal or excess weight. It is possible that the high leptin levels in people with sufficient body fat indicate leptin resistance, but it is equally likely that leptin action is not important in individuals with enough fat. In obese people, central regulatory systems may be responding to other factors, and the leptin hormone signal is being overridden. Peripheral leptin administration to normal and overweight humans has not produced significant weight loss.

Monogenic causes of obesity are also found in humans and animals with abnormalities in the melanocortin signaling pathway from the arcuate nucleus to the paraventricular nucleus in the hypothalamus, which is described below. Other monogenic obesities have been identified only in experimental animals. These abnormal genes affect other brain mechanisms, adipose tissue differentiation and function, and intermediary metabolism.

In most humans, a complex, polygenic contribution of inheritance to obesity is likely. The proportion of the population affected by a polygenic sensitivity to obesity is still being established, but it is likely to be substantial. The techniques of population genetics allow an estimation of the number of contributing genes. These estimates range from as low as 10 to as high as 40.

The best evidence for a strong genetic influence on the development of human obesity comes from studies of twins, that is, monozygotic versus dizygotic twins and twins reared together versus twins reared apart. The studies of Stunkard and others indicate that between 33% and 60% of the variance in body weight is due to genetic influences. Recent work from Bouchard and colleagues has confirmed a familial predisposition to obesity and indicates that fat distribution (upper body vs. lower body) is genetically influenced. Studies suggest that metabolic rate is also partially genetically determined. Obesity is increased when those who are genetically predisposed to obesity express behavior associated with obesity, including increased food intake and decreased energy expenditure.

ENVIRONMENT

The prevalence of obesity in the U.S. population has experienced explosive growth in the last 25 years. The prevalence of obesity is also increasing rapidly worldwide. The very rapid accumulation of obesity is not consistent with genetic change. However, it is not clear which components of the environment are most important in producing the propensity for obesity. People in the United States have the highest per capita calorie consumption of any people on earth, and it is likely that growth in per-capita calorie consumption is an important contributor to obesity. It is also likely that reductions in physical labor and activity that have accompanied shifts in the work force and lifestyle contribute to obesity. For example, there is some evidence that obesity is related to increased time spent watching television and to reductions in physical activities in schools. Other possible environmental causes of obesity are listed in Table 10-4. These include food intake driven by hunger, desire for food created by advertising, and the increase in sedentary activities such as using computers. There is a strong inverse relationship between

Table 10-4. Probable Causes of Obesity

EXCESS FOOD INTAKE	REDUCED ENERGY EXPENDITURE
Genetic	Genetic
Abnormal neural regulation	Abnormal neural regulation
Learned behavior	Physical impairments and injuries
Social pressure	Automobile-based society
Wide availability of attractive foods	Sedentary occupations
Marketing of foods	Sedentary leisure activity
Boredom	
Depression	

socioeconomic status and prevalence of obesity in the United States. This contrasts sharply with the strong direct relationship between socioeconomic status and obesity in the developing world.

The issue of whether diet composition plays a role in the development of obesity has provoked considerable debate. Fat has greater energy density (9 kcal/gm) compared to protein or carbohydrate (4 kcal/gm), and it costs less energy to store ingested fat than to synthesize fat from ingested carbohydrate. Fat in the diet has been considered a problem, independent of any relationship to obesity, because saturated fat down-regulates low-density lipoprotein receptors and increases blood cholesterol. Individuals have reported reduced fat consumption over the last few decades, and yet obesity has increased. The validity of the self-reported data has been questioned because data from the food industry show no decline in per-capita fat consumption.

Dietary carbohydrate has also been proposed as a cause for obesity. Carbohydrate consumption provokes insulin release, which lowers blood glucose, thus provoking further consumption. However, strong evidence is lacking that insulin secretion provoked by meals drives additional eating. There are indications that carbohydrates can be behaviorally reinforcing, so individuals may be motivated to seek more carbohydrates after sufficient exposure.

Protein ingestion provokes insulin secretion, but protein also causes secretion of glucagon, which blunts the hypoglycemic effect of insulin. There is evidence in animals and humans that protein may produce more satiety than the same amount (on a weight basis) of carbohydrate or fat.

With respect to diet composition, definitive data regarding which macronutrient is the biggest contributor to obesity are not available. However, it is absolutely clear that the total caloric intake is determinant of body weight.

The most desirable macronutrient (fat, carbohydrate, and protein) content of the diet for prevention and treatment of obesity is not known, but it is absolutely clear that total caloric intake is a determinant of body weight.

ADIPOSE TISSUE HORMONES

The discovery of leptin reinforced the understanding that adipose tissue is not just a depot for triglyceride storage during feeding and release of fatty acids during fasting. As indicated above, adipose-tissue leptin secretion is correlated with the total amount of adipose tissue. Different fat stores produce leptin at varying rates, so it is likely that fat in some locations is more important with respect to leptin signaling than others.

Adiponectin is a polypeptide secreted by adipose tissue in substantial amounts. Plasma levels of adiponectin are reduced in obesity and associated conditions such as type 2 diabetes, and decreased adiponectin is correlated with increased insulin resistance. There is evidence linking reduced blood levels of adiponectin to inflammation and atherosclerosis. Weight loss increases plasma levels of adiponectin.

Adipose tissue also secretes tumor necrosis factor α, (TNFα). TNFα increases insulin resistance and may be a link between obesity and diabetes and heart disease. Other proteins secreted by fat tissue include adipsin, acylation-stimulating protein, angiotensinogen, and plasminogen activator inhibitor-1. The role of these adipose-derived signal molecules is still being defined, but secretion of these molecules is abnormally regulated when fat mass is abnormal.

Adipose tissue is a metabolically active tissue that secretes hormones such as *leptin* and adipocytokines such as *adiponectin*. Leptin levels are correlated with fat mass and are increased in obesity. Adiponectin levels are correlated with insulin sensitivity and are decreased in obesity.

Brain Centers

The brain is the target of many hormonal signals related to appetite and body weight (Fig. 10-2). Leptin is an indicator of fat mass. Another hormone, ghrelin, is secreted by cells in the stomach fundus. Under normal circumstances, plasma levels of ghrelin are high before meals and decline after meals. There are receptors for ghrelin in the hypothalamus, just as there are for leptin, and ghrelin action on the hypothalamus results in increased food intake. Evidence that ghrelin plays a role in obesity is inconsistent, but it is clear that ghrelin represents one source of information about food ingestion. Insulin receptors are

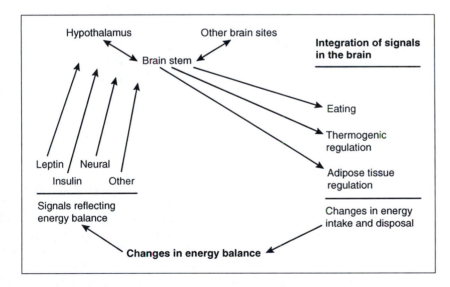

Fig. 10-2. Integration of Signals Thought to Regulate Feeding and Energy Metabolism

found in the brain. The role of insulin may be similar to that of leptin in that insulin levels are highest among those with the greatest amounts of fat.

The richest source of information about body energy status is provided by the nervous system, particularly by the vagus nerve. Information about the status of the stomach, intestine, and liver travels via the vagus nerve and is received first in the brainstem. Information being transmitted includes the stretch of the stomach, the activity of the intestine, and the energy state of hepatocytes. Finally, critical energy metabolism molecules such as glucose are sensed directly in a number of brain locations. Fatty acids and metabolism of fatty acids are also likely to be sensed by the brain at certain sites.

The hypothalamus is a particularly important structure in appetite and body weight regulation. Classic experiments showed that elements in the hypothalamus are associated with hunger and satiety. Damage to the ventromedial hypothalamus produced obesity, while damage to the lateral hypothalamus produced lack of hunger and starvation.

Recent studies have provided more information about regulation in the hypothalamus. Leptin receptors are expressed on two sets of neurons located in the arcuate nucleus of the hypothalamus (Fig. 10-3). One set

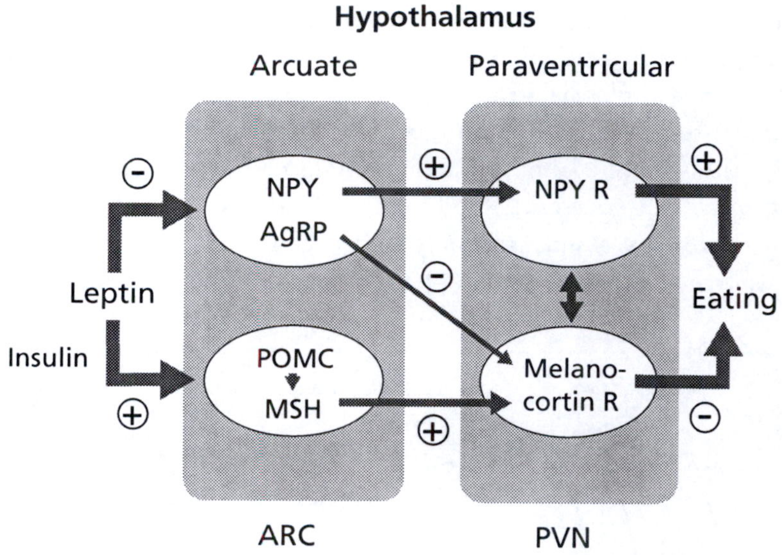

Fig. 10-3. Action of Leptin at the Hypothalmus

Leptin interaction with its receptors in the arcuate nucleus suppresses NPY-producing neurons and stimulates other neurons to increase MSH production from its precursor POMC. NPY interaction with its receptors in the paraventricular nucleus increases food intake. MSH interaction with the melanocortin receptor reduces food intake. This system is modified by agouti-related protein, an MSH antagonist produced by NPY neurons. The effects of insulin are similar to those of leptin. NPY = neuropeptide Y; R = receptor; AgRP = agouti-related protein; MSH = melanocyte-stimulating hormone; POMC = proopiomelanocortin; ARC = arcuate nucleus in the hypothalamus; PVN = paraventricular nucleus in the hypothalamus; + = stimulation; − = inhibition.

of neurons produces a hormone known as neuropeptide Y (NPY), which acts principally in the paraventricular nucleus of the hypothalamus to increase food intake. The other set of arcuate neurons produces melanocyte-stimulating hormone (MSH) from its precursor pro-opiomelanocortin (POMC). MSH acts at melanocortin receptors in the paraventricular nucleus to decrease food intake. Leptin normally suppresses NPY-producing neurons and stimulates MSH-producing neurons, and food intake is reduced. In the absence of leptin, the NPY system is activated, the MSH system is suppressed, and food intake increases. This coordinated regulation is amplified by an additional component, an MSH antagonist known as agouti-related protein (AgRP), which is produced by NPY neurons. Alterations in MSH, AgRP, and melanocortin receptors can produce obesity in animals and humans.

Leptin Action in the Hypothalamus

NPY stimulates food intake.

Leptin suppresses NPY secretion.

MSH reduces food intake.

Leptin stimulates MSH.

Net result: food intake decreases.

Other areas of the brain also receive information related to food intake from the environment. There is strong, consistent evidence that dopamine levels in the nucleus accumbens are responsive to rewarding stimuli, including food intake, and opioid levels in limbic structures are responsive to preferred foods. Thus, there are brain mechanisms underlying food choices. A substantial proportion of food intake may be related to the search for pleasure instead of basic provision of calories and nutrients. The habitual level of activity, choices to exercise, and resting metabolic rate are also partly responsive to neural mechanisms.

All of this information must be integrated by the brain to produce eating behavior, energy balance, and body weight. Complexity and overlapping functions tend to produce some overall stability, which is reflected in the periods of stable body weight that most people experience. Obesity results from the interaction of genetic and other physiologic mechanisms with the environment, and the brain is the most obvious point of intersection for these factors.

ENDOCRINE SYSTEM

Endocrine causes of obesity are unusual. Hyperthyroidism is associated with excessive catabolism and weight loss. The lost weight is regained when the hyperthyroidism is treated. However, the common perception that hypothyroidism causes obesity is not supported by evidence. Cushing syndrome results in central obesity, which resolves when

CASE STUDY: *CONTINUED*

This patient has a strong family history of obesity. He does little physical activity at home or at work. Although he denied eating excessively, his caloric intake must exceed his energy expenditure, as he gained weight steadily over the years. The combination of hypertension, obesity, and hyperglycemia in this patient suggests that he has the metabolic syndrome, which is closely associated with central obesity.

hypercortisolism is treated. Androgens promote central fat deposition, but androgens alter the distribution of body fat more than the content.

Increased carbohydrate intake results in increased insulin secretion. Insulin suppresses hormone-sensitive lipase and promotes uptake of free fatty acids into adipose tissue for fat synthesis. Injected insulin can also result in increased intake, which is probably due to hypoglycemia.

Endocrine causes of obesity are very rare. Cushing syndrome and certain hypothalamic injuries cause obesity. Hypothyroidism does not cause obesity.

Treatment of Obesity

Behavioral modifications, that is, permanent reduction in caloric intake and increased physical activity, remain the mainstays of therapy. These are very difficult to maintain, partly because behavior patterns are difficult to alter and partly because homeostatic mechanisms operate to sustain usual weight. Calorie reduction leading to weight loss is accompanied by a slight reduction in basal metabolic rate, which makes it more difficult to sustain the weight loss. Fortunately, weight loss of 5% to 10% improves glucose tolerance, hyperlipidemia, and hypertension, even if weight remains far above the "ideal" level.

Recommendations for Treatment of Obesity

Diet and **exercise** remain the cornerstones of obesity therapy.
Reduce calorie consumption by 500 to 1000 cal/day
Reduce saturated fat intake
Increase vegetable and fiber intake
Engage in at least 30 min/day of moderate activity (e.g., walking)

In general, lifestyle changes are recommended for patients in the overweight category with no comorbid conditions (Table 10-5). Even

Table 10-5. Matching Therapy to Risk

BMI (KG/M²)	COMORBIDITIES	TREATMENT
Greater than 25	Yes or No	Education about permanent lifestyle changes
Greater than 30	No	Education and behavior modification program
Greater than 30	Yes	Education and behavior modification program; consider drugs
Greater than 35	Yes or no	Drugs appropriate; seek other more aggressive intervention such as very low-calorie diet
Greater than 40	Yes	All of the above and consider surgery

simple changes like increasing walking or fidgeting and restricting television viewing can help by increasing energy expenditure and decreasing exposure to food-related advertising. More rigorous attempts at behavior modification are indicated for patients who are obese, depending on their willingness to engage in such behavior changes. Drug therapy can be added for patients with a BMI above 27 and a comorbid condition, but in general, medications should be reserved for those in the obese category with a BMI above 30, especially if they have a comorbid condition. Surgery may be appropriate for those with a BMI greater than 40 or those with a BMI greater than 35 and associated comorbidity. A combination of diet and exercise modification should continue even if additional therapy is required.

Very low-calorie diets (VLCDs) can be effective and safe under the supervision of a physician for the short-term management of severe obesity. Treatment with these diets for more than a few weeks at a time can rarely be justified, except at specialized centers. Most authorities believe that an adequate protein source is needed to ensure safety. Monitoring of fluid intake, muscle cramping, muscle strength, electrolytes, uric acid, and the Q-T interval on the ECG is recommended.

Choosing pharmacological intervention for obesity is a risk-benefit decision. Most of the drugs are associated with significant side effects.

The drugs used for the treatment of obesity can be associated with significant side effects. Therefore, drug treatment should be reserved for patients whose obesity is medically threatening. The difficulty lies in identifying when obesity represents a serious threat for an individual patient. Drug treatment for patients with no comorbid conditions can be considered if the BMI is at least 30 but is more likely to be considered if the BMI is greater than 35. The existence of comorbid conditions such as diabetes or sleep apnea that respond to weight loss may lower the threshold for treatment.

Notes

PHARMACOLOGIC TREATMENT

Pharmacologic management of obesity falls into three broad categories: (1) anorectic agents, which suppress appetite; (2) thermogenic agents, which increase metabolic rate, energy expenditure, or both; and (3) malabsorptive agents, which interfere with the absorption of food.

Pharmacologic Treatments of Obesity

Anorectics suppress appetite.

Thermogenics increase metabolic rate or energy expenditure.

Malabsorptives interfere with food absorption.

Anorectic Agents

Serotonergic Anorectics. Sibutramine has both serotonergic and noradrenergic stimulatory properties. The mechanism in each case is blockade of the presynaptic reuptake of the neurotransmitters serotonin and norepinephrine. The parts of the brain in which these drugs work are not clearly understood, but there is evidence in humans and in animals that serotonergic and noradrenergic stimulation enhances the sensation of satiety. Sibutramine has been shown to cause anorexia and weight loss in animal and human studies. There is also evidence in animals that sibutramine enhances energy expenditure and thermogenesis. In clinical trials lasting up to 1 year, sibutramine was associated with a sustained loss of 10% of body weight. In other human trials, sibutramine increased weight loss, which was maintained for up to 2 years. The Food and Drug Administration (FDA) has approved sibutramine for long-term treatment of human obesity.

The principal side effect of sibutramine is hypertension. Many patients experience only mild increases (a few mm Hg) in blood pressure, but a few patients experience more severe increases, which are unacceptable. Some patients have no increase in blood pressure, but sibutramine blunts the expected reduction in blood pressure with weight loss. Other side effects of sibutramine include somnolence, fatigue, abdominal discomfort, and diarrhea. Most patients regain whatever weight was lost if sibutramine is discontinued.

Sibutramine, an anorectic agent, can induce loss of as much as 10% of body weight. Side effects include hypertension, fatigue, diarrhea, and abdominal discomfort.

Other serotonergic agents, particularly those used for management of depression, occasionally have been associated with changes in appetite and weight loss. In general, these responses are feeble and not useful clinically.

Noradrenergic Anorectics. These agents act at norepinephrine synapses within the brain and produce greater satiety. Phentermine is the main example of this type of drug. This class of agent is related to earlier amphetamine anorectics. Amphetamines clearly produce a reduction in appetite and possibly an increase in energy expenditure. However, the true amphetamines are associated with unacceptable side effects such as drug dependence, and their use in obesity management is now either discouraged or illegal. The attenuated amphetamines currently available for this type of treatment, such as phentermine, do have some stimulatory effects, but there is little or no potential for abuse. There is short-term evidence for weight loss with phentermine, but evidence of long-term effectiveness is lacking. The FDA has approved phentermine only for short-term obesity therapy.

Other Approaches to Anorectic Therapy. There was great interest in the therapeutic potential of leptin, the protein hormone from adipose tissue that appears to signal the brain that there is enough (or too much) fat. Leptin decreases food intake and increases energy expenditure in animals. However, obese humans have high leptin levels, and studies of their sensitivity to pharmacologic doses of leptin have not been promising.

A variety of brain neurotransmitters stimulate or suppress feeding, and vigorous attempts are being made to exploit these pharmacologically. For example, attempts are being made to produce antagonists to neuropeptide Y, a brain neurotransmitter which is a major stimulator of food intake. The success of this approach has yet to be determined.

Thermogenic Agents

These agents enhance energy expenditure and thus promote weight loss without affecting appetite. Thyroid hormone in pharmacologic doses was used for this purpose in the 1960s. Treatment with thyroid hormone did produce weight loss, indicating the potential for this style of therapy, but the side effects were unacceptable. These side effects were those expected with hyperthyroidism: cardiac arrhythmias, high output heart failure, bone loss, muscle wasting, and mental disturbances.

The pharmaceutical industry is attempting to exploit a novel adrenergic receptor, the β-3 adrenergic receptor, to enhance thermogenesis. This β-3 receptor was found originally on brown adipose tissue in animals. Humans have β-3 responsiveness, but whether this occurs in brown adipose tissue is still uncertain. Agents that stimulate the β-3 receptor with minimal stimulation of classic adrenergic receptors do appear to be thermogenic in animal and human trials. It is not yet clear whether the enhanced thermogenesis will lead to long-term weight loss in humans, or whether these agents are sufficiently specific for the β-3 receptor that they will not stimulate β-1 and β-2 receptors and cause cardiac dysrhythmias.

The combination of caffeine or theobromine with ephedrine was noted to cause weight loss when it was used in Europe for management of asthma. Studies indicate that these drugs are thermogenic in humans, but evidence regarding effectiveness and safety of these agents for weight loss is lacking.

Malabsorptive Agents

These agents prevent ingested food from being absorbed into the body. Orlistat is the principal agent in this class. Orlistat produces partial malabsorption of fat (about 30% of ingested fat) by blocking the action of intestinal lipase. The major drawback for this approach is that the fat that is not absorbed in the small intestine is usually metabolized by bacteria in the large bowel, resulting in flatulence, diarrhea, and cramping. This drawback is also an advantage, since it reminds patients to restrict their intake of fat. The combination of induced malabsorption and facilitated behavior change produces weight loss. Human studies have documented the potential for loss of approximately 10% of body weight, with sustained effectiveness for up to 2 years. The FDA has approved orlistat for long-term management of obesity. The side effects of orlistat are directly related to the induced malabsorption. Patients taking orlistat long-term may have only marginal plasma levels of fat soluble vitamins and should receive oral vitamin supplements.

Orlistat is a malabsorptive agent that can induce loss of 10% of body weight. Side effects include flatulence, cramping, loose bowel movements, and diarrhea.

Acarbose inhibits α-glucosidase, the enzyme that degrades starch to glucose. Acarbose delays and partially blocks carbohydrate absorption in the small bowel, but the undigested starch is metabolized by bacteria in the large intestine, and some of these metabolites and their associated calories are absorbed. Acarbose is available but has not been shown to cause weight loss.

SURGICAL TREATMENT

Concerns about the safety of obesity surgery, significant costs and risks, and the feeling that artificial willpower is not the business of the physicians have limited acceptance of obesity surgery in the medical community. However, current evidence indicates that surgery is the best long-term method of ameliorating medically serious obesity until better medical therapies become available. Weight loss in the range of 100 pounds or more is possible by this approach.

Obesity surgery falls into three broad categories: (1) gastric restriction; (2) gastric bypass, which includes a partial duodenal bypass; and

(3) more aggressive malabsorptive procedures. Current evidence favors the gastric bypass as the approach indicated for most patients. In many cases this can be done by a laparoscopic approach. The role of more aggressive procedures has not been established.

Surgery is appropriate for selected patients with medically severe obesity.

REVIEW QUESTIONS

Directions: For each of the following questions, choose the *one best* answer.

1 Aggressive treatment of obesity is not completely effective and may have risks. Which of the obese patients listed below is the most likely candidate for aggressive treatment?

  A A 55-year-old woman with a body mass index (BMI) of 29 kg/m² who has tried many diets
  B A 32-year-old man with type 2 diabetes whose identical twin also has morbid obesity
  C A 60-year-old man with depression who has a waist circumference of 36 inches
  D A 40-year-old woman with heartburn who has a waist circumference of 31 inches

2 A 30-year-old woman complains of fatigue. On physical examination the physician notes the following: height 5'6", weight 210 lb, and blood pressure 140/95 mm Hg. In the course of the evaluation the physician remarks on the patient's weight. The patient states that she does not want to do anything about her weight. Which of the following facts would most strengthen the physician's case that she would benefit from weight reduction?

A She has a high leptin level
B She has a high adiponectin level
C Her waist circumference is 36 inches
D There is a family history of obesity

3 The attorney general asks a physician for help in evaluating the advertising of a local weight loss business. Based on current data, which of the following claims is likely to be true?

A The diet used by the weight loss program increases energy expenditure by suppressing the effects of seratonin
B The weight loss program is 85% successful in decreasing body weight by 50% and maintaining this weight loss for several years
C In this weight loss program, patients lose weight due to a combination of decreased caloric intake and exercise
D The weight loss program converts android (upper body) obesity into less threatening gynoid (lower body) obesity

4 A 58-year-old man with severe obesity has lost 20 lb with a combination of behavior modification and increased exercise. He has been unable to decrease his caloric intake further and cannot increase his exercise due to severe degenerative arthritis in his shoulders and knees. He asks his physician for a medication that will help him lose additional weight. Which of the following is correct?

A Sibutramine, an anorectic that suppresses seratonin and norepinephrine secretion, is associated with hypotension
B Phentermine is an attenuated amphetamine that acts at noradrenergic synapses and has high potential for abuse
C Thyroid hormone increases energy expenditure, reduces bone mass, lowers cardiac output, and increases muscle hypertrophy
D Orlistat, a pancreatic lipase inhibitor, is associated with malabsorption of fat soluble vitamins

5 A 49-year-old woman comes to her physician for help with weight loss. Her mother, two brothers, and a sister are also obese. Physical examination reveals a height of 5′4″, weight 192 lb, and a body mass index (BMI) of 33 kg/m². Waist circumference is 34 inches. Blood pressure is 145/95 mm Hg; heart rate is 64 beats/min. Her thyroid gland is difficult to palpate. The remainder of her examination is within normal limits. If her obesity has a genetic component, it is most likely to be due to

A polygenetic obesity
B a mutation in her leptin receptor
C deletion of her gene for neuropeptide Y (NPY)
D autoimmune hypothyroidism
E familial Cushing syndrome

References

Allison DH, Fontaine KR, Manson JE, et al: Annual deaths attributable to obesity in the United States. *JAMA* 282: 1530–1538, 1999.

Flegal KM, Carroll MD, Ogden CL, et al: Prevalence and trends in obesity among US adults, 1999–2000. *JAMA* 288: 1723–1727, 2002.

Lustig RH: The neuroendocrinology of obesity. *Endocrinol Metab Clin N Am* 30: 765–785, 2001.

National Institutes of Health: Clinical guidelines on the identification, evaluation, and treatment of overweight and obesity in adults: the evidence report. *Obes Res.* 6 Suppl 2: 51S–209S, 1998.

National Task Force on Prevention and Treatment of Obesity: Overweight, obesity and health risk. *Arch Int Med* 160: 898–904, 2000.

Ogden CL, Flegal KM, Carroll MD, et al: Prevalence and trends in overweight among US children and adolescents, 1999–2000. *JAMA* 288: 1728–1732, 2002.

Ukkola O, Santaniemi M: Adiponectin: a link between excess adiposity and associated comorbidities? *J Mol Med* 80: 696–702, 2002.

Wing RR, Hill JO: Successful weight loss maintenance. *Annu Rev Nutr* 21: 323–341, 2001.

Yanovski SZ, Yanovski JA: Drug therapy. Obesity. *N Engl J Med* 346: 591–602, 2002.

11

Endocrinology of Male Reproduction

Charles P. Billington, M.D.

▪ CHAPTER OUTLINE ▪

▪ LEARNING OBJECTIVES ▪

At the completion of this chapter, the student will:
1. be able to describe the physiological effects of androgens.
2. understand the components of the male hypothalamic-pituitary-gonadal axis.
3. be aware of defects affecting the male reproductive system at the chromosomal, hypothalamic, pituitary, gonadal, and peripheral levels.
4. be able to describe the clinical manifestations of defects at each level.
5. understand the evaluation and testing of defects at each level.
6. understand the rationale for medical treatments directed at each level.

CASE STUDY: *INTRODUCTION*

The patient is a 51-year-old man who presented with impotence. He reported approximately 10 years of nearly absent sexual function with a gradual decline in erection capability before that. He has been married for 25 years, and he and his wife have no children. Although working full time, he complained of muscular weakness and general fatigue. His history included an assortment of minor surgeries and a bout with mumps at age 21 while in the military. His examination was remarkable for markedly reduced pubic and other body hair, eunuchoid fat distribution (fat around the hips rather than around the abdomen), and very small testicles. Laboratory examination revealed a very low testosterone level and high luteinizing hormone (LH) and follicle-stimulating hormone (FSH) levels.

Androgen Functions

The principal effects produced by the male reproductive axis result from gonadal androgen production and action. The androgens are classic steroid hormones. They are synthesized primarily in the testes (adrenals contribute only a small fraction in men) and travel in the circulation mostly bound to carrier proteins. The major androgen produced by the testes is testosterone, which can be converted to the more active dihydrotestosterone (DHT) in target tissues and to estradiol in adipose tissue (Figure 11-1). Approximately 60% of the testosterone in the circulation is bound to sex hormone–binding globulin (SHBG) produced by the liver, and approximately 38% is bound to albumin. The remaining 2% is unbound. The free testosterone, plus some testosterone that dissociates from its binding proteins, can enter target cells and bind to the androgen receptor (AR) in the cytoplasm. The complex is translocated to the nucleus where interaction with DNA results in messenger RNA (mRNA) synthesis and, eventually, protein synthesis.

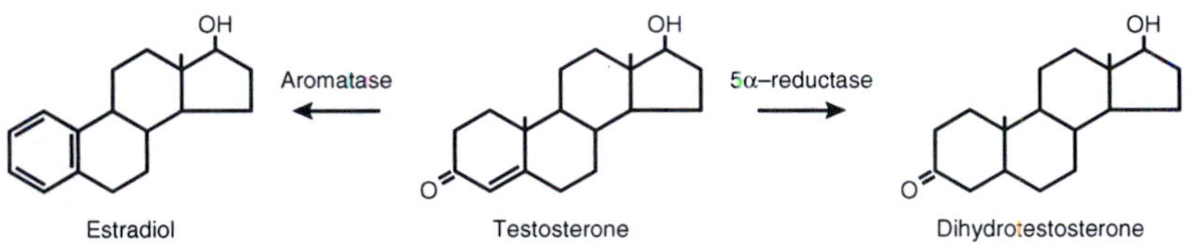

Fig. 11-1. Testosterone Can Be Converted to Dihydrotestosterone or Estradiol

Androgens Produce the Male Phenotype

Male genitalia
Male body hair pattern
Male fat pattern (central fat deposition)
More muscle
Deeper voice
Bigger bones
Acne
Male sexual behavior

At various points in development, androgens produce the male phenotype: male internal genitalia, penis, scrotum and descended testicles, male pattern body hair, male fat pattern (central or intra-abdominal fat deposition), increased muscle mass, vocal cord elongation and thickening, and increases in bone mass. Androgens appear to be largely responsible for the skin changes resulting in acne. In addition there are androgen effects on sexual behavior and on behavior in general.

Time Course of Androgen Effects

Fetus: development of internal and external genitalia
Puberty: maturation of genitalia, secondary sex characteristics, growth spurt, and epiphyseal closure
Adult: maintenance of libido, potency, fertility, strength, and bone mass

The critical function of the male gonadal system, from a species perspective, is the androgen contribution to fertility and conception. Testosterone from the testes is essential for maintaining the germinal structures in which the sperm develop and mature. Hypogonadal men typically experience fertility disorders.

Once androgenization has been produced, the phenotypic changes tend to persist even if androgen levels decrease later. However, prolonged hypoandrogenization reduces male pattern body hair, muscle mass, and fat pattern and may reduce the efficiency of erection, libido, and other sexual behaviors.

Hypothalamic-Pituitary-Gonadal Axis

The principal components of the male endocrine system—the hypothalamic-pituitary-gonadal (HPG) axis—are indicated in Fig. 11-2. Hormone released from the hypothalamus stimulates hormone output

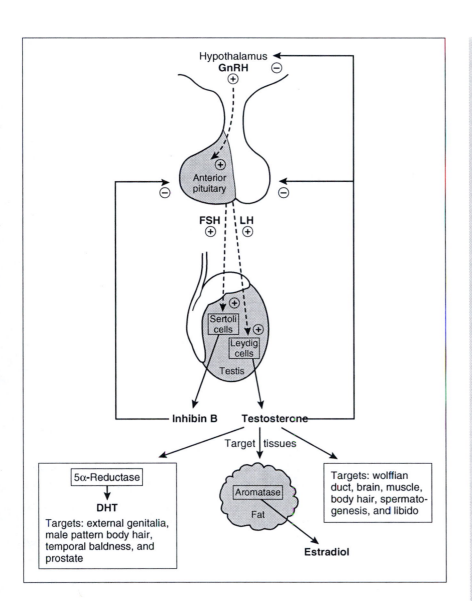

Fig. 11-2. Hypothalamic-Pituitary-Gonadal Axis in Men, Androgen Target Tissues, and Additional Metabolism of Testosterone

The pulsatile release of gonadotropin-releasing hormone (GnRH), follicle-stimulating hormone (FSH), and luteinizing hormone (LH) is represented by the dotted lines. Note that testosterone exerts negative feedback on the pituitary and hypothalamus. Inhibin B exerts negative feedback on the pituitary. DHT = dihydrotestosterone.

from the anterior pituitary gland. These hormones stimulate the testes to produce testosterone, smaller amounts of other androgens, and inhibin B, which elicit responses in their target tissues. Testosterone and inhibin B exert negative feedback on both the pituitary gland and the hypothalamus. Pituitary hormones and input from higher centers in the central nervous system (CNS) also exert feedback on the hypothalamus. Defects at each point in the pathway illustrate the operation of that component and its contribution to the overall HPG axis.

In the fetus and newborn infants the HPG axis is quite active, and testosterone levels can be close to adult levels. After 6 months of age the HPG axis becomes quiescent, even though GnRH is still present. At puberty GnRH pulses increase again, and LH and FSH pulses resume during sleep and then reach adult levels.

Levels of Testicular Failure (Hypogonadism)

Problem at the level of the testes—primary hypogonadism

Problem at the level of the pituitary—secondary hypogonadism

Problem at the level of the hypothalamus—tertiary hypogonadism

---

Hypothalamus

PHYSIOLOGY

Gonadotropin-releasing hormone (GnRH), also known as luteinizing hormone–releasing hormone (LHRH) is synthesized in the hypothalamus and is secreted into the hypothalamic-pituitary portal system. Within the hypothalamus, GnRH neurons develop in the olfactory placode and migrate by way of the olfactory bulb to their final destination, mostly in the paraventricular nucleus of the hypothalamus. Migration of GnRH cells and the olfactory epithelium is regulated by anosmin, the product of the KAL gene. GnRH neurons also receive modulatory input from other sites within the central nervous system. Negative feedback on the hypothalamus is provided by testosterone from the testes (Fig. 11-3).

Hypothalamic gonadotropin-releasing hormone must be secreted in pulses to be effective. Pulses are secreted every 90 to 120 minutes.

One feature of the HPG axis that deserves special mention is the intrinsic rhythmic activity of GnRH neurons, referred to as the hypothalamic pulse generator, which causes GnRH to be released into the hypothalamic-pituitary portal system in bursts. Pulsatile GnRH elicits pulsatile release of the gonadotropins LH and FSH from the anterior pituitary. Frequent sampling of GnRH from the pituitary portal system would reveal a pattern of serum concentrations like that shown in Fig. 11-4. Men lacking normal pulse frequency or amplitude may be hypogonadal or infertile.

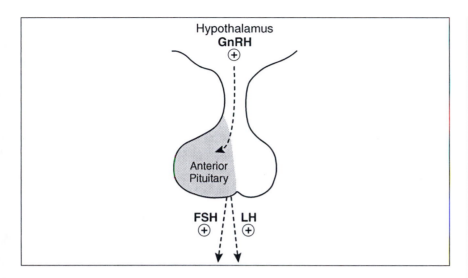

Fig. 11-3. Hypothalamic-Pituitary Level of the Hypothalamic-Pituitary-Gonadal Axis in Men

The pulsatile release of gonadotropin-releasing hormone (GnRH), follicle-stimulating hormone (FSH), and luteinizing hormone (LH) is represented by the *dotted lines*.

The HPG axis is functionally down-regulated during extreme conditions, such as starvation and severe illness. Input from the CNS is thought to mediate this response.

HYPOTHALAMIC DEFECTS

Congenital abnormalities of the hypothalamus, which can be autosomal recessive, autosomal dominant, or X-linked, result in absent or defective GnRH or in abnormal GnRH pulses. Deletions of the KAL

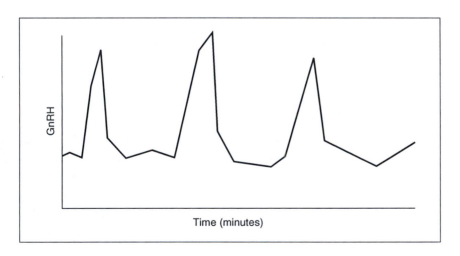

Fig. 11-4. Pattern of Pulsatile Release of Hypothalamic Gonadotropin-Releasing Hormone

gene result in X-linked Kallman syndrome, the combination of hypogonadotropic hypogonadism and an absent or defective sense of smell.

Acquired hypothalamic defects can be caused by tumors such as craniopharyngioma or metastatic tumors, injury from head trauma or radiation therapy, inflammation resulting from sarcoidosis, or infection such as tuberculosis. High levels of prolactin from any cause inhibit GnRH secretion. Severe illness and weight loss below the critical level needed to maintain the hypothalamic pulse generator also result in GnRH deficiency.

Major Causes of Hypothalamic Defects

Congenital abnormalities

Starvation or severe illness

Tumors (large pituitary tumors, craniopharyngioma, metastatic tumors)

Trauma

Inflammation (arteritis, sarcoidosis)

Infection

Radiation therapy

High prolactin

Manifestations of Hypothalamic Disorders

GnRH levels outside of the hypothalamic-pituitary portal system are too low to measure reliably. Defects at the hypothalamic level result in low or low-normal gonadotropin (LH and FSH) levels and low testosterone production. These "low-normal" gonadotropin values are inappropriately low, considering that testosterone levels are low. If the feedback response mechanisms were normal, FSH and LH levels would be high. The clinical consequences depend on whether the hypogonadism is complete or partial and the time of onset (prenatally, before puberty, or after puberty).

Defects at the hypothalamic level lower all hormones of the HPG axis.

Treatment Directed at the Hypothalamic Level

If it is not necessary to restore fertility, patients usually are treated with testosterone. Full treatment, which includes restoring fertility, in hypogonadal men involves administration of pulsatile GnRH by a pump. GnRH cannot be given orally because peptide hormones are digested in the gastrointestinal tract. Patients with inadequate GnRH pulses due to severe illness or weight loss respond to treatment of the underlying disease and to weight gain.

Administration of GnRH continuously produces down-regulation of GnRH receptors and LH and FSH secretion. This property has been

---

CASE STUDY: *CONTINUED*

The patient has obvious symptoms (muscle weakness, fatigue) and signs (impotence, reduced pubic and other body hair, female-type distribution of body fat, small testicles) of androgen deficiency. This was confirmed by his low level of testosterone. He has no features suggesting that his androgen deficiency is due to an abnormality at the level of the hypothalamus. He has no history of trauma or irradiation. There is no history of headache or fever to suggest an enlarging central tumor or a central inflammatory process. He had normal sexual function until sometime in his 30s, which makes a congenital syndrome like Kallman syndrome unlikely. The patient's elevated gonadotropin levels confirm his testicular failure and also indicate that the hypothalamus is functioning.

---

exploited clinically. Long-acting *GnRH agonists* are used to produce chemical castration in men with prostate cancer because prostate cancer is androgen dependent. GnRH agonists are also used to treat central precocious puberty (see Chapter 14).

GnRH antagonists have been developed for use in many of the same situations. The antagonists may lower gonadotropin levels more effectively than the long-acting agonists. A combination of a GnRH antagonist and testosterone has the potential of functioning as a male contraceptive. The GnRH antagonist turns off spermatogenesis, which requires FSH, while the testosterone component preserves libido and potency.

Pituitary

PHYSIOLOGY

The gonadotropins LH and FSH are released from anterior pituitary gonadotroph cells in response to pulsatile stimulation by GnRH (Fig. 11-3). LH and FSH are glycoproteins that share a common α-subunit but have unique β-subunits. Low-frequency GnRH pulses preferentially stimulate the FSH β-subunit gene; more frequent pulses or higher amplitude pulses stimulate the LH β-subunit gene. The GnRH receptor is one of the G-protein-linked hormone receptor family. LH has a shorter half-life than FSH, so plasma levels of FSH are more stable. LH and FSH are named for their actions on the ovary during the menstrual cycle. The structure of these hormones is the same in both sexes, and they function as tropic hormones for the gonads in both sexes. LH stimulates the Leydig cells of the testes to produce testosterone, and FSH stimulates the Sertoli cells of the testes to produce inhibin B. Negative feedback by testosterone suppresses LH secretion, and negative feedback by inhibin B suppresses FSH secretion. FSH β-subunit synthesis is also controlled by peptide hormones made within the pituitary such as activin, which antagonizes inhibin, and follistatin, which antagonizes activin.

PITUITARY DEFECTS

Pituitary cells secreting gonadotropins are very sensitive to damage, so FSH and LH secretion is often lost when normal pituitary tissue is compressed by a pituitary adenoma, a craniopharyngioma, or a metastatic tumor. Prolactin-producing pituitary tumors are particularly likely to interfere with the HPG axis because prolactin inhibits LH and FSH release by suppressing the hypothalamic GnRH pulse generator.

The pituitary is very susceptible to damage by chronic meningitis because it is located at the base of the brain. Tuberculosis and fungal infections also cause pituitary failure. Chronic inflammation due to arteritis or sarcoidosis, infiltrative disorders such as hemochromatosis, trauma from a basilar skull fracture, and radiation exposure when radiation treatment is given for other disorders are other causes of inadequate gonadotropin production.

Major Causes of Pituitary Defects

Tumors (pituitary adenoma, craniopharyngioma, metastatic tumors)

Trauma

Inflammation (arteritis, sarcoidosis)

Infection

Infiltration (hemochromatosis)

Infarction

Radiation therapy

It is very rare for a pituitary adenoma to oversecrete functional gonadotropins. Some adenomas secrete the α-subunit, which is common to both FSH and LH, but this is not active without the β-subunit.

Manifestations of Pituitary Disorders

Defects at the pituitary level result in secondary hypogonadism, with either low or inappropriately "normal" gonadotropin levels and low testosterone. As with hypothalamic lesions, clinical consequences depend on whether the hypogonadism is complete or partial and the time of onset (prenatally, before puberty, or after puberty). A prolactin level should be measured if a pituitary disorder is suspected. If pituitary damage is extensive, patients may also have symptoms and signs of hypothyroidism (see Chapter 3), adrenal insufficiency (see Chapter 5), or both as a result of a lack of TSH and ACTH.

Defects at the pituitary level lower FSH, LH, and testosterone concentrations.

> ### CASE STUDY: *CONTINUED*
>
> This patient's laboratory values were not consistent with an abnormality at the pituitary level. The pituitary gland should respond to lack of negative feedback from testosterone by increasing output of LH and FSH, and the patient's high gonadotropin levels indicate that his pituitary gland was responding normally.

Treatment Directed at the Pituitary Level

If fertility is not a concern, men with secondary hypogonadism can be treated with testosterone. Men who are seeking fertility can be treated with episodic injections of gonadotropins. The usual preparation used is human chorionic gonadotropin (HCG), a placental hormone with actions similar to those of LH. HCG may be augmented with human menopausal gonadotropin (HMG), a mixture of LH and FSH.

Testicles

PHYSIOLOGY

In the testes, LH stimulates Leydig cells to produce testosterone. FSH stimulates Sertoli cells to produce androgen-binding protein, which binds testosterone from the Leydig cells within the seminiferous tubules. FSH also stimulates inhibin B secretion from Sertoli cells. Inhibin B in turn regulates FSH synthesis by negative feedback (Fig. 11-5). Both FSH and high local concentrations of testosterone are

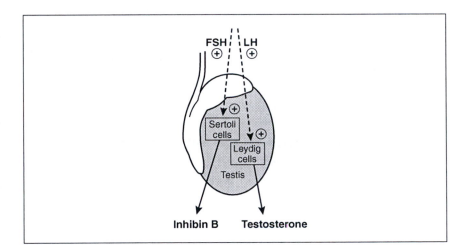

Fig. 11-5. Action of Pituitary Gonadotropins on Target Cells Within the Testes

The pulsatile release of follicle-stimulating hormone (FSH) and luteinizing hormone (LH) is represented by the *dotted lines*.

necessary for spermatogenesis and fertility, but libido and sexual performance respond only to testosterone. The mass of Leydig cells is small. Most of the testicular volume is made up of seminiferous tubules, which contain the maturing sperm, germinal epithelium, and the Sertoli cells. Small testes generally indicate a deficiency in these elements.

TESTICULAR DEFECTS

Developmental disorders such as Klinefelter syndrome, the result of nondisjunction during meiosis leading to a 47,XXY male (see Chapters 13 and 14), other types of gonadal dysgenesis, cryptorchidism (testes fail to descend into the scrotum), gonadotropin resistance due to abnormal LH receptors or Leydig cell failure, enzymatic defects of testosterone synthesis, and myotonic dystrophy all result in primary hypogonadism.

Acquired testicular disorders cause primary hypogonadism by several mechanisms. Testicular tumors can damage testicles directly. Hypogonadism can also occur as a result of chemotherapy or radiation treatment. Testicles are more susceptible to trauma than many organs because of their exposed location. Testicular torsion results in twisting of the artery supplying the testicle. Some viral infections, especially mumps in a postpubescent man, and bacterial infections can produce orchitis (inflammation of the testes) severe enough to produce hypogonadism. Orchitis can also be caused by autoimmune disease. Hypogonadism associated with an episode of orchitis may not become manifest until years later.

In the absence of illness or testicular trauma, men do not have an abrupt decline in Leydig cell function with age, equivalent to menopause in women. In healthy men testosterone levels decline slowly with age, and free testosterone levels may fall by 40%. Levels often remain within the normal range. However, this range is very broad, and lower values in this range may not be normal for young, healthy men or optimal for older men. Men whose aging changes are more severe can develop hypogonadism.

Major Causes of Testicular Defects

Developmental disorders
Tumors
Chemotherapy
Radiation therapy
Orchitis (infection, autoimmunity)

Manifestations of Testicular Disease

Testicular defects result in low testosterone levels. LH and FSH levels are high because the pituitary is no longer suppressed by negative feedback. As with hypothalamic and pituitary disorders, symptoms and signs depend on the degree of androgen deficiency.

Testicular defects result in low testosterone with high TSH and LH levels.

If congenital disorders are partial or worsen slowly, early development can be normal. Men with Klinefelter syndrome develop normally until after puberty when the testes fail. The increase in LH and FSH cannot elicit adequate Leydig cell testosterone synthesis or seminiferous tubule and germ cell development (see Chapters 13 and 14), and LH and FSH remain high. The testes remain small and become fibrotic. Body hair and external genitalia mature to varying degrees. Since the phenotype is so variable, a karyotype is required to confirm the diagnosis. Gynecomastia (increased breast tissue), impotence, and infertility are common complaints. Men who go untreated develop osteopenia because they produce too little testosterone to maintain bone mass.

In men whose aging changes are severe enough to produce hypogonadism, testosterone levels are low or low-normal. LH levels can be high but often remain within the normal range, possibly at somewhat higher than previous levels.

Treatment of Gonadal Disorders

Most men with testicular failure are treated with testosterone. Testosterone replacement can restore libido and sexual function, increase muscle mass, reduce fatigue, and maintain bone mass. Testosterone contributes to the pubertal growth spurt in boys but also causes closure of the epiphyses. Therefore, boys who develop gonadal failure before puberty are usually not treated with testosterone until they are around 13 years old to avoid premature epiphyseal closure resulting in short stature.

CASE STUDY: *CONTINUED*

The patient most likely has a testicular abnormality. His testosterone level was low, and his gonadotropin levels high, indicating an unsuccessful attempt by the hypothalamic-pituitary system to correct his hypogonadism. This patient's hypogonadism was most likely due to orchitis caused by his mumps infection many years before. He might also have Klinefelter syndrome or another form of gonadal dysgenesis. In some cases, adolescent males with Klinefelter syndrome have normal pubertal development with testicular failure manifested later. A karyotype would be necessary to confirm this diagnosis.

Androgen therapy is contraindicated in some men with prostate hyperplasia and in men with prostate cancer. Androgen replacement therapy does not cause prostate cancer but stimulates growth of hormone-sensitive cancers already present.

Androgen Target Tissues

PHYSIOLOGY

Two types of androgen target tissues exist—those that respond primarily to testosterone and those that require 5α-reductase action to convert testosterone to DHT for normal androgen action. Examples of these two types of tissues are shown in Fig. 11-6. Testosterone and DHT bind to the same androgen receptor. DHT has much greater affinity for the androgen receptor than does testosterone, so tissues possessing an active 5α-reductase system show greater androgen effect.

Testosterone vs. Dihydrotestosterone (DHT)

Both bind to the same androgen receptor.

Testosterone is required for development of internal genitalia (epididymis, vas deferens, seminal vesicles).

DHT has greater receptor affinity and more androgen effect.

DHT is required for development of external genitalia (penis, scrotum, prostate).

Androgens such as testosterone can also be converted to estrogen. This requires the enzyme aromatase, which is found in adipose tissue. Much of the estrogen found in men is thought to be derived from this pathway. Estrogens can exert negative feedback on the hypothalamus and pituitary.

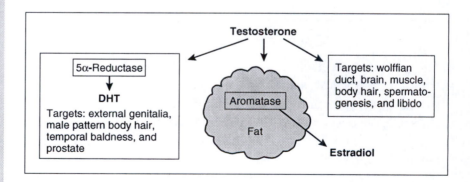

Fig. 11-6. Testosterone Action

Note the enzymatic conversion of testosterone to dihydrotestosterone (DHT) and estrogen.

Fates of Testosterone in Target Tissues

Interacts directly with androgen receptor

Converted to DHT (requires 5a-reductase)

Converted to estradiol (requires aromatase)

ANDROGEN TARGET TISSUE DEFECTS

The most dramatic target tissue disorders result from gene mutations that reduce androgen-receptor function or reduce the efficiency of 5α-reductase so that conversion of testosterone to the more potent androgen DHT is decreased.

Excess conversion of testosterone to estrogen by aromatase in men with excess adipose tissue is the most common target tissue abnormality. Although their testosterone levels remain much higher than their estrogen levels, these men show extra estrogen effects because the ratio of estrogen to androgen is increased above the normal range.

Gene mutations resulting in loss of aromatase (loss of estrogen synthesis) or nonfunctional estrogen receptors (loss of estrogen action) were thought in the past always to be lethal. A man with a mutation in the estrogen receptor gene, who was totally resistant to estrogen, was described in 1994. His estrogen levels were high, but he was not able to respond to endogenous or exogenous estrogen. A man without functional aromatase was identified in 1995. His plasma estrogen levels were very low, but he responded to exogenous estrogen because his estrogen receptors were normal.

Androgen Target Tissue Disorders

Androgen receptor deficiency

5α-reductase deficiency

Gynecomastia

Aromatase deficiency

Estrogen receptor deficiency

Manifestations of Target Tissue Defects

Clinical manifestations of abnormal androgen action can be dramatic. Men with a severe deficit or defect in androgen receptors are phenotypic females, and the disorder is called "testicular feminization." They have high gonadotropin levels because the abnormal receptors in the pituitary cannot recognize testosterone feedback. Testosterone levels are high because the testes respond appropriately to high gonadotropin levels. Estrogen levels are high because the excess testosterone is converted to estrogen by aromatase in adipose tissue. This leads to breast development. These men have female external genitalia, a vagina ending in a blind pouch, and no internal genitalia except testes. They have sparse body hair because development of body hair depends on androgen action. Milder defects result in an androgynous phenotype (see Chapters 13 and 14).

A child with 5α-reductase deficiency appears female or has ambiguous external genitalia at birth. A blind vaginal pouch is present. LH, FSH, and testosterone levels are near normal, and the internal genitalia develop normally. DHT levels are low so masculinization of the external genitalia is incomplete. At puberty the level of testosterone rises dramatically. Secondary male sex characteristics develop, and the external genitalia become masculinized (see Chapters 13 and 14). The ratio of DHT to testosterone remains abnormally low. Affected individuals do not have acne or male pattern balding, and body hair is reduced. In areas where this genetic defect is common, a change from female to male gender identity at the time of puberty is accepted surprisingly well.

Gynecomastia is common in men of all ages, especially during puberty (see Chapter 14) and in men who are obese. True gynecomastia refers to the presence of firm ductal tissue under the areola; gynecomastia does not refer to fat in the breast area. Benign gynecomastia can be unilateral. LH, FSH, and testosterone levels in most men with gynecomastia are normal. Their estrogen levels are within the normal range but are thought to be increased relative to testosterone levels. The abnormality may be subtle.

Hypogonadal men who have low testosterone levels also have relatively increased estrogen levels, especially if they are obese. These men often have gynecomastia. Other causes of gynecomastia include drugs such as cimetidine, spironolactone, and flutamide, which are androgen-receptor blockers; hyperprolactinemia, which suppresses the hypothalamic pulse generator and decreases LH and testosterone production; and some systemic diseases. Testicular tumors and feminizing adrenal tumors can cause gynecomastia, but these are rare.

The men described above with the aromatase and estrogen receptor mutations have normal adult male sexual development. They have normal or high testosterone levels, and yet their FSH and LH levels are high. This indicates that estrogen action is necessary for normal feedback inhibition of pituitary gonadotrophs in men. The young men with these conditions are very tall, with unfused epiphyses, low bone density, and high bone turnover characteristic of osteoporosis. Estrogen apparently is necessary for normal bone maturation in men as well as in women.

Treatment of Target Tissue Defects

Defects in 5 α-reductase activity usually produce their effects in utero. Full treatment would require prenatal diagnosis and a fetal DHT delivery system (or gene therapy), which is not available. Treatment depends on the degree of virilization (see Chapter 14).

There is no therapy that restores androgen receptors. In individuals with testicular feminization, the phenotype and gender assignment are female. The testes must be removed because malignancy is likely to arise in intra-abdominal testes. Estrogen treatment is given so that secondary sexual characteristics develop.

Gynecomastia is usually asymptomatic and benign and needs no treatment except stopping the causative agent, if possible. Weight loss may help, since estrogen is produced from androgens in adipose tissue. Testosterone-deficient men are treated with testosterone. If gynecomastia is painful, unilateral, and not centrally located under the nipple, or develops rapidly, a mammogram should be obtained to rule out malignancy.

Pharmacologic Treatment: Androgens and Antiandrogens

TESTOSTERONE REPLACEMENT THERAPY

Testosterone cannot be given orally because it is degraded quickly as it passes through the liver. When given orally, 17α-alkylated testosterone derivatives are active but cause liver toxicity. Less water soluble 17β-testosterone esters such as testosterone enanthate and testosterone cypionate have a much longer duration of action. These testosterone esters can be given intramuscularly at 2 to 3 week intervals. This often results in peak plasma levels above the normal range initially and trough levels below the normal range later.

Testosterone can be delivered more uniformly in transdermal patches, although skin reactions to these patches can be a problem; in gels that are applied to the skin; and in capsules that adhere to the buccal mucosa. Testosterone pellets, which are planted subcutaneously, provide normal testosterone, DHT, and estradiol levels for several months. They are rarely used in the United States because of the need for implantation and because pellets can be extruded spontaneously.

Testosterone causes increased growth of body hair and can cause acne and fluid retention resulting in leg edema. Whether testosterone replacement causes a significant lowering of HDL cholesterol in hypogonadal men is not known.

The prostate must be monitored in men given testosterone replacement therapy. A hemoglobin level should be monitored, especially in men likely to have hypoxemia (smokers and men with chronic obstructive lung disease or sleep apnea) because testosterone also stimulates synthesis of erythropoietin.

ANABOLIC USES OF ANDROGENS

Androgens cause nitrogen retention, increase protein synthesis, increase muscle mass, and stabilize bone mass in hypogonadal men. It is not clear whether androgens, alone or in combination with another anabolic hormone such as growth hormone, would benefit men with muscle wasting or bone loss due to underlying diseases or aging.

Androgens are used by athletes who are not hypogonadal, with the hope of increasing their muscle mass and strength to supranormal levels. These men usually use some form of testosterone or a testosterone derivative. In most cases the doses used are several orders of magnitude higher than replacement doses of testosterone. The high doses suppress the hypothalamus and pituitary, which can lead to a low sperm count or testicular atrophy or both. Liver diseases, including tumors, have been reported in association with this abuse.

ANTIANDROGEN THERAPY

In some clinical situations the goal is to block androgen action at the target tissue level with antiandrogen therapy. Flutamide is an androgen receptor blocker that is used in the treatment of prostate cancer. Cyproterone acetate, another androgen receptor inhibitor, is not available in the United States. Finasteride, an inhibitor of 5α-reductase, is used for treatment of prostate cancer and prostatic hypertrophy. Finasteride inhibits DHT production but does not affect LH or testosterone levels.

Androgen Blockade

Androgen receptor blockers

5-α reductase blockers

TREATMENT OF IMPOTENCE

Penile erection depends on adequate arterial dilatation for blood flow into the corpora cavernosa. This is affected by neurologic, vascular and hormonal disorders and systemic illness. Impotent men should be tested for testosterone deficiency, although most impotent men are not hypogonadal, and not all hypogonadal men are impotent. Impotence due to hypogonadism can be treated with testosterone. Men who are not hypogonadal should be tested for thyroid disorders, hyperprolactinemia, and diabetes.

Drugs contributing to impotence should be stopped, if possible. These include alcohol, opiates, estrogens, anti-androgens, spironolactone (inhibits androgen binding to the androgen receptor), and antidepressants, including selective seratonin reuptake inhibitors [SSRIs]. Antihypertensive drugs reduce blood pressure in patients who already have compromised blood flow. Smoking also contributes to importence.

Neurologic or vascular disorders that impair blood flow to the penis can be treated with vasoactive drugs. Nitric oxide (NO) activates guanylate cyclase, resulting in more cyclic guanosine monophosphate (cGMP), which produces smooth muscle relaxation in the corpora cavernosa and inflow of blood. Sildenafil and related drugs increase NO by inhibiting phosphodiesterase type 5, the enzyme that degrades cGMP. Alprostadil (prostaglandin E_1) relaxes trabecular smooth muscle and dilates cavernosal arteries when introduced into the urethra or injected into the cavernosa. Other treatments include vacuum devices that produce engorgement of the penis by reducing the surrounding pressure and surgically implanted penile prostheses.

REVIEW QUESTIONS

Directions: For each of the following questions, choose the *one best* answer.

1 A 20-year-old man complains of lack of energy and impotence. He has little beard growth or body hair. Laboratory evaluation reveals a low testosterone level and high levels of luteinizing hormone (LH) and follicle-stimulating hormone (FSH). This patient is most likely to have

A sarcoidosis of the hypothalamus
B craniopharyngioma compressing the pituitary
C history of head trauma
D Klinefelter syndrome (47,XXY)
E congenital hypogonadotropic hypogonadism

2 A man presents in clinic with impotence, decreased libido, listlessness, and muscular weakness. His laboratory examination shows low testosterone levels and low gonadotropin levels. This picture is consistent with a history of

A treatment with a 5α-reductase inhibitor
B mumps orchitis
C prostate cancer treatment with androgen-receptor blockade
D a pituitary tumor
E Sertoli cell damage from chemotherapy

3 A medical researcher finds a new, potent, and long-lasting gonadotropin-releasing hormone (GnRH) agonist. Which of the following hormone patterns is consistent with the effects of this drug?

A Low testosterone and low gonadotropins
B High testosterone and low gonadotropins
C Low testosterone and high gonadotropins
D High testosterone and high gonadotropins

4 During a clinical trial of drug xx, many subjects have developed gynecomastia. The medical researcher's review indicates that many men treated with the drug have elevated testosterone levels associated with elevated levels of luteinizing hormone (LH) and follicle-stimulating hormone (FSH). Which of the following is consistent with this finding?

A Drug xx activates the androgen receptor
B Drug xx blocks the androgen receptor
C Drug xx activates the estrogen receptor
D Drug xx blocks the estrogen receptor

5 A physician who sees a patient with malnutrition would expect which of the following laboratory results?

A Increased testosterone and decreased luteinizing hormone (LH)
B Increased testosterone and increased LH
C Decreased testosterone and decreased LH
D Decreased testosterone and increased LH

6 A 17-year-old boy was raised as a female until puberty when his testicles descended, his voice deepened, and he developed a male body habitus, a sparse beard, and penile enlargement. LH and FSH are within normal limits. This individual is most likely to have

A aromatase deficiency
B anosmin deficiency
C estrogen receptor deficiency
D inhibin B deficiency
E 5α-reductase deficiency

References

AACE Guidelines: AACE clinical practice guidelines for the evaluation and treatment of male sexual dsfunction. *Endocr Prac* 4: 220–234, 1998.

Bagatelle CJ, Bremner WJ: Androgens in men: uses and abuses. *N Engl J Med* 334: 707–714, 1996.

Bulun SE: Aromatase deficiency in women and men: would you have predicted the phenotypes? *J Clin Endocrinol Metab* 81: 867–871, 1996.

Goldstein I, Lue TF, Padma-Nathan H, et al: Oral sildenafil in the treatment of erectile dysfunction *N Engl J Med* 338:1397–1404, 1998.

Griffin JE: Androgen resistance: the clinical spectrum *N Engl J Med* 326: 611–618, 1992.

Harman SM, Metter EJ, Tobin J, et al: Longitudinal effects of aging on serum total and free testosterone levels in healthy men. *J Clin Endocrinol Metab* 86: 724–731, 2001.

Hayes FJ, Seminara SB, Crowley WF: Hypogonadotropic hypogonadism. *Endocrinol Metab Clin North Am* 27: 739–762, 1998.

Lue TF: Erectile dysfunction. *N Engl J Med* 342: 1802–1813, 2000.

Quigley CA, de Bellis A, Marschke KB, et al: Androgen receptor defects: historical, clinical and molecular perspectives. *Endocr Rev* 16: 271–321, 1995.

Smyth CM, Bremner WJ: Klinefelter syndrome. *Arch Int Med* 158: 1309–1314, 1998.

Tenover JL: Male hormone replacement therapy including "andropause". *Endocrinol Metab Clin North Am* 27: 969–978, 1998.

12

Endocrinology of Female Reproduction

Virginia R. Lupo, M.D. and Catherine B. Niewoehner, M.D.

■ CHAPTER OUTLINE ■

■ LEARNING OBJECTIVES ■

At the completion of this chapter, the student will:
1. understand the hypothalamic-pituitary-ovarian hormone axis and its regulation by feedback mechanisms.
2. understand the ovarian events of the menstrual cycle.
3. understand the endometrial phases of the menstrual cycle.
4. understand how the menstrual cycle can be disturbed at the level of the hypothalamus, pituitary, ovary, uterus, and outflow tract.
5. be aware of the mechanisms of hormonal contraception.
6. understand the evaluation and approach to treatment of amenorrhea.
7. be aware of the causes and consequences of excess androgen production and action.
8. recognize the events of menopause and the consequences of estrogen deficiency and hormone replacement therapy.

CASE STUDY: *INTRODUCTION*

J. Martin is a 22-year-old woman who came to the clinic because she has not had a menstrual period for 2 years. A long-distance runner on her college cross-country running team, this young woman is concerned because a recent x-ray of an injured left foot revealed several old stress fractures and loss of bone mineralization throughout her foot. She has always been healthy and active. She experienced menarche at the age of 13, and her periods were regular, occurring every 28 days, until she began training for a marathon 3 years ago. Her menses ceased for several months but resumed after the marathon. Six months later she began long-distance running again, and her menses ceased. She has a good appetite but maintains her weight with low-fat foods. She has not been sexually active during the past year. Her mother had autoimmune hypothyroidism and experienced menopause early. Her father and sister are well.

Physical examination revealed that her height was 5'6" and her weight was 98 lb. Four years earlier her weight was 118 lb. Breast development and body hair distribution were normal. Her pelvic exam was normal except for vaginal dryness and an atrophic vaginal mucosa. Cervical mucus was decreased and did not fern.

Hypothalamic-Pituitary-Ovarian Hormone System

The cyclic rise and fall of hormones resulting in ovulation and the potential for pregnancy each month is the result of intricately coordinated hormone secretion by the hypothalamus, pituitary, and ovaries and the responses of the reproductive tract to these hormones (Fig. 12-1).

HYPOTHALAMIC HORMONE SECRETION

The hypothalamic hormone regulating the pituitary-ovarian axis is gonadotropin-releasing hormone (GnRH), a 10–amino acid peptide synthesized in the arcuate nucleus of the medial-basal hypothalamus and in the preoptic area of the ventral hypothalamus. GnRH is transported by a network of portal veins to the anterior pituitary, where it binds to cell membrane receptors on gonadotropin-producing cells (gonadotrophs) [see Chapter 2]. GnRH regulates the synthesis and release of the gonadotropins follicle-stimulating hormone (FSH) and luteinizing hormone (LH). GnRH secretion is pulsatile, and GnRH action depends on the frequency and amplitude of these pulses.

Variations in GnRH pulsatility determine whether the pituitary releases primarily FSH or LH into the general circulation.

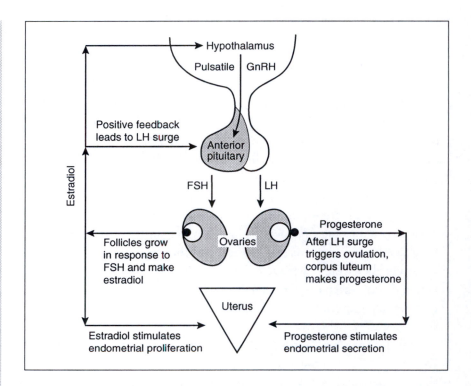

Fig. 12-1. Hypothalamic-Pituitary-Ovarian Axis and the Uterus

The uterus is the target organ for ovarian hormones. Most of the time high levels of estrogen and progesterone inhibit follicle-stimulating hormone (FSH) and luteinizing hormone (LH) secretion by negative feedback. However, there is a period during the first half of the menstrual cycle when estrogen exerts positive feedback. GnRH = gonadotropin-releasing hormone.

Native GnRH has a half-life of several minutes, but substitutions of the amino acid at the sixth position markedly prolong the half-life of GnRH. Modification of other amino acids produces GnRH agonists or antagonists. Agonists increase gonadotropin secretion if they are administered in a pulsatile fashion, but sustained administration soon down-regulates GnRH receptors, and release of FSH and LH is suppressed.

PITUITARY HORMONE SECRETION

FSH and LH are glycoprotein hormones produced in the gonadotrophs of the anterior pituitary. They have a common alpha chain, which is also shared by another anterior pituitary hormone, thyroid-stimulating hormone (TSH), and by human chorionic gonadotropin (HCG), which is produced by the placenta during pregnancy. Each hormone has a unique beta chain, which binds to a specific receptor and accounts for the characteristic action of the hormone. The beta chains of LH and HCG are similar, but the beta chain of HCG is distinguished by a carboxy terminal tail of 24 extra amino acids. FSH and LH are secreted into the circulation in pulses in response to pulsatile secretion of GnRH. They stimulate production of ovarian hormones.

OVARIAN HORMONE SECRETION

Estrogen and progesterone are the major hormones secreted by the ovaries in response to FSH and LH stimulation. Synthetic pathways for these steroid hormones are shown in Figure 12-2. The ovarian stroma cells also produce androgens in response to LH stimulation. Some ovarian androgens are secreted into the circulation, but most are converted to estrogens in the ovarian granulosa cells. The most active estrogen is estradiol, which is derived from testosterone by the enzymatic action of aromatase (see Fig. 12-2). Since conversion of androgens to estrogens also occurs in adipose tissue, obese women often have higher estrogen levels than lean women.

Ovarian steroid hormones travel in the circulation mostly bound to carrier proteins. All of the hormones bind to albumin, but one third of estrogen is bound to sex hormone–binding globulin (SHBG). The most active androgens, testosterone and dihydrotestosterone, are bound primarily to SHBG. Only the small fraction of free hormone is active.

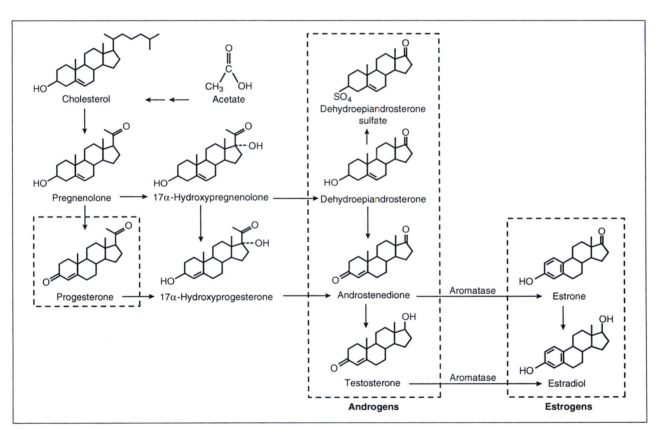

Fig. 12-2. Pathways of Ovarian Hormone Synthesis

Although pathways are shown as unidirectional for simplicity, steps from pregnenolone forward are reversible. The enzyme aromatase converts androgens into estrogens. Androgens also are converted to estrogens in peripheral tissues, especially adipose tissue. Testosterone is converted into the more active dihydrotestosterone by the enzyme 5α-reductase in peripheral tissues.

Table 12-1. Major Actions of Estrogens

Pubertal growth spurt	Maintain normal vasculature
Closing of epiphyses at puberty	Decrease bone resorption
Pubertal maturation of uterus, vagina	Reduce bowel motility
Proliferation of endometrial lining	Increase blood-clotting factors
Breast development	Increase blood coagulation
Pigmentation of breasts and pubic area	Increase HDL cholesterol
Female distribution of body fat	Increase triglyceride turnover
Influence libido	Increase hepatic-binding protein synthesis
Maintain normal skin	Increase renin substrate

Notes

Estrogen and progesterone have wide-ranging effects on tissues and metabolic processes. The major effects of these hormones are listed in Tables 12-1 and 12-2. Circulating estrogen and progesterone concentrations also regulate GnRH pulses and FSH and LH secretion by the pituitary (see Events in the Ovary). Ovarian androgens increase strength and libido and contribute to hair growth.

The ovaries also produce growth factors and polypeptide hormones such as inhibins, activins, and relaxin. They affect pituitary hormone secretion (inhibin decreases FSH secretion; activin increases FSH secretion) and modulate hormone action. Their physiologic roles are not well understood.

Normal Menstrual Cycle

During childhood the hypothalamus and the pituitary gland are very sensitive to negative feedback by circulating estrogen, and LH and FSH concentrations are low. As puberty approaches, this is no longer true (see Chapter 14). GnRH pulses increase in frequency and amplitude and FSH and LH secretion rises. As puberty advances, the interplay between hypothalamic, pituitary, and ovarian hormones results in the series of events in the ovary and endometrium known as the menstrual cycle (Fig. 12-3).

EVENTS IN THE OVARY

The ovary is composed of three areas: (1) the outer cortex containing the follicles and germinal epithelium; (2) the central stroma; and (3) the hilum, where the ovary attaches to the mesovarium. Hilum interstitial cells are similar to the testosterone-producing Leydig cells

Table 12-2. Major Actions of Progesterone

Breast development	Contributes to insulin resistance
Endometrial gland maturation	Increases body temperature
Maintains uterus during pregnancy	Increases minute ventilation
Inhibits lactation during pregnancy	

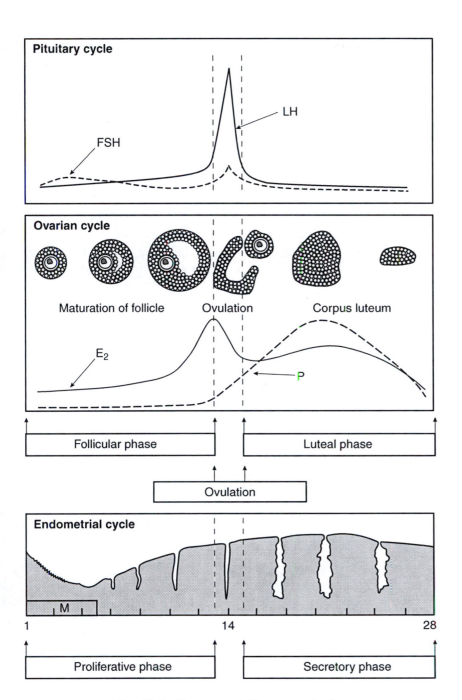

**Fig. 12-3. Hormonal Changes during
Normal Menstrual Cycle**

The changes in pituitary hormone secretion, ovarian follicle development, hormone secretion, and the endometrial responses to ovarian hormones are shown. FSH = follicle-stimulating hormone; LH = luteinizing hormone; E2 = estradiol; P = progesterone; M = menses (days of menstrual bleeding).

of the testes. The oocytes are enclosed in follicles embedded in stromal tissue in the inner part of the cortex. All of the ova that a woman will ever have are formed by the time she is a fetus at 20 weeks' gestation. At that time she has approximately 6 million primary oocytes with nuclei arrested in the diplotene phase of the first meiotic division.

These oocytes do not proceed through meiosis until fertilization occurs, sometimes as long as 45 or more years later. The fact that these eggs have been exposed to environmental stresses for many years may explain the increase in poor reproductive function as women age and the exponential rise in chromosomal aneuploidy after the age of 35.

During gestation primary oocytes are incorporated into the basic unit of the ovary, the primordial follicle. A primordial follicle consists of a primary oocyte surrounded by a layer of granulosa cells held within a basement membrane (Fig. 12-4). Stromal tissue surrounds the follicle. From midgestation through childhood, a few primordial follicles develop into primary follicles with growing oocytes and then undergo atresia. Of the 6 million original primordial follicles, approximately

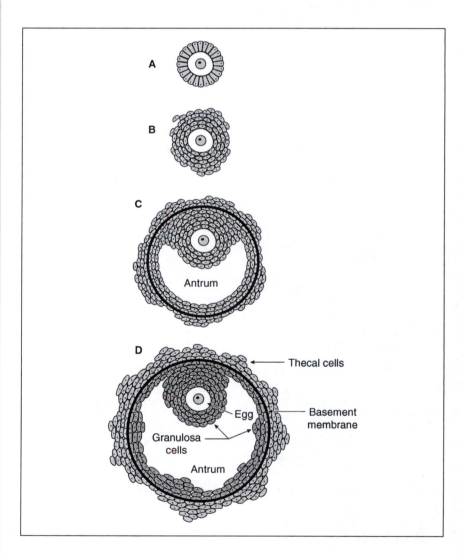

Fig. 12-4. Maturation of Selected Dominant Follicle Prior to Ovulation

Schematic representation of (A) a primordial follicle, (B) an enlarging follicle surrounded by increasing numbers of granulosa cells, (C) an antral follicle, and (D) a fully developed follicle prior to ovulation. Note the development of the fluid-filled cavity in C and the thecal cells surrounding the follicle in B–D.

2 million are still present at birth. By the onset of menses during puberty (menarche), only 500,000 primordial follicles remain.

Woman's Age	Number of Oocytes (approx.)
20 weeks' gestation	6,000,000
Birth	2,000,000
Menarche	500,000
55	0

Menarche is the onset of the first menses during puberty.

After menarche many primordial follicles emerge from the resting phase every month, probably due to changes in the local environment induced by FSH. Although the beginning of a menstrual cycle is defined arbitrarily as the first day of menstrual blood flow, FSH levels actually begin to rise slightly before menses under the influence of tonic secretion of GnRH at a rate of one pulse per hour. As the level of FSH increases, a single dominant follicle is selected from the group of maturing, emerging primordial follicles. This follicle matures fully as it progresses toward ovulation (Fig. 12-4). The other emerging follicles undergo atresia. The factors responsible for selection of the dominant follicle are not understood.

From menarche to menopause, approximately one follicle per month develops to maturity and ovulation (a total of approximately 400 follicles).

Stimulation of the selected follicle by FSH causes granulosa cells to proliferate into a multilayered covering for the ovum. Fluid appears between the granulosa cells. This coalesces to form a fluid-filled cavity called the antrum. At the same time, the stromal cells around the follicle become more distinct, and a layer of stromal cells known as theca interna cells can be seen immediately adjacent to the basal lamina around the granulosa cells. A more loosely structured layer of stromal cells, the theca externa, forms the outermost layer of the follicle (Fig. 12-4). At the level of the ovary, the first half of the menstrual cycle is called the *follicular phase* because of the development of the dominant follicle (Table 12-3).

FSH stimulates estrogen production by the granulosa cells. The rise in estrogen suppresses pituitary FSH secretion by negative feedback, and by day 10 the FSH level begins to decline. However, since estrogen also induces the development of FSH receptors, FSH action is more efficient despite the lower FSH level, and estrogen production by the ovary continues to rise. The follicle continues to enlarge.

Table 12-3. Phases of Menstrual Cycle

TIME OF MENSTRUAL CYCLE	OVARY	ENDOMETRIUM	MAJOR HORMONE
First half	Follicular phase	Proliferative phase	Estrogen
Second half	Luteal phase	Secretory phase	Progesterone

Notes

The rapid rise in estrogen secretion by the ripe ovarian follicle triggers a change in the pattern of GnRH secretion to rapid pulses. These rapid pulses stimulate the gonadotrophs to produce a surge of LH. There is a brief period of positive feedback, when the rising estrogen level also stimulates a midcycle rise in FSH. The LH surge is followed by ovulation within the next 24 hours. At the time of ovulation, the follicle ruptures and the egg is extruded into the peritoneal cavity. Rupture of the follicle is not due to pressure, but to proteolytic digestion of the follicle wall.

The rise in estrogen, which peaks at ovulation, increases production and causes thinning of cervical mucus, which allows sperm to penetrate the cervix more easily. At this time a drop of mucus on a slide dries in a ferning pattern (Fig. 12-5), and a drop of mucus suspended between two glass slides can stretch as much as 10 cm without breaking. The ability of cervical mucus to stretch is referred to as *spinnbarkeit*. Ferning and spinnbarkeit are clinical signs of ovulation, which can be used to time intercourse for increased likelihood of conception or for contraception.

Some women note a sharp pain due to peritoneal irritation, which follows rupture of the ovarian follicle. This pain of ovulation occurring

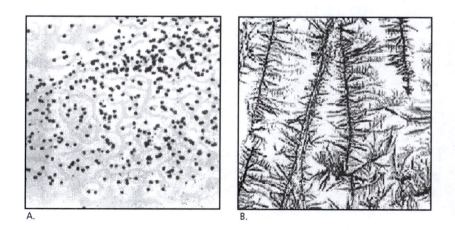

A.   B.

Fig. 12-5. Ferning of Cervical Mucus

(A) A smear of cervical mucus obtained from a normally menstruating woman on day 5 of the menstrual cycle. Lack of ferning is compatible with the low estrogen level at this time of the cycle. (B) A smear of cervical mucus obtained from the same woman just before ovulation when the estrogen level is high shows a ferning pattern.

at midcycle is called *mittelschmerz*. Some women note an increase in libido due to increased ovarian androgen production induced by the LH surge before ovulation. A rise in basal body temperature immediately after rising in the morning can be observed in 95% of women who have just ovulated. This subtle sign of increased circulating progesterone confirms ovulation. Intercourse at the time of the temperature rise does not result in pregnancy as often as might be expected because maximal fertility occurs immediately *before* ovulation.

Signs Indicating Ovulation

Mittelschmerz (pain due to follicle rupture)
Ferning of cervical mucus (estrogen effect)
Increased spinnbarkeit (estrogen effect)
Rise in basal body temperature (progesterone effect)
Increased libido (androgen effect)

Maturation and ovulation of two follicles that are subsequently fertilized results in fraternal twins. There is a familial predisposition to multiple ovulation. Women prone to multiple gestations may have higher FSH levels or more sensitive FSH receptors. Administration of high doses of exogenous gonadotropins in an attempt to induce fertility often results in maturation of several follicles. Identical twinning is not increased by exogenous gonadotropins.

After ovulation the follicle antrum is filled with blood and lymph, and the wall of the follicle collapses. Blood vessels from the surrounding thecal layer invade the follicle. The granulosa cells remaining in the ruptured follicle enlarge and produce progesterone in response to the high level of circulating LH. These progesterone-rich cells appear yellow, or luteinized. The luteinized granulosa cells together with the surrounding thecal cells form the corpus luteum, meaning "yellow body." At the level of the ovary, the period of the menstrual cycle after ovulation is called the *luteal phase* (see Table 12-3).

Estrogen dominates the proliferative phase of the menstrual cycle. The estrogen level remains high after ovulation, but progesterone dominates the luteal phase. Progesterone converts the lining of the uterus into an environment that can sustain a pregnancy (see Events in the Endometrium). Progesterone reduces production and causes thickening of cervical mucus, even if estrogen is present.

During the luteal phase, pituitary secretion of LH and FSH becomes suppressed by the high levels of progesterone and estrogen (negative feedback). However, the corpus luteum cannot be sustained long without LH and FSH support. The corpus luteum involutes, leaving a small white scar called the corpus albicans. When the corpus luteum fails, estrogen and progesterone levels fall, the hypothalamus and pituitary gland are released from feedback inhibition, and FSH starts to rise again. The endometrium cannot be sustained without progesterone; the endometrial lining is sloughed, and another menstrual cycle begins.

If conception occurs, the placenta produces human chorionic gonadotropin (HCG), a hormone that acts like LH. HCG sustains the corpus luteum, which continues to produce progesterone to support the endometrium, and menstrual bleeding does not occur (see Chapter 15).

In many women the menstrual cycle begins every 28 days. Variation in the length of a menstrual cycle is almost always due to variation in the length of the follicular phase, not the luteal phase. The time from ovulation until beginning of menses is usually 14 days. Variations resulting in a short luteal phase are a rare but treatable cause of infertility.

EVENTS IN THE ENDOMETRIUM

The cyclic rise and fall of estrogen and progesterone has predictable effects on the inner lining of the uterus (the endometrium), and it is the uterine response that determines the dating of the menstrual cycle (see Fig. 12-3). Day 1 is the date of the onset of menses. At this time, the endometrial lining is being sloughed because estrogen and progesterone levels are too low to maintain it. However, FSH levels are rising and estrogen levels soon increase in response.

At the end of menstrual blood flow, a thin basal layer of endometrium remains. Under the influence of rising estrogen levels during the ovarian follicular phase, endometrial glands proliferate from the stumps of glands remaining in the basal layer. Estrogen causes the glands to enlarge and become coiled, and the thickness of the lining of the uterus increases tenfold. Growth of the glands is accompanied by growth of the stroma and proliferation of spiral arteries from remaining basal arteries. A rich capillary network forms. All this occurs in preparation for implantation of a fertilized egg. At the level of the uterus, the phase of the menstrual cycle preceding ovulation is called the *proliferative phase* (see Table 12-3).

After ovulation the effects of progesterone on the endometrium predominate. Progesterone halts further growth in thickness and causes solidification and maturation of the endometrium. The endometrial glands cease to proliferate and begin secreting glycoproteins into the uterine cavity to create a favorable environment for implantation of the fertilized egg. At the level of the endometrium, the phase of the menstrual cycle from ovulation to menses is called the *secretory phase* (see Table 12-3).

The changes in endometrial histology caused by estrogen and progesterone are sufficiently distinct to allow dating of the menstrual cycle that is usually accurate to within 48 hours.

If conception does not occur and the corpus luteum involutes, progesterone levels fall precipitously, and there is no longer sufficient hormonal support for the spiral arterioles. The arterioles constrict, causing necrosis of the endometrial lining. Tissue sloughs off, resulting in blood loss referred to as a menstrual period. In most women, bleeding lasts for 5 days. The average volume of blood lost during menses is 30 mL. Loss of more than 80 mL of menstrual blood each month usually results in anemia.

DYSMENORRHEA AND PREMENSTRUAL SYNDROME

In some women dysmenorrhea (painful menses) without any underlying pathology occurs during ovulatory menstrual cycles. The pain is cramping in nature and is thought to be due to uterine contractions caused by prostaglandins released as the endometrium is sloughed. Treatment includes inhibitors of prostaglandin release, suppression of ovulation with oral contraception, or both. Dilatation of the cervix during menses is also perceived by some women as cramping.

Premenstrual syndrome is a collection of recurrent symptoms (fatigue, irritability, mood swings, anxiety, depression, insomnia) that occur in some women mostly during the luteal phase of ovulatory menstrual cycles, although symptoms can persist into the follicular phase. The cause is uncertain. Although the luteal phase is associated with marked changes in the levels of FSH, LH, estrogen, and progesterone, no hormonal abnormalities have been identified in women with this syndrome.

Menstrual Cycle Dysfunction

Normal menstrual cycles require normal function of the hypothalamus, pituitary, ovaries, and outflow tract. Failure of menses (amenorrhea) can be due to a problem at any of these levels. Causes of primary amenorrhea (failure of menses to occur at puberty) and secondary amenorrhea (cessation of menses after it has been established) are somewhat different. However, there is a great deal of overlap in the differential diagnosis (Table 12-4).

Table 12-4. Major Causes of Amenorrhea

HYPOTHALAMIC LEVEL	OVARY LEVEL
Failure to attain or maintain critical level of body fat	Ovarian dysgenesis (Turner syndrome)
Severe stress	Testicular feminization syndrome
Severe systemic illness	Chemotherapy
Syndrome of anosmia and GnRH deficiency	Radiation damage
	Autoimmune disease
PITUITARY LEVEL	**OUTFLOW TRACT LEVEL**
Large pituitary tumors	Congenital obstruction
Hyperprolactinemia	Müllerian agenesis
Postpartum necrosis	Recurrent endometrial infections
	Overvigorous curettage (Asherman syndrome)

PRIMARY AMENORRHEA

In the United States, the onset of first menses (menarche) occurs at an average age of 12 years and 8 months. Primary amenorrhea is defined as no menses by the age of 14 in the absence of development of secondary sex characteristics (breast budding, pubic hair, axillary hair) *or* no menses by the age of 16 regardless of the presence or absence of secondary sex characteristics.

Primary Amenorrhea

No menses and no development of secondary sex characteristics by age 14 years

No menses by age 16 years

If a young woman appears healthy and has a family history of delayed sexual maturation, investigation may reveal that her pubertal development is just delayed (Chapter 14). If secondary sex characteristics have developed, it is essential to be sure that the patient is not pregnant.

Hypothalamic Level

Hypothalamic primary amenorrhea is most often due to failure to accumulate enough body fat to reach the set point required for menarche. Body fat must reach this critical level for GnRH pulses of sufficient frequency and amplitude to stimulate pituitary gonadotropin release. The mechanism by which the adipose tissue level regulates hypothalamic function is uncertain; the interaction of the adipose tissue hormone leptin with the central nervous system is undergoing intense evaluation at this time (see Chapter 10). Hypothalamic primary amenorrhea is not unusual in teenage athletes, especially gymnasts, dancers, and young women running more than 20 miles per week. Hypothalamic amenorrhea is common in young women with anorexia nervosa who have very low levels of body fat due to a combination of starvation and exercise.

CASE STUDY: *CONTINUED*

Since Ms. Martin's height, breast development, body hair, age of first menses, and earlier menstrual cycles were normal, it was unlikely that her amenorrhea was due to a developmental abnormality. Her cervix and vagina were patent. She had obvious signs of estrogen deficiency, including vaginal dryness, an atrophic vaginal mucosa, and decreased cervical mucus that did not fern. A pregnancy test was negative, as expected in view of the clinical evidence for estrogen deficiency. Additional tests were ordered to determine whether the problem was at the level of her hypothalamus, pituitary gland, or ovaries.

Patients experiencing severe stress or severe systemic illness are also at increased risk of developing hypothalamic amenorrhea. Sexual maturation and menses usually respond promptly to decreased exercise, weight gain, or both, and to resolution of underlying stress or illness.

A rare CNS defect results in the combination of anosmia (absent sense of smell) and GnRH deficiency, which is analogous to Kallman syndrome in men (see Chapter 11). FSH and LH levels and ovarian hormone levels are low in these women. These patients respond to GnRH agonists given in a pulsatile regimen to prevent down-regulation of receptors.

Pituitary Level

Craniopharyngiomas and other large pituitary tumors that destroy the pituitary gland by mass effects can cause primary amenorrhea. Patients with these tumors have low or low-normal FSH and LH levels and may have symptoms and signs of other pituitary hormone deficiencies as well (see Chapter 2). Treatment is directed toward removal of the underlying tumor whenever possible and estrogen and progesterone replacement.

Even small prolactin (PRL)-producing pituitary tumors can cause primary amenorrhea because high PRL levels interfere with GnRH pulses. There are many other causes of hyperprolactinemia, including renal failure, medications like the phenothiazines, and primary hypothyroidism. Phenothiazines suppress hypothalamic production of dopamine, which is a physiological inhibitor of prolactin secretion (see Chapter 2). Patients with primary hypothyroidism have high levels of both thyrotropin-releasing hormone (TRH) and thyroid-stimulating hormone (TSH). Normal TRH levels have little effect on PRL, but high levels of TRH stimulate prolactin release. Hyperprolactinemia can usually be suppressed with dopamine agonists if treatment of the underlying disorder is not possible. This restores GnRH pulses and gonadotropin secretion.

Ovarian Level

If primary amenorrhea is due to absence or destruction of the ovaries, estrogen levels are low and FSH and LH levels are high due to the absence of negative feedback by ovarian hormones.

Turner syndrome or gonadal dysgenesis (karyotype 45,XO) is the most common congenital cause of primary amenorrhea. Loss of the second X chromosome results in ovaries that are fibrous streaks with few, if any, germ cells present at puberty. The pubertal growth spurt and secondary sexual characteristics do not develop in the absence of ovarian follicles, which are needed to synthesize estrogen. Although the outflow tract is intact, the uterus is usually quite small. Some other clinical features of this syndrome include short stature, a webbed neck, a shield chest, and an abnormal carrying angle (valgus deformity of the elbows) [see Chapters 13 and 14]. A karyotype is necessary to confirm the diagnosis, since the clinical features are quite variable, especially in women who are mosaics with karyotype 45,XX/45,XO.

Testicular feminization syndrome (karyotype 46,XY) is another congenital disorder that presents with primary amenorrhea. Patients with this disorder have a male genotype but a female phenotype due to absence of functional androgen receptors. They have high FSH, LH, and testosterone levels because the pituitary lacks the receptors to recognize testosterone. Estrogen levels are high because testosterone is converted to estrogen in peripheral tissues. These patients have female external genitalia and female breast development but no ovaries or uterus and little body hair (see Chapters 13 and 14).

Environmental insults causing premature death of ovarian follicles and primary amenorrhea include radiation therapy and chemotherapy given for childhood malignancies.

Amenorrhea due to ovarian failure is treated with estrogen and progesterone replacement.

Outflow Tract Level

If the problem is at the level of the outflow tract, secondary sex characteristics develop normally because hypothalamic-pituitary-ovarian feedback loops are normal. Obstruction of menstrual flow can occur at several levels. An imperforate hymen results in monthly discomfort, which becomes progressively worse due to buildup of menstrual blood behind the intact hymen. Eventually a bulge can be noted on the perineum. This is an infrequent but easily corrected problem.

Disorders of müllerian duct development are of more concern. There may be no vaginal orifice. In these cases surgical correction can be immensely rewarding, even if reproduction is not possible. Complete müllerian agenesis results in congenital absence of the uterus and proximal vagina.

SECONDARY AMENORRHEA

Secondary amenorrhea refers to amenorrhea occurring in a nonpregnant woman who has previously had menses and who is not expected to be experiencing menopause. Many of the conditions that cause primary amenorrhea can also cause secondary amenorrhea. As with primary amenorrhea, the problem can be at the level of the hypothalamus, the pituitary, the ovaries, or the outflow tract.

Hypothalamic Level

Lack of body fat, anorexia nervosa, weight loss, stress, or systemic illness can cause secondary amenorrhea as well as primary amenorrhea (see Primary Amenorrhea: Hypothalamic Level).

Pituitary Level

The same tumors that cause primary amenorrhea can cause secondary amenorrhea. Since mass lesions often affect the gonadotrophs before the cells producing TSH and ACTH, women with these tumors may not have symptoms and signs of other pituitary hormone deficiencies. Hyperprolactinemia, which disrupts GnRH pulses, is a common cause of secondary amenorrhea. As indicated above, hyperprolactinemia can be due to a pituitary tumor, dopamine-suppressing drugs such as the phenothiazines, renal failure, and hypothyroidism, which results in an increase in TRH sufficient to stimulate PRL secretion.

Amenorrhea following childbirth can be due to postpartum necrosis of the pituitary gland. The pituitary gland normally hypertrophies during pregnancy because the rise in estrogen stimulates lactotrophs. If postpartum hemorrhage results in hypotension, the pituitary may undergo acute infarction due to lack of blood flow. Patients present with inability to lactate, since milk production requires prolactin from the anterior pituitary (see Chapter 15). With modern obstetric care this catastrophe is rare.

Women with secondary amenorrhea due to pituitary disorders have low or low-normal FSH and LH levels. Treatment is the same as the treatment for primary amenorrhea at the pituitary level (see Primary Amenorrhea: Pituitary Level).

Ovarian Level

Women with Turner syndrome can present with secondary amenorrhea rather than primary amenorrhea if follicle atresia is sufficiently delayed to allow the women to go through puberty. This is especially likely if women with this syndrome are mosaics of 45,XX and 45,XO. Premature ovarian failure (premature menopause) refers to ovarian failure in a woman under the age of 35. This can be due to autoimmune disease, chemotherapy, or radiation therapy, but the cause is frequently unknown.

If amenorrhea is due to ovarian failure, FSH and LH levels are high due to absence of negative feedback by estrogen and progesterone. Ovarian failure is treated with estrogen and progesterone replacement.

Outflow Tract Level

Recurrent infections that destroy the endometrial cavity and overvigorous curettage that denudes the endometrial lining result in scarring and amenorrhea if the endometrial glands are damaged too severely to respond to estrogen (Asherman syndrome). The uterus is especially sensitive to vigorous curettage during the month after childbirth, when the uterus is vascular and hypertrophied. Asherman syndrome is treated by resecting some of the scar tissue and giving large doses of estrogen in an effort to stimulate regrowth of the endometrial lining.

EVALUATION AND TREATMENT OF AMENORRHEA

A flow diagram for evaluation of amenorrhea is shown in Fig. 12-6. After completing the history and physical examination to be sure that ovaries, a uterus, and a vagina are present and that the outflow tract is patent, a pregnancy test should be obtained regardless of the sexual history. A serum TSH level and a PRL level should be obtained even if other symptoms and signs of hyperprolactinemia and hypothyroidism are absent. These are common causes of amenorrhea, and

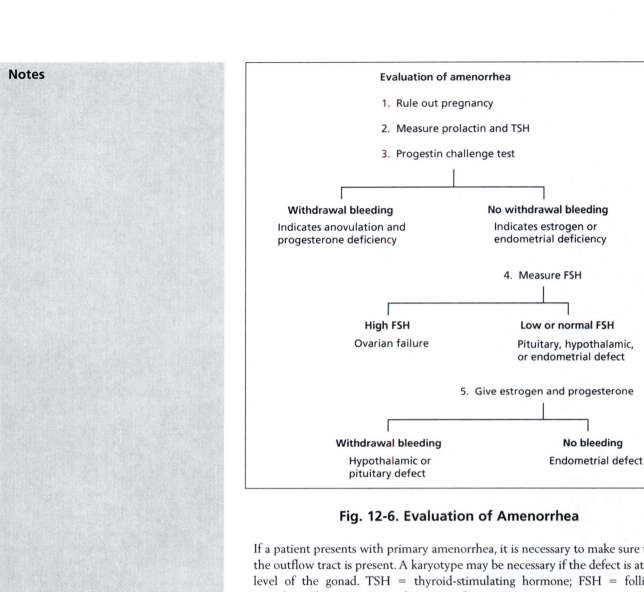

Fig. 12-6. Evaluation of Amenorrhea

If a patient presents with primary amenorrhea, it is necessary to make sure that the outflow tract is present. A karyotype may be necessary if the defect is at the level of the gonad. TSH = thyroid-stimulating hormone; FSH = follicle-stimulating hormone; LH = luteinizing hormone.

other symptoms and signs may not appear until later in the course. Subtle elevations of TRH can stimulate enough PRL secretion to disrupt GnRH pulses in patients who are clinically euthyroid.

If the pregnancy test is negative, and TSH and prolactin levels are within the normal range, a *progestin challenge* can be given to test for adequate estrogen activity. Progesterone or another oral progestin is given for several days and then withdrawn. Withdrawal bleeding occurring several days later indicates that enough estrogen is available to prepare the endometrium for the progesterone. The availability of estrogen indicates that the hypothalamus and pituitary are producing GnRH pulses and gonadotropins. Withdrawal bleeding also confirms that the endometrium is able to respond to estrogen and that the outflow tract is patent. If withdrawal bleeding occurs after a progestin challenge, amenorrhea is likely due to anovulation and progesterone deficiency.

If amenorrhea is due to estrogen depletion, there will be no primed endometrium to respond to a progesterone challenge. A serum FSH

Table 12.5. Amenorrhea: Hormone Relationships

LEVEL OF FAILURE	FSH	LH	ESTROGEN
Hypothalamus	Low*	Low*	Low
Pituitary	Low*	Low*	Low
Ovary	High	High	Low
Uterus	Normal	Normal	Normal

Note. FSH = follicle-stimulating hormone; LH = luteinizing hormone.
* Value may be low-normal.

level will help to determine whether this is due to ovarian incompetence or to a problem at the pituitary or hypothalamic level. The FSH level will be low or low-normal if the problem is at the pituitary or hypothalamic level. The FSH level will be high if the problem is due to ovarian failure (Table 12-5). If the FSH level is high, it may be necessary to obtain a karyotype to diagnose Turner syndrome or to rule out the presence of a Y chromosome remnant. If a karyotype reveals a Y chromosome remnant, the removal of the patient's gonads is required because remnants are likely to become neoplastic.

If the FSH level is normal, the problem may be the endometrium itself. If the endometrium is able to respond to estrogen stimulation, priming the endometrium with estrogen for 3 weeks and then giving and withdrawing progesterone should result in withdrawal bleeding.

Specific treatment of the underlying cause of amenorrhea is ideal but not always possible. Estrogen replacement stimulates development of secondary sex characteristics and growth in girls with incomplete pubertal maturation. Progesterone is added to prevent the endometrial hyperplasia that results if estrogen replacement is given alone. Women without a uterus need not be given progesterone. Patients with Turner syndrome can be given growth hormone (GH) therapy to increase final height. GH is given prior to estrogen replacement because estrogen stimulates closure of the epiphyses. Ovarian androgens are usually not replaced because they do not provide any additional increase in height, and virilizing side effects are common.

Even if sexual development is not an issue, hormone replacement is recommended for most women of premenopausal age with hypogonadism, regardless of whether the underlying problem is at the level of the hypothalamus, the pituitary gland, or the ovaries. Lack of estrogen results in osteopenia, and fractures may occur despite excellent physical conditioning. Women with hypogonadism also experience other consequences of estrogen deficiency that are common in postmenopausal women (see below).

If ovarian follicles are present, and the goal is ovulation and pregnancy, treatment with gonadotropins or pulsatile GnRH might be necessary. If the FSH and LH levels are consistently high, follicles are probably absent and the woman is sterile.

Disorders of Androgen Excess

Women produce androgens, including androstenedione, dehydroepiandrosterone (DHEA), and testosterone, in the ovaries and the adrenal glands. Dehydroepiandrosterone sulfate (DHEAS) is made in the adrenal glands. Testosterone is converted to DHT in peripheral tissues by the enzyme 5α-reductase, and both hormones share the same androgen receptor. Androstenedione, DHEA, and DHEAS are not true androgens because they do not interact with the androgen receptor. However, they can be converted to testosterone, and overproduction of any of these hormones can lead to symptoms and signs of androgen excess. DHEAS has no androgen effect.

Androgen	Relative Potency
Dihydrotestosterone	2.5
Testosterone	1.0
Androstenedione	0.15
DHEA	0.05

Most testosterone and DHT in the circulation are bound to SHBG. Since androgens decrease hepatic synthesis of SHBG, androgen overproduction increases the proportion of the free hormone, which is the

---

CASE STUDY: *CONTINUED*

The differential diagnosis for Ms. Martin's amenorrhea included hypothalamic amenorrhea, hypothyroidism, hyperprolactinemia, a pituitary tumor, or premature ovarian failure. Her thyroid function tests and TSH level were normal. Her PRL level was also within normal limits. A progestin challenge was not followed by withdrawal bleeding, indicating that her endometrium had not been prepared by estrogen.

Her FSH level should have been high in the absence of estrogen feedback, but the FSH level was low. This indicated that the hypothalamus or pituitary was the source of the problem, not the ovaries. Her clinical picture suggested hypothalamic amenorrhea due to loss of the critical fat mass required for normal GnRH pulses.

She was not willing to change her food intake or moderate her level of activity, so she was treated with an oral contraceptive containing estrogen and progesterone. After graduation from college she obtained a job as a marketing executive with an athletic shoe company. She decreased her running to 18 miles per week and stopped her oral contraceptive. Her weight increased to 115 lb, and her menstrual periods resumed. Subsequently she had two normal pregnancies.

active form. Ingestion or application of anabolic steroids has the same effect as increasing endogenous androgen production. Estrogen increases SHBG production.

It is possible to have increased androgen action even if circulating androgen levels are normal, if a high level of 5a-reductase activity results in increased conversion of testosterone to the more active DHT. An increase in the number of tissue androgen receptors can also result in increased androgen action.

Factors Affecting SHBG

Decreased SHBG Synthesis	Increased SHBG Synthesis
Androgens	Estrogens
Obesity	Pregnancy
Hypothyroidism	Hyperthyroidism
Glucocorticoid excess	

Even mild androgen excess can cause hirsutism (excess hair growth) and acne. Some women develop oligomenorrhea (infrequent menstrual flow) or amenorrhea. Higher androgen levels result in temporal balding, deepening of the voice, clitoromegaly, and development of a male body habitus.

OVARIAN ANDROGEN OVERPRODUCTION

Ovarian androgen overproduction most often occurs in women with polycystic ovary syndrome (PCOS), although benign ovarian cysts are also sources of androgens. Ovarian androgen-secreting tumors, which can produce very high androgen levels, are rare.

Causes of Increased Androgen Effect

Increased endogenous androgen production (ovarian, adrenal or both)

Exogenous androgen (anabolic steroids)

Decreased androgen binding (low SHBG)

Increased conversion of testosterone to dihydrotestosterone

Increased androgen receptor number or sensitivity

Polycystic Ovary Syndrome

PCOS is a combination of androgen excess and chronic anovulation that occurs in the absence of specific underlying ovarian or adrenal disease. The syndrome is associated with altered regulation of the pituitary-ovarian axis (Fig. 12-7) and insulin resistance. PCOS is common, with a prevalence of 6% in women of reproductive age. The underlying cause is unknown, but PCOS appears to be a complex multifactorial disorder with a strong familial component.

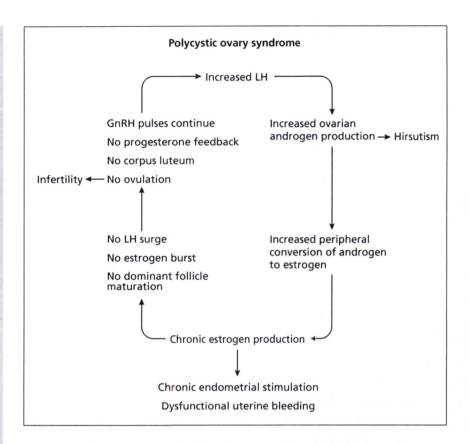

**Fig. 12-7. Metabolic Abnormalities of Polycystic
Ovary Syndrome**

The underlying cause of the syndrome is uncertain. Note that once the syndrome is established, a vicious cycle perpetuates the anovulation and hirsutism. LH = luteinizing hormone; GnRH = gonadotropin-releasing hormone.

LH pulse amplitude and frequency are increased. LH levels are increased, although not necessarily above the normal range. FSH levels are normal or low, so the LH to FSH ratio is high compared to the ratio in the early follicular phase in young women without PCOS. In response to LH, ovarian theca cells increase androgen production. The androgens are converted to estrogen in granulosa cells and in peripheral tissues. Estrogen production is chronic, not cyclic. The estrogen level remains in the early to middle follicular phase range, a level that continues to stimulate GnRH pulses. There is no late follicular phase burst of estrogen, no LH surge, no ovulation, and no corpus luteum to produce progesterone. With ongoing GnRH pulses and insufficient progesterone feedback, LH secretion continues. The result is a vicious cycle resulting in menstrual irregularities and infertility. The continuous production of estrogen unopposed by progesterone results in endometrial hyperplasia. Bleeding occurs erratically as areas of the hyperplastic endometrial lining are sloughed. Low-level estrogen production and continuous androgen overproduction result in decreased

SHBG, which also increases the free androgen level. Some women also have increased adrenal androgen production. Although women with PCOS have increased acne and hirsutism, they usually do not have more severe signs of androgen excess.

Signs of Androgen Excess

Hirsutism
Acne
Temporal balding
Deeper voice
Clitoromegaly
Male body habitus

The insulin resistance associated with PCOS is present in muscle, adipose tissue, and liver. The cause is uncertain, but many women with PCOS have a postreceptor defect in insulin signaling. Women with PCOS develop hyperinsulinemia in an attempt to overcome insulin resistance. Insulin decreases production of SHBG by the liver. Insulin also acts synergistically with LH to stimulate androgen production by ovarian theca cells. Insulin resistance is greater in obese women with PCOS but is present in lean women with PCOS as well. Impaired glucose tolerance, type 2 diabetes, and hyperlipidemia are more common in patients with PCOS than in weight-matched controls.

Continuous LH stimulation results in hypertrophied theca cells and enlarged ovaries. Since a dominant follicle is not selected each month, multiple 2 to 5 mm follicles remain in the early developmental stages. Many small ovarian cysts often are present, but multiple cysts are not needed to make the diagnosis, and polycystic morphology is found in regularly ovulating women without PCOS.

TSH, PRL, and FSH should be measured to rule out other causes of anovulation. Women with moderate or severe hyperandrogenism should have 17α-hydroxyprogesterone, testosterone, and DHEAS levels measured to rule out congenital adrenal hyperplasia or an androgen-secreting tumor.

Women with PCOS are treated with low-dose oral contraceptives or periodic progestin therapy to interrupt continuous stimulation of the endometrium by unopposed estrogen. Oral contraceptive treatment also slows hair growth. (Other treatments for hirsutism are described below.) Women who wish to become pregnant are treated with an antiestrogen such as clomiphene citrate to reduce estrogen feedback, or with exogenous gonadotropins or pulsatile GnRH to override the PCOS cycle and allow the arrested menstrual cycle to proceed to ovulation. Drugs that reduce insulin resistance, such as metformin (see Chapter 8), increase the likelihood of ovulation. If present, obesity, hyperlipidemia, and impaired glucose tolerance also require treatment.

ADRENAL ANDROGEN OVERPRODUCTION

Congenital Adrenal Hyperplasia (CAH)

This is the most common cause of adrenal androgen excess. CAH is caused by decreased activity of one of the enzymes required for production of cortisol (Fig. 12-8; see Chapter 5). When plasma cortisol is low, the pituitary increases production of ACTH, which increases flux through the metabolic pathway leading to cortisol synthesis. Metabolites proximal to the dysfunctional or absent enzyme accumulate and are diverted into pathways leading to androgen synthesis. The most common enzymatic defect is 21-hydroxylase deficiency; followed by 11β-hydroxylase deficiency and 3β-hydroxysteroid dehydrogenase deficiency (Fig. 12-8). If the enzymatic defect is severe, virilization of the genitalia occurs in utero and is apparent at birth. If the enzymatic defect is mild, patients present later with hirsutism alone or hirsutism coupled with abnormal menstrual cycles. Treatment with cortisol suppresses ACTH.

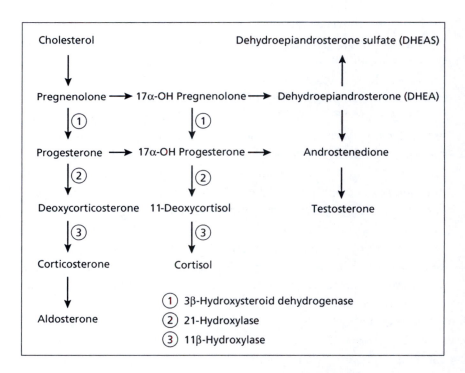

Fig. 12-8. Adrenal Steroid Hormone Synthesis

Pathways of adrenal steroid hormone synthesis are shown as unidirectional for simplicity, but steps from pregnenolone forward are reversible. Although a defect or deficiency of any of the enzymes shown can lead to congenital adrenal hyperplasia (CAH), the most common cause is 21-hydroxylase deficiency. This results in decreased cortisol synthesis and a compensatory increase in pituitary adrenocorticotropic hormone secretion, which leads to the accumulation of 17α-hydroxyprogesterone. Some of the excess 17α-hydroxyprogesterone is diverted to excess androgen synthesis.

Pituitary tumors producing ACTH (Cushing disease) and tumors producing ectopic ACTH (Cushing syndrome) also increase flux into adrenal androgen synthesis. Treatment of these disorders is discussed in Chapter 5. Adrenal androgen-secreting tumors, which can secrete very high levels of androgens, are rare.

HIRSUTISM

Hirsutism, the presence of excessive body hair, is one of the earliest signs of increased androgen action. It is very difficult to differentiate between normal and excessive hair growth. Women develop more face and body hair as estrogen levels decline with age and the ratio of circulating androgen to estrogen increases. Even a slight increase in body hair is very distressing for some women.

Hirsutism is the presence of excessive body hair in women.

Androgen-responsive hair growth results from the interaction of DHT with its receptors in hair follicles. Before puberty most body hair is the fine, nonpigmented vellus hair, which is found all over the body. Terminal hair, which is coarse, pigmented, and responsive to androgens, is found only in the eyebrows and scalp. At the time of puberty, androgen levels increase dramatically, and vellus hair is converted to terminal hair. In women this occurs mostly in the axillary and pubic regions, but if DHT production is excessive or the skin is unusually responsive to DHT, terminal hair appears on the lower face, periareolar areas of the breast, the chest, back, lower abdomen, and the inner thighs.

Most women with hirsutism have a combination of increased androgen production and increased hair follicle sensitivity to DHT. Women can also develop hirsutism if estrogen production is decreased by hyperprolactinemia or premature ovarian failure, which leaves the action of adrenal androgens relatively unopposed. Drugs such as minoxidil, phenytoin, diazoxide, cyclosporin, and danazol also stimulate hair growth.

Evaluation

The history and physical examination can be very helpful in the evaluation of hirsutism (Table 12-6). Benign forms of hirsutism often begin around the time of puberty, when gonadotropin production increases dramatically, and gradually become worse over time. Often there is a family history of hirsutism. Women who have mild, slowly developing hirsutism and regular menses are especially likely to have a benign underlying cause. Women with previously normal menstrual cycles who have rapidly developing hirsutism unrelated to puberty are more likely to have androgen-secreting tumors.

Laboratory evaluation of hirsutism should include measurement of serum testosterone; a very high level suggests an androgen-secreting

Table 12-6. Evaluation of Androgen Excess

HISTORY	PHYSICAL EXAMINATION	LABORATORY (SERUM VALUES)
Duration and severity of symptoms and signs	Body habitus	Testosterone
Relationship to onset of puberty	Obesity	FSH and LH
Family history	Acne	Prolactin
Frequency of menses	Breast development	17α-hydroxyprogesterone
	Body hair: amount and distribution	Dexamethasone suppression test (if hypercortisolism is suspected)
	Clitoromegaly	DHEAS
	Signs of hypercortisolism	

Note. FSH = follicle-stimulating hormone; LH = luteinizing hormone; DHEAS = dehydroepiandrosterone sulfate.

tumor. LH and FSH are measured as indicators of pituitary-ovarian coordination and ovarian failure. Women with PCOS are likely to have a relatively fixed LH to FSH ratio of approximately 3 to 1. A PRL level is needed to rule out hyperprolactinemia. A 17α-hydroxyprogesterone level is obtained to rule out CAH caused by 21-hydroxylase deficiency (see Chapter 5). If signs of hypercortisolism are present, a workup for Cushing syndrome with a dexamethasone suppression test should proceed as described in Chapter 5. A high DHEAS level suggests that the excess androgen is of adrenal origin.

Treatment

Treatment should be directed at the underlying cause of the hirsutism, if one can be found (Table 12-7). However, in many women it is difficult to determine whether the excess androgen is produced by the ovaries, the adrenals, or both.

Treatment of hirsutism involves suppressing androgen secretion, blocking conversion of testosterone to dihydrotestosterone or blocking androgen receptors.

Table 12-7. Treatment of Hirsutism

Gonadotropin Suppression	Antiandrogens
Oral contraceptives	Spironolactone
GnRH analogs	Flutamide
	Cyproterone acetate*
Adrenal Androgen Suppression	
Glucocorticoids	**5α-Reductase linhibitors**
	Finasteride

Note. GnRH = gonadotropin-releasing hormone.
* Not available in the United States

Gonadotropin-stimulated ovarian androgen overproduction can be treated with oral contraceptives to suppress LH and FSH production. The estrogen component of oral contraceptives also stimulates SHBG synthesis so that less free androgen is available to interact with androgen receptors on hair follicles. Oral contraceptives with the least androgenic progestins should be used.

Continuous administration of a GnRH analog decreases LH and FSH production by down-regulating pituitary GnRH receptors. Estrogen replacement must be added to prevent the consequences of estrogen deficiency, and a progestin must be added to prevent unopposed estrogen stimulation of the endometrium. A glucocorticoid, which inhibits ACTH production by negative feedback on the pituitary gland, is used to treat women with CAH.

Antiandrogens such as spironolactone, flutamide, and cyproterone acetate inhibit androgen binding to its receptors. Spironolactone is an aldosterone antagonist, which also interacts with the androgen receptor. Spironolactone does cause more frequent menses, but this can be controlled with an oral contraceptive. Flutamide is more expensive and more hepatotoxic. Cyproterone acetate is a potent progestin as well as an antiandrogen. It is available in Europe and Canada but not in the United States.

Finasteride prevents conversion of testosterone to DHT by inhibiting 5α-reductase. Finasteride should not be given to women who can become pregnant because in animal studies it causes ambiguous genitalia in male offspring.

It is easier to suppress new hair growth than to eradicate established hirsutism. Most patients have some response to medical therapy, but this can take months to develop. All medications have dose-related side effects, so low-dose combined therapy may be better than high-dose monotherapy. Scoring systems to monitor treatment have been devised, but these are subjective or difficult to carry out accurately. It is just as helpful to ask whether a patient requires less shaving, plucking, waxing, or electrolysis to remove unwanted hair.

Hormonal Contraception

MECHANISMS OF ACTION

Hormonal contraception involves regular administration of estrogen, progestin, or both to prevent pregnancy, either by preventing ovulation or by creating an unfavorable climate for fertilization and implantation within the reproductive tract. A combination of estrogen and a progestin is usually given orally. The estrogen component suppresses pituitary FSH secretion by negative feedback. This prevents development of a dominant follicle, thereby suppressing ovulation. Estrogen also increases the number of progesterone receptors, making the progesterone component more effective. Cyclic estrogen also stabilizes the endometrium to prevent irregular bleeding.

Oral Contraceptives

The **estrogen** component suppresses FSH secretion and increases progesterone receptors. The **progestin** component suppresses LH secretion, decreases fallopian tube motility, opposes estrogen action on the endometrium, and decreases and thickens cervical mucus.

Naturally occurring estrogens are ineffective when given orally because they are metabolized rapidly by the liver. Synthetic ethinyl estradiol is used in almost all combined oral contraceptive preparations. The dose of ethinyl estradiol has fallen almost fivefold since oral contraceptives were introduced in the 1960s, and today women rarely take more than 35 mcg/d.

The progesterone component of contraceptives acts at several levels. Progesterone suppresses pituitary LH secretion, which inhibits ovulation. Progesterone decreases fallopian tube motility, limiting the ability of a fertilized ovum to progress into the endometrial cavity and implant. Progesterone prevents estrogen-induced hyperplasia of the endometrium, making the uterine lining unfavorable for implantation of the fertilized ovum. Progesterone also causes cervical mucous to be tenacious and thick, which prevents sperm from penetrating into the endometrial cavity.

Progesterone-only contraceptives offer hormonal contraception without exposure to estrogen. Progesterone does not suppress FSH, so estrogen levels are not suppressed, and ovulation occurs in some women. Contraception depends on the effects of progesterone on cervical mucus and on the endometrium.

Progesterone contraception can be given orally, intramuscularly, or in subcutaneous depot form. Naturally occurring progesterone is metabolized rapidly by the liver when given orally, but many synthetic forms of progesterone are available. The newest progestins have very potent contraceptive action but have less androgen activity and fewer masculinizing side effects than the progestins originally used.

Progesterone provides highly effective contraception for 3 months when given intramuscularly. When placed subcutaneously in pellets, progesterone is effective for up to 5 years. Progesterone can also be administered via a progesterone-impregnated intrauterine device or a vaginal ring. Resumption of regular ovulation may be delayed following use of depot forms of progesterone, so these should not be used in women who want only short-term contraception. Progesterone antagonists such as mifepristone, which produce a hostile environment for pregnancy by blocking the effects of progesterone on the uterus, are not available in the United States.

Long-acting GnRH agonists initially stimulate FSH and LH secretion but then down-regulate GnRH receptors. Secretion of FSH and

LH is suppressed and ovulation is inhibited. GnRH agonists are effective but expensive, and prolonged use of this therapy alone results in a continuous low estrogen state with deleterious effects on bone mass.

Most women take pills containing both estrogen and progesterone for 21 days each month. This interval is followed by 7 days with no medication to allow withdrawal bleeding. Fixed dose pills provide the same dose of estrogen and progesterone each day for 21 days. Variable dose pills alter the estrogen or progesterone doses every 10 days or every 7 days to minimize side effects while maintaining contraception. Emergency postcoital contraception requires a large dose of estrogen or combined estrogen and progestin, which probably prevents implantation.

SIDE EFFECTS

Many side effects of oral contraceptives are related to metabolic effects on the liver. Oral estrogen results in increased hepatic synthesis of clotting factors II and X and plasminogen and decreased synthesis of antithrombin. Estrogens also increase platelet aggregation (prostacyclin production is reduced). Since aging and cigarette smoking also result in a more hypercoagulable state, the risk of thromboembolic events caused by exogenous estrogen increases markedly in women over age 35 who smoke. The risk of cerebrovascular disease and myocardial infarction is also higher in this group. Women with a previous history of thrombophlebitis are usually not given oral estrogen.

Contraindications to Estrogen-Containing Oral Contraceptives

Previous thromboembolic disease
Estrogen-sensitive malignancy
Known or suspected pregnancy
Unexplained vaginal bleeding
Smoking over age 35

Estrogen causes mild fluid retention, nausea, headache or breast pain in some women. Estrogen increases plasma renin activity and salt and water retention, which exacerbates hypertension. Estrogen decreases low-density lipoprotein (LDL) cholesterol and increases high-density lipoprotein (HDL) cholesterol levels, which is beneficial, but estrogen also increases triglyceride and very low-density lipoprotein (VLDL) synthesis, which can exacerbate underlying hypertriglyceridemia. Estrogen reduces bile flow and can cause cholestasis.

Progestins cause weight gain, and some women experience progestin-induced depression and fatigue. Older progestins decrease HDL cholesterol, but newer progestins with little androgen activity have less effect. Progesterone-only regimens are associated with irregular menstrual bleeding. Oral contraceptives cause a mild, often transient, increase in insulin resistance similar to that seen in pregnancy (see Chapter 15).

Most studies show no effect of oral contraceptives on breast cancer and a protective effect on cancer of the ovary and the endometrium. The effect on cervical cancer is uncertain.

The estrogen component of most pills is the same, but many progestins with different androgenic and metabolic side effects are available. Minor side effects of oral contraceptives are most pronounced during the first two cycles. Adjustments in the balance of estrogen and progestin and in the type of progestin should not be made until a period for acclimation has passed. Most women eventually find an oral contraceptive that works well for them.

Menopause

Menopause is the permanent cessation of menses, which occurs when the ovaries can no longer produce estrogen due to exhaustion of ovarian follicles. As indicated above, oocyte depletion is a lifelong process. Subtle ovulatory dysfunction is common after the age of 30, and fertility drops markedly as ovulation becomes less frequent after the age of 40. The follicular phase of the menstrual cycle becomes shorter, levels of FSH increase as estrogen production drops, and luteal phase defects become more and more frequent. Irregular uterine bleeding is common. Uterine bleeding may decrease due to decreased estrogen production or increase if the remaining estrogen action is not opposed by adequate progesterone production during anovulatory cycles.

The *climacteric* is the entire period during which estrogen production is decreasing, starting with the first decrease in ovulation frequency and ending with generalized atrophy of all estrogen-sensitive

---

CASE STUDY: *CONTINUED*

At the age of 33, Ms. Martin's menstrual flow became lighter and more irregular. She returned to the clinic at the age of 34 having had no menses for 8 months. She was running approximately 14 miles per week. She complained of fatigue and episodes of feeling too warm. Her libido had not changed, but intercourse had become painful because of vaginal dryness.

Her height was 5'6" and her weight was 120 lb. Her blood pressure was 110/60 mm Hg, and her heart rate was 60 beats/min. Significant findings during her physical examination included dry skin and a slightly enlarged thyroid gland. Her breast examination was normal. Her pelvic examination revealed atrophic vaginal mucosa, scant cervical mucous, which did not fern, and a normal uterus. Her ovaries were not palpable. A pregnancy test was negative. TSH and PRL levels were within normal limits. A progestin challenge was not followed by withdrawal bleeding.

tissues. Menopause is the specific point in time during the climacteric at which cessation of menses occurs.

If lack of menses is the diagnostic criterion, menopause can be ascertained only in retrospect. Usually the diagnosis is made after 6 to 12 months of amenorrhea in a woman who is over 45 years of age. A serum FSH level that is markedly elevated due to lack of estrogen feedback helps to confirm the diagnosis. The average age of menopause in the United States is 52 years. In general, menopause occurs later in obese women who have higher estrogen levels due to conversion of androgens to estrogen in body fat. Menopause occurs earlier in women who smoke cigarettes, perhaps because they tend to be thinner.

Ovarian failure is considered premature if menopause occurs prior to the age of 35. This can be caused by an autoimmune process directed at some component of the ovarian follicles or by radiation or chemotherapy. Often the cause is unknown.

EARLY CONSEQUENCES OF ESTROGEN DEPLETION

Episodes of vasomotor instability called hot flashes, or hot flushes, occur in 70% to 80% of women during the perimenopausal period (Table 12-8). Women note sudden onset of flushing involving the head, neck, and chest. This is accompanied by a sensation of intense body heat, which is followed by perspiration. The core temperature increases by approximately 0.2°C, which elicits reflex vasodilatation followed by sweating. The heart rate increases slightly, and some women complain of palpitations. The duration of these episodes is highly variable. The flush lasts from a few minutes to an hour. Some women experience hot flashes for less than 1 year; others have hot flashes for 5 to 10 years. The severity of the associated symptoms ranges from barely noticeable to incapacitating.

Hot flashes are caused by the declining estrogen level at menopause, which somehow stimulates central thermoregulatory centers.

It is the declining estrogen level that stimulates central thermoregulatory centers and release of GnRH. Women who have always been estrogen deficient do not have hot flashes unless estrogen replacement is

Table 12-8. Consequences of Estrogen Depletion

EARLY CONSEQUENCES		LONG-TERM CONSEQUENCES
Vasomotor instability (hot flashes)	Urogenital atrophy	Loss of bone mass
Flushing	Atrophic vaginitis and cystitis	Osteoporotic fractures
Sweating	Painful intercourse	Increased central obesity
Increased heart rate	Thin skin that is less firm	
Sleep disturbance and fatigue	Decreased axillary and pubic hair	

withdrawn. Hot flashes are correlated with surges in serum LH levels, but LH secretion is not the cause of vasomotor instability. Women with a surgically absent hypothalamus do not produce LH, but they still experience hot flashes. GnRH agonists given continuously down-regulate GnRH receptors and suppress LH release but do not affect the incidence of hot flashes.

Hot flashes are frequently nocturnal. They cause sleep disturbances by rousing a woman completely or by altering her sleep state and limiting the adequacy of her sleep time. The sleep disruption is thought to be responsible for much of the fatigue, irritability, and depression experienced by some women at the time of the menopause. Hot flashes seem to be more severe in women who undergo surgical oophorectomy and have a rapid decline in estrogen levels as compared to women who undergo gradual ovarian decline with aging.

Estrogen depletion also causes urogenital atrophy. Many women develop atrophic urethritis and cystitis, with itching and burning and sometimes urinary frequency and incontinence. Vulvar and vaginal atrophy along with decreased mucus production can result in burning, itching, painful intercourse, and vaginal bleeding related to a thin epithelium. Skin and hair are also affected by estrogen depletion. Skin becomes thinner and more wrinkled, and axillary and pubic hair become sparser.

LONG-TERM CONSEQUENCES OF ESTROGEN DEPLETION

In premenopausal women, estrogen exerts a protective effect on bone mass (see Table 12-8). Estrogen suppresses parathyroid hormone-induced cytokine release by mononuclear cells, which decreases cytokine-mediated activation of osteoclasts. After the loss of estrogen at menopause, bone turnover increases and osteoclasts dig more and deeper resorption cavities, which are not filled completely by osteoblasts. Estrogen deficiency is responsible for 75% of bone loss within the first 15 years of menopause. Thereafter, most bone loss occurs due to the aging process. Trabecular bone is more vulnerable to estrogen depletion than cortical bone, but both decrease markedly during the first decade after menopause. The loss of bone mass is associated with increased risk of fractures of the wrist, spine, and hip (see Chapter 7).

In premenopausal women, estrogen acts on endothelium and vascular smooth muscle to increase vasodilatation and blood flow. These effects are lost after menopause. Loss of estrogen results in lower HDL cholesterol and higher LDL cholesterol levels. After menopause women lose lean body mass. They develop more central obesity, which is associated with increased insulin resistance and with increased atherosclerotic vascular disease.

HORMONAL TREATMENT OF MENOPAUSE

Estrogen replacement therapy after menopause decreases the vasomotor symptoms associated with hot flashes and reduces the symptoms and signs of urogenital atrophy. Estrogen replacement also helps stabilize bone mass and prevents osteoporotic fractures (see Chapter 7). Lower doses of estrogen are used for hormone replacement now than in the past. The dose of estrogen required for vasomotor symptom relief and osteoporosis prevention is almost sixfold lower than the estrogen content in the lowest dose oral contraceptives. Circulating estrogen levels during hormone replacement therapy (HRT) are similar to the lowest estrogen levels during a typical menstrual cycle.

Unopposed estrogen replacement causes hyperplasia of the endometrium, which advances to adenocarcinoma in a small number of women. A progestin is added to stabilize the endometrium and prevent hyperplasia unless a woman has had a hysterectomy.

Estrogen and progesterone can be given continuously or intermittently. If given intermittently, withdrawal bleeding occurs when the progestin is withdrawn. Continuous combined therapy results in endometrial atrophy and cessation of uterine bleeding after 1 year in most women, but breakthrough bleeding occurs during the initial months.

Earlier observational and case-control studies indicated that postmenopausal women who took HRT had a lower risk of heart disease and strokes. However, the Heart and Estrogen/Progestin Replacement Study (HERS), a randomized, controlled trial in women with pre-existing heart disease, showed more early cardiovascular events in women treated with HRT. The Women's Health Initiative (WHI), a very large, randomized, controlled trial of HRT in postmenopausal women, most of whom did not have heart disease, also showed no reduction in cardiovascular risk. Combined HRT was associated with more venous thromboembolic events and strokes and, after 4 to 5 years, an increase in invasive breast cancer. Women taking HRT had fewer hip fractures and a lower risk of colorectal cancer. The number of events was small, and there was no difference in mortality in women given HRT versus placebo. Nevertheless, the combined HRT arm of the WHI was stopped early, after 5 years. The increased risks were not observed in women treated only with estrogen because they had had a hysterectomy. This stydy arm also has been stopped.

At this time HRT is recommended only for women with troubling vasomotor symptoms, which often abate within 2 to 3 years after menopause. HRT is contraindicated for women with a history of venous thromboembolism, atherosclerotic vascular disease, or breast cancer and for women who have a first degree relative with breast cancer. Women with persistent vasomotor symptoms or risk for osteoporosis who cannot tolerate other therapies (see Chapter 7) must weigh the risks and benefits of continuing HRT on an individual basis.

Postmenopausal HRT is available in oral, transdermal, and intravaginal forms. Vaginal estrogen preparations or nonestrogen lubricants may be sufficient for women who want relief only for urogenital symptoms. Whether transdermal HRT and oral estrogens and progestins other than those used in the WHI have the same risks is not known.

CASE STUDY: *RESOLUTION*

Ms. Martin's symptoms and signs indicated new estrogen deficiency, which was confirmed by absence of withdrawal bleeding after a progestin challenge. Her FSH and LH levels were very high, in the postmenopausal range, indicating loss of almost all ovarian follicles. Her episodes of feeling too warm probably were hot flashes. The cause of her premature ovarian failure is not certain, but a familial autoimmune disorder is likely in view of her mother's autoimmune thyroid disease and early menopause.

Ms. Martin was started on daily estradiol and was given progesterone for 10 days/month to counteract the effects of estrogen on the endometrium. On this regimen she had regular withdrawal bleeding. Her fatigue improved, and her episodes of warmth, vaginal dryness, and discomfort during intercourse disappeared. She agreed to have a pelvic examination and a mammogram each year. She was particularly concerned about preventing osteoporotic fractures because demineralization and stress fractures in her left foot had been noted years before during her intense exercise. She planned to continue her current level of exercise and to increase her calcium intake.

Selective estrogen receptor modulators (SERMs) are synthetic compounds that take advantage of the different milieu around estrogen receptors in different tissues. They function as estrogen agonists in bone but do not stimulate the uterus or the breast. The SERM raloxifene decreases vertebral fractures but not hip fractures. Raloxifene causes hot flashes and, like estrogen, increases the risk for venous thromboembolism.

Phytoestrogens are weak estrogen agonists derived from plants (soy and others). They reduce vasomotor symptoms in some women but have not been shown to reduce osteoporotic fractures. Long-term safety and efficacy of these compounds is not known.

Ovarian androgen production also decreases after menopause. Testosterone replacement improves libido, sexual function, and bone mass in women who have undergone bilateral oophorectomy, but long-term safety is unknown.

REVIEW QUESTIONS

Directions: For each of the following questions, choose the *one best* answer.

Questions 1 and 2

A young woman, Anita G., comes to the clinic for a physical examination in order to obtain health insurance.

1 Based on her history of regular menses, it is most likely that she is in the *late proliferative phase* of her menstrual cycle. If so the physician would expect her to have

A a high progesterone level, proliferative endometrium, and a suppressed luteinizing hormone (LH) level

B a high progesterone level, secretory endometrium, and a developing corpus luteum

C low estrogen and progesterone levels, many follicles developing, and a rising follicle-stimulating hormone (FSH) level

D a high estrogen level, a well-developed dominant follicle, and a rising LH level

E a low estrogen level, a well-developed corpus luteum, and a high FSH level

2 Several months later Ms. G. returns to the clinic having had no menses for 6 weeks. Her pregnancy test is positive. If her pregnancy is to develop normally, which of the following must occur?

A The pituitary must secrete high levels of human chorionic gonadotropin (HCG) to sustain the corpus luteum

B The placenta must secrete high levels of LH and FSH to sustain the ovary

C The corpus luteum must secrete high levels of progesterone to sustain the endometrium

D The placenta must secrete high levels of estrogen to sustain the fetal pituitary

E The pituitary must secrete high levels of prolactin to sustain the placenta

3 An 18-year-old woman has never had a menstrual period. Her vagina and uterus are patent. A pregnancy test is negative. Thyroid function and the prolactin (PRL) level are normal. No bleeding follows a progesterone challenge test. Based on this information, the physician is certain that

A her LH level is high but her FSH level is low

B her müllerian duct inhibitory hormone level is high

C her human chorionic gonadotropin (HCG) level is high

D her estrogen level is low

E her gonadotropin-releasing hormone (GnRH) pulse generator is abnormal

4 Jennifer L. is a 32-year-old woman who had normal menstrual periods until she developed amenorrhea 6 months ago. She complains of fatigue, frequent flu-like illnesses, dry skin, and vaginal dryness during intercourse. Cervical mucus is scant and does not fern. Laboratory evaluation revealed the following: follicle-stimulating hormone (FSH), 3 IU/L (normal: 3–20 IU/L); luteinizing hormone (LH),

7 IU/L (normal: 8–28 IU/L); estradiol, 90 pmol/L (normal: 108–360 pmol/L); testosterone, 15 ng/dL (normal: 20–80 ng/dL); free thyroxine, 0.4 ng/dL (normal: 0.7–1.81 ng/dL); and thyroid stimulating hormone (TSH), 1 μU/mL (normal: 0.5–6.0 μU/mL). The most likely cause for her amenorrhea is

A congenital adrenal hyperplasia (CAH)
B a large pituitary tumor
C primary hypothyroidism
D GnRH failure due to stress
E chromosomal XO/XX mosaic

5 Sara T. is a 22-year-old woman who has always had irregular menstrual bleeding. She has had acne, increased hair on her upper lip and chin, and a male escutcheon (hair extending from pubis to umbilicus) for several years. She has no temporal balding or clitoromegaly. Laboratory tests reveal the following: luteinizing hormone (LH), 25 IU/L (normal: 8–28 IU/L); follicle-stimulating hormone (FSH), 6 IU/L (normal: 3–20 IU/L); free testosterone, modestly elevated; 17α-hydroxyprogesterone, normal; and dehydroepiandrosterone sulfate (DHEAS), normal. She most likely has

A polycystic ovary syndrome (PCOS)
B an adrenal androgen-producing tumor
C congenital adrenal hyperplasia (CAH)
D an ovarian androgen-producing tumor
E testicular feminization (testosterone receptor deficiency)

6 Julia R. consults her physician because an evaluation for infertility indicates that she has polycystic ovary syndrome (PCOS). Which of the following factors is consistent with this diagnosis?

A Decreased insulin resistance
B Morbid obesity due to high progesterone production
C Bone loss due to constant estrogen and androgen secretion
D Increased luteinizing hormone (LH) pulses and ovulation frequency
E Endometrial hyperplasia due to chronic estrogen secretion

Questions 7 and 8

Marion Z. is a previously healthy 52-year-old woman who has had no menses for 9 months. She is experiencing hot flashes and disturbed sleep and asks about hormone replacement therapy.

7 Further evaluation is most likely to reveal

A high levels of follicle-stimulating hormone (FSH) and luteinizing hormone (LH)

B 50% of her ovarian follicles remain

C absent gonadotropin-releasing hormone (GnRH) pulses

D a low estrogen but a high progesterone level

8 Risks and benefits of hormone replacement therapy for Ms Z. include which of the following?

A High incidence of urethritis and more vaginal atrophy

B Lower osteoporosis risk but higher risk of venous thromboembolism

C Higher level of low-density lipoprotein (LDL) cholesterol and lower level of high-density lipoprotein (HDL) cholesterol

D Fewer hot flashes but more sleep disturbance

E Restoration of regular cycles and fertility

References

Baird DT, Glasier AF: Hormonal contraception. *New Engl J Med* 328: 1543–1549, 1993.

Dunair A: Insulin action in the polycystic ovary syndrome. *Endocrinol Metab Clin North Am* 28: 341–359, 1999.

Gruber CJ, Tschugguel W, Schneeberger C, Huber JC: Production and actions of estrogens. *N Engl J Med* 346: 340–352, 2002.

Haseltine FP, Wentz AC, Redmond GP, et al (eds). Proceedings of a symposium. An NICHD conference: androgens and women's health. *Am J Med* 98 (suppl 1A): 1S–143S, 1995.

Hulley S, Grady D, Bush T, et al: Randomized trial of estrogen plus progestin for secondary prevention of coronary heart disease in postmenopausal women. Heart and estrogen/progestin replacement study (HERS) research group. *JAMA* 280: 605–613, 1998.

Kronenberg F, Fugh-Berman A: Complementary and alternative medicine for menopausal symptoms: a review of randomized, controlled trials. *Ann Int Med* 137: 805–813, 2002.

Murkies AL, Wilcox G, Davis SR: Phytoestrogens. *J Clin Endocrinol Metab* 83: 297–303, 1998.

Prior JC: Perimenopause: the complex endocrinology of the menopausal transition. *Endocr Rev* 19: 397–428, 1998.

Rittmaster RS: Medical treatment of androgen-dependent hirsutism. *J Clin Endocrinol Metab* 80: 2559–2563, 1995.

Seibert C, Barbouche E, Fagan J, et al: Prescribing oral contraceptives for women older than 35 years of age. *Ann Int Med* 138: 4–64, 2003

Shifren JL, Braunstein GD, Simon JA, et al: Transdermal testosterone treatment in women with impaired sexual function after oophorectomy. *N Engl J Med* 343: 682–688, 2000.

Riggs BL, Hartmann LC: Selective estrogen-receptor modulators— mechanisms of action and application to clinical practice. *N Engl J Med* 348: 618–629, 2003.

Taylor AE: Polycystic ovary syndrome. *Endocrinol Metab Clin North Am* 27: 877–902, 1998.

Notes

Vandenbroucke JP, Rosing J, Bloemenkamp S, et al: Oral contraceptives and the risk of venous thrombosis. *N Engl J Med* 344: 1527–1535, 2001.

Writing Group for the Women's Health Initiative Investigators: Risks and benefits of estrogen and progestin in healthy postmenopausal women. *JAMA* 288: 321–222, 2002.

13

Growth

Erica A. Eugster, M.D., and Joseph J. Sockalosky, M.D.

▪ CHAPTER OUTLINE ▪

▪ LEARNING OBJECTIVES ▪

At the completion of this chapter, the student will:
1. be aware of important growth parameters and the use of standardized growth charts.
2. understand the concept of growth velocity and its importance in evaluation of growth.
3. understand the different phases of growth and the primary endocrine mediators of each phase.
4. understand the role of growth hormone and insulin-like growth factors in the promotion of linear growth.
5. recognize normal variants of growth that result in short stature.
6. understand the endocrine causes of short stature and tall stature in children and the approaches to treatment.

303

> ## Case Study 1: *Introduction*
>
> A 6-year-old boy is referred to the growth clinic for evaluation of short stature. Six months ago his height was measured at 102 cm (less than the 5th percentile), and his weight was 16 kg. He has always been healthy. His birth history, growth, and development have reportedly been normal. Family history reveals that the mother is 5′1″ tall and had menarche at 13.5 years. The father is 5′5″ and entered puberty at an "average" age. Physical examination reveals a normally proportioned boy with a height of 105 cm (thus his growth velocity is 3 cm in 6 mo = 6 cm/yr), weight of 17 kg, and no abnormal findings.

Growth Parameters

Growth is a complex process resulting from the dynamic interaction of numerous factors, both endocrine and nonendocrine. An aberration in growth may be the first or only manifestation of a pathologic process. Body size and proportions have an important impact on an individual's psychological health and well-being.

Careful measurement and plotting of growth parameters on a standardized growth chart (Fig. 13-1) at regular intervals are essential components of pediatric care. Height and weight are measured throughout childhood and adolescence. Head circumference is usually measured only during the first 3 years of life.

Height

Of all growth parameters, height is the one most affected by endocrine abnormalities. The most important factor in the evaluation of linear growth is the *growth velocity*, or rate of growth over time.

A **normal growth velocity** implies that there is no pathologic process interfering with growth.

Weight

Failure to thrive and obesity are the extremes of abnormal weight in children.

Failure to Thrive

Poor weight gain in infancy and early childhood is termed failure to thrive. The causes are many and are usually not endocrine; two exceptions are adrenal insufficiency and hyperthyroidism. Most cases of failure to thrive can be accounted for by malnutrition, chronic disease, congenital anomalies, or psychosocial deprivation (Table 13-1).

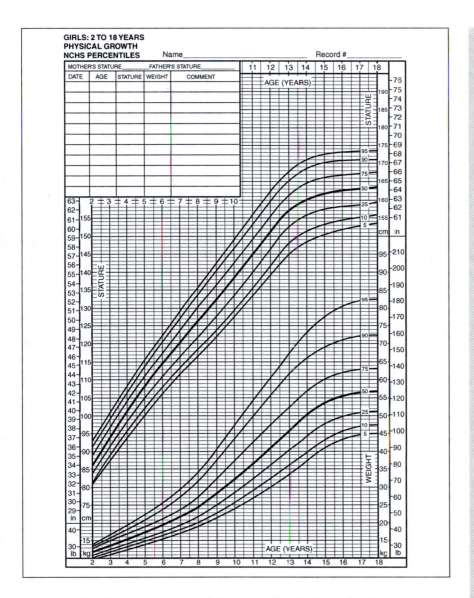

Fig. 13-1. Example of Standardized Growth Chart

NCHS = National Center for Health Statistics.

Obesity

An imbalance between energy intake and energy utilization results in obesity. In most cases obesity is due to a combination of genetic and environmental factors (so-called exogenous obesity), rather than to hormonal imbalance or disease process (Table 13-1). Children with exogenous obesity often have a strong family history of obesity.

Obese children generally have tall stature, but the weight percentile is higher than the height percentile. These children may have lower energy needs or "slower metabolism" than the general population, but even if this is true, they consume more calories than their bodies require. In the case of very young children, caretakers are providing them with these calories.

Table 13-1. Major Causes of Abnormal Weight in Children

FAILURE TO THRIVE	OBESITY
Malnutrition	**Exogenous obesity**
Inadequate intake	**Syndromes**
Malabsorption	Prader-Willi
Gastroesophageal reflux	Lawrence Moon Biedl
Chronic disease	**Hormonal abnormalities**
Cystic fibrosis	Glucocorticoid excess
Congenital heart disease	Polycystic ovarian syndrome
Inborn errors of metabolism	Pseudohypoparathyroidism
Congenital anomalies	**Hypothalamic lesions**
Chromosomal abnormalities	
Syndromes	
Neurologic disorders	
Psychosocial deprivation	
Hormonal	
Hyperthyroidism	
Adrenal insufficiency	

Notes

First Law of Thermodynamics

$\Delta U = Q - W$

ΔU = stored energy (fat)

Q = intake (calories consumed)

W = work (calories burned)

Obesity is also seen in association with a number of genetic syndromes. Affected individuals tend to have short stature, dysmorphic features, hypogonadism, or mental retardation. Examples of such syndromes include Prader-Willi and Lawrence-Moon-Biedl syndromes.

Obesity in childhood is rarely due to a hormonal disorder other than glucocorticoid excess. Growth hormone (GH) deficiency and thyroid hormone deficiency usually do not result in significant obesity. Endocrine causes of obesity in children are usually associated with decreased linear growth.

Short or poorly growing obese children are more likely to have an endocrine disorder or a syndrome than are tall or normally growing obese children.

Obesity can be due to a hypothalamic abnormality. In these cases overeating is thought to be due to a lesion in the satiety center in the brain. Both congenital and acquired conditions cause this kind of obesity.

HEAD CIRCUMFERENCE

Growth of the head is determined primarily by growth of the brain, which requires adequate nutrition and a favorable environment (normal calvarium and sutures, blood flow, and oxygen). Hormones such as thyroid hormone are important for brain differentiation and development but not brain size. Microcephaly and macrocephaly represent the two extremes of head size.

Microcephaly is defined as head size >2 standard deviations (SD) below the mean head size for age. It is often associated with structural or functional abnormalities of the brain and reduced intellectual potential. *Macrocephaly* is defined as head size >2 SD above the mean head size for age. The major causes of abnormal head size are listed in Table 13-2.

Microcephaly = head size >2 SD below the mean for age
Macrocephaly = head size >2 SD above the mean for age

BONE AGE

A bone age x-ray is used to determine skeletal maturation, which is then compared to chronologic age. An x-ray of the left hand and wrist is matched to standardized radiographs representing different ages for boys and girls (Fig. 13-2). An x-ray of the hemiskeleton is used in the first 1 to 2 years of life. Normal bone age (bone age = chronologic age) implies absence of a pathologic process affecting growth.

In children over the age of 7, adult height can be predicted by using a **bone age x-ray** with the current height.

Table 13-2. Causes of Abnormal Head Circumference

MICROCEPHALY	MACROCEPHALY
Genetic factors	**Hydrocephalus**
Chromosomal abnormalities	**Infection**
syndromes	Abscess
Intrauterine factors	Subdural effusion
Exposure to toxins	**Toxic or metabolic factors**
infection	Lead
Perinatal or postnatal insult	Hypervitaminosis A
Ischemia	Mucopolysaccharidosis
Trauma	**Trauma**
Infection	Subdural hematoma
Severe malnutrition	Hygroma
	Congenital anomalies
	Syndromes
	Familial

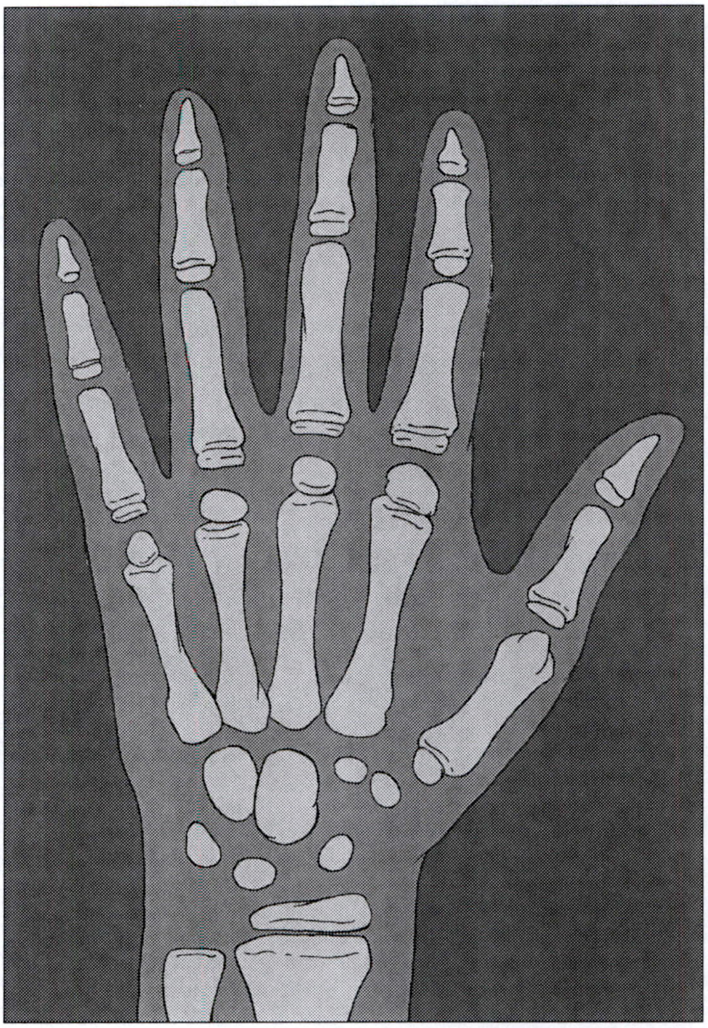

Fig. 13-2. Example of Bone Age X-Ray

This is the standard for girls aged 5 years, 9 months.

Phases of Growth

Linear growth can be thought of as occurring in three distinct phases—prenatal, postnatal, and pubertal—each of which has unique characteristics.

PRENATAL GROWTH

Growth of the fetus is influenced by genetic make-up, environmental conditions, and the hormonal milieu (Table 13-3).

Genetic Factors

Genetic factors include race and gender, parental size, and chromosomal abnormalities. Genetic forces tend to be more important after birth than during the prenatal period.

Table 13-3. Major Influences on Linear Fetal Growth

Genetic factors	**Hormones**
Intrauterine environment	Insulin
Placental function	Insulin-like growth factor I (IGF-I)
Multiple gestation	IGF-II
Infection	IGF-binding proteins
Exposure to toxins and teratogens	Chorionic somatomammotropin
Maternal factors	Other growth factors
Body size	
Parity	
Nutrition and general health	
Smoking	

Environmental Factors

Environmental influences are the result of combined maternal and intrauterine forces. Maternal nutrition, alcohol use, smoking, and infections and other diseases have a strong impact on size at birth. The size of the mother is more important than the size of the father. This is also true in other species. For example, when Shetland ponies are bred with Shire horses, the foal size is average for Shetlands if the mother is a Shetland pony. The foal size is average for Shires if the mother is a Shire horse (Fig. 13-3).

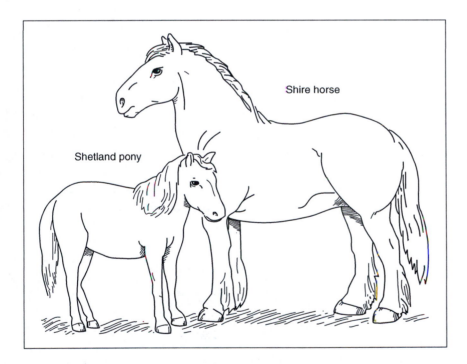

Fig. 13-3. The Effect of Maternal Size on Birth Weight was Demonstrated by Breeding Shetland Ponies and Shire Horses

Foal size is average for Shetlands if the mother is a Shetland pony. Foal size is average for Shires if the mother is a Shire horse.

Hormones and Growth Factors

Our understanding of growth factors is expanding rapidly. As the list of known growth factors increases, so does our appreciation of the complexity of their actions and interactions in the promotion of growth. Hormones that are known to have a major impact on fetal somatic growth include insulin and insulin-like growth factors I and II (IGF-I and IGF-II).

In general, hormones that are essential for normal linear growth after birth (thyroid hormone, GH, and others) do not have a significant role in the somatic growth of the fetus. However, these hormones have other important functions in fetal development. Thyroid hormone plays an important role in central nervous system (CNS) development and skeletal maturation. Glucocorticoids are necessary for pulmonary maturation, and androgens are essential for normal male sexual differentiation. Metabolic effects of GH are listed in Table 13-4.

Insulin

Insulin exerts its influence through a number of anabolic actions, primarily in the last trimester of pregnancy (Table 13-4). The importance of insulin is demonstrated by situations of insulin deficiency and excess. Infants with pancreatic agenesis have intrauterine growth retardation. Infants with leprechaunism (Donahue syndrome) have an abnormal insulin receptor, resulting in lack of insulin action and severe growth retardation. These infants are short, with a skinny, wizened appearance as a result of a lack of subcutaneous fat. In contrast, infants born to diabetic mothers have macrosomia due to excess fetal insulin, which is secreted in response to the increase in maternal glucose crossing the placenta.

Insulin-Like Growth Factors

IGF-I and IGF-II are potent growth-promoting polypeptides in the fetus independent of growth hormone. These proteins have striking structural homology to proinsulin, and they have insulin-like metabolic actions. IGF-I and IGF-II and their receptors are widely expressed in a variety of fetal tissues throughout gestation and are believed to have both autocrine and paracrine actions. Decreased placental expression of IGF-II has been found in animal studies of restricted fetal growth.

Table 13-4. Metabolic Effects of Insulin and Growth Hormone (GH)

	INSULIN	GH
Protein synthesis	Increases	Increases
IGF-I synthesis		Increases
Fat synthesis	Increases	Decreases
Lipolysis	Decreases	Increases
Glycogen synthesis	Increases	
Glycogenolysis	Decreases	Increases
Gluconeogenesis	Decreases	Increases

IGF-I promotes differentiation of many different tissue types. At birth, serum levels of IGF-I have been found to correlate with birth weight.

IGF Binding Proteins (IGFBPs)

The IGFs circulate 99% bound to a family of six IGFBPs, which have important regulatory effects on the IGF system. They prolong the plasma half-life of the IGFs, and by controlling the availability of the IGFs to their receptors, they act as a reservoir of growth factors. These binding proteins have been shown to augment or diminish the activity of the IGFs in vitro. IGFBP-1 levels are increased in infants with intrauterine growth retardation and have been found to be inversely correlated with birth weight. IGFBP-3 is the major binding protein for IGF-I in postnatal life.

Chorionic Somatomammotropin

The placental hormone chorionic somatomammotropin (CS), also known as human placental lactogen, has 96% homology to GH. Fetal size at birth is normal when this hormone is missing, but evidence points to a direct role for CS in the promotion of fetal growth. CS increases DNA synthesis in fetal fibroblasts, myoblasts, and hepatocytes. Serum concentrations of CS are correlated with the size of the placenta and with fetal insulin-like growth factor levels. In animal studies maternal malnutrition is associated with a decrease in the number of CS receptors in the fetal liver.

Other Growth Factors

Epidermal growth factor (EGF) and transforming growth factor α (TGFα) belong to a family of related growth factors that exert their effects through EGF receptors that are widely expressed in placental and fetal tissues. Although these growth factors are present in many tissues, their roles in human development are not well understood. Less well-characterized growth factors thought to be important in fetal growth include erythropoietin, fibroblast growth factor, nerve growth factor, platelet-derived growth factor, hematopoetic growth factor, and vascular endothelial growth factor.

Linear growth velocity in the fetus reaches a peak of 2.5 cm/week during the second trimester. If this were to continue, the linear growth rate would be more than 4 ft/yr.

POSTNATAL GROWTH: PREPUBERTAL

After birth, infants often change percentiles on the growth chart by accelerating upward or by shifting downward in order to reach their genetically programmed growth channel. This process is usually complete by 2 years of age. Once children establish their position on the growth chart, they grow at predictable rates throughout childhood and adolescence. Since minor fluctuations in growth are normal, measurements should be obtained at no less than 6-month intervals. Growth rates also show seasonal variations, with highest growth velocities occurring in the spring and summer.

From the age of 4 until puberty, children should grow at a rate of at least 4.5 cm/yr.

Nonendocrine Factors

Important nonendocrine influences during the growing years include genetics, nutrition, general health, and psychosocial factors.

Endocrine Factors

Endocrine factors influencing prepubertal growth include GH, IGF-1, thyroid hormone, and insulin.

Growth Hormone

After the first 6 to 9 months of life, growth hormone is the primary mediator of linear growth. GH is a 191–amino acid polypeptide hormone of 22 kD secreted by the somatotrophs of the anterior pituitary gland. The gene for GH is on chromosome 17. GH exists in both free and bound forms. In the bound form, it is coupled to growth hormone–binding protein (GHBP), which is identical in structure to the extracellular domain of the GH receptor.

Growth hormone secretion is controlled by both inhibitory and stimulatory factors and is modulated by feedback interactions within the GH axis (Fig. 13-4). The primary stimulus for GH secretion is the hypothalamic peptide GH-releasing hormone (GHRH).

Numerous other substances stimulate GH secretion including neurotransmitters, exercise, hypoglycemia, and sleep deprivation (Table 13-5). Growth hormone is secreted in pulsatile fashion, with the highest pulses occurring during sleep. The amplitude of the pulses increases during puberty (Fig. 13-5). The primary inhibitor of GH secretion is somatostatin (SS), also secreted by the hypothalamus.

Testing for **GH deficiency** involves administration of a substance known to stimulate GH release, such as clonidine, arginine, or L-dopa, with subsequent measurement of GH response.

GH has important physiologic effects on many different tissues. Primary sites of GH action are shown in Fig. 13-6. Direct metabolic consequences of GH action include production of IGF-I in liver and nonhepatic tissues, increased protein synthesis, lipolysis, and glucose

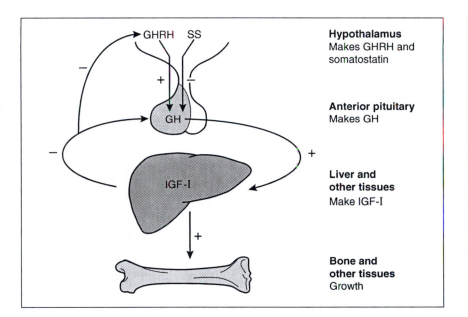

Fig. 13-4. Growth Hormone Feedback Regulation

GHRH = growth hormone–releasing hormone; SS = somatostatin; GH = growth hormone; IGF-I = insulin-like growth factor I.

transport. Growth hormone helps maintain normal blood sugar by stimulating hepatic gluconeogenesis and glycogenolysis (see Table 13-4). GH affects mineral metabolism, leading to increased sodium retention and increases in intracellular potassium, magnesium, and phosphorous. GH also increases skeleton and muscle mass. Many of the effects of GH occur via the IGF system.

Neonates with GH deficiency may present with hypoglycemia because GH is important in glucose homeostasis. Their size is normal, indicating the absence of GH effect on prenatal linear growth.

Table 13-5. Factors Regulating Production of Growth Hormone (GH) and Insulin-Like Growth Factor-1 (IGF-1)

STIMULATORS OF GH SECRETION	INHIBITORS OF GH SECRETION	INHIBITORS OF IGF-1 SECRETION	INHIBITORS OF IGF-1 ACTION
Deep sleep	Obesity	Malnutrition	IGF-1 receptor deficiency
α-Adrenergic stimulation	β-Adrenergic stimulation	Acute illness	
Fasting	High free fatty acids	Chronic illness	
Hypoglycemia	Hyperglycemia	GH receptor deficiency	
Amino acids	IGF-1 (negative feedback)	GH receptor antibodies	
Stress	Glucocorticoids		
Sex steroids	Hypothyroidism		

Note. Factors affecting GH secretion act at higher cortical centers and the hypothalamus. Factors affecting IGF-1 secretion act at the liver and other tissues.

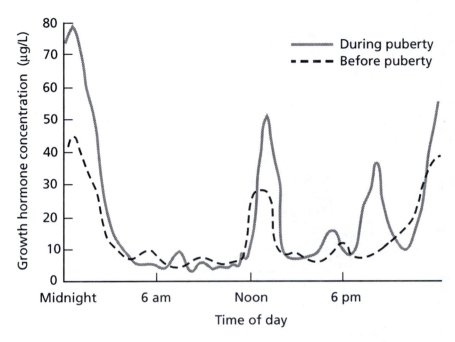

Fig. 13-5. Pulsatile Secretion of Growth Hormone (GH) in Prepubertal and Pubertal Males

This figure shows the highest pulses occurring during sleep, and increased pulse amplitude during puberty.

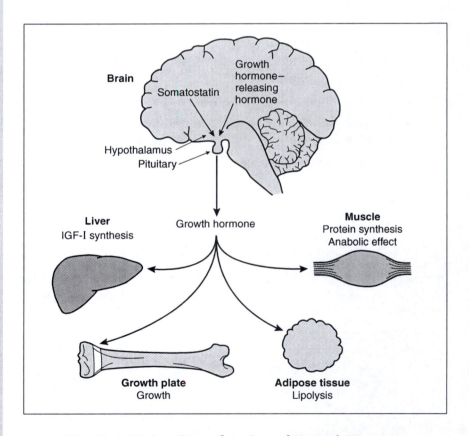

Fig. 13-6. Major Sites of Action of Growth Hormone

IGF-I = insulin-like growth factor I.

IGF-I and IGF-II

Postnatally, IGF-I and IGF-II are secreted in direct response to GH. These polypeptide growth factors have endocrine, paracrine, and autocrine actions. In addition, they exert negative feedback on the secretion of GH by acting at the pituitary and hypothalamus. Although GH levels fluctuate widely, the IGFs are present at sustained concentrations.

Serum levels of IGF-I rise slowly throughout childhood. IGF-I stimulates proliferation and differentiation of many different cell types. Together with GH, IGF-I stimulates skeletal growth directly by promoting differentiation and proliferation of chondrocytes within the growth plate. This process is thought to be initiated by the binding of GH to prechondrocytes, with subsequent production of IGF-I (Fig. 13-7). Levels of IGF-I are decreased by malnutrition and are altered by a variety of disease states (see Table 13-5). Because of its insulin-like actions, IGF-I can cause hypoglycemia when given acutely.

Serum levels of IGF-I and IGFBP-3 are strongly correlated with GH secretion and can be useful in the diagnosis of GH deficiency.

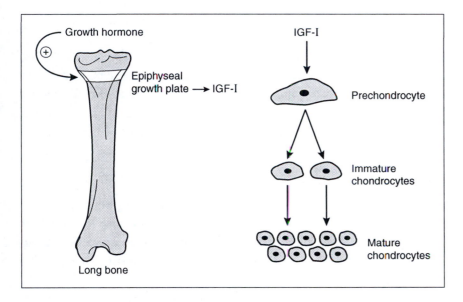

Fig. 13-7. Role of Growth Hormone (GH) and Insulin-Like Growth Factor-I (IGF-I) in the Differentiation and Proliferation of Chondrocytes in the Epiphyseal Growth Plate

GH interaction with its receptors in the epiphyseal growth plate results in increased IGF-I messenger RNA and increased IGF-I. Increased IGF-I stimulates proliferation and maturation of chondrocytes.

IGF-II has 70% homology with IGF-I. IGF-II also causes differentiation and proliferation of cells. Serum levels decrease progressively after birth, and its postnatal importance is uncertain.

Thyroid Hormone

Normal levels of thyroid hormone are essential for normal linear growth and skeletal maturation. The growth-promoting actions of thyroid hormone occur via permissive effects on the GH/IGF axis, as well as through direct effects of thyroid hormones at the level of the growth plates. Thyroid hormone and growth hormone have a synergistic effect on growth.

Major Factors Affecting Growth from Birth to Puberty

Nonendocrine	Endocrine
Genetics	Insulin
Nutrition	GH
Physical health	IGF-I
Psychosocial factors	Thyroid hormone

PUBERTAL GROWTH

The growth spurt of puberty is associated with an increase in the pulse amplitude of GH secretion and production of androgens and estrogens. Sex steroids increase the production of GH. Sex steroids also increase muscle mass, adipose tissue, and bone density and stimulate the development of primary and secondary sexual characteristics. By the end of puberty, boys have more lean tissue mass than girls, while girls have more adipose tissue mass than boys. Sex steroids also stimulate increased IGF-I production in cartilage and the maturation of osteoblasts. Estrogen is the hormone that is responsible for eventual fusion of the epiphyseal growth plates in both boys and girls. Thyroid hormone is also necessary for normal growth during puberty. The pubertal growth spurt occurs earlier in girls than in boys (see Chapter 14).

CESSATION OF GROWTH

Linear growth velocity gradually decreases after the pubertal growth spurt, and linear growth ceases when epiphyseal closure is complete. This occurs earlier in girls, who achieve approximately 95% of their adult height by the age of 13. Boys do not achieve approximately 95% of their adult height until the age of 14.5 years.

A child's final adult height can be estimated, if the heights of his or her parents are known, by calculating a mid-parental height range. Whether a child achieves or exceeds this range depends on the timing and rate of progression of puberty and the presence of any conditions that might have an adverse effect on growth. The earlier puberty occurs, and the more rapidly puberty progresses, the shorter the final adult height is likely to be.

Approximately 95% of total adult height has been reached when the bone age is 13 years in girls and 14.5 years in boys.

Short Stature

NORMAL VARIANTS

Many referrals to pediatric endocrine clinics are made for short stature. In most cases no pathologic cause for short stature can be identified. The most common causes for short stature are simply variations of normal growth for the population.

Genetic Short Stature

Children with genetic short stature have heights that are at or below the 3rd percentile for age. Their growth velocity is normal and their bone age is also normal (equal to chronologic age). The onset of puberty occurs at a normal age. Their parents are short. Children with genetic short stature achieve a final adult height that is short for the general population but normal for their families.

Midparental Height Range Calculation

Girls: ([father's height − 5″] + mother's height) ÷ 2 = mean adult height ± 2″

Boys: ([mothers height + 5″] + fathers height) ÷ 2 = mean adult height ± 2″

Constitutional Delay of Growth

Constitutional delay of growth is a common variation of normal growth. Children with constitutional delay have slow growth velocity during the first few years of life, causing them to shift downward on the growth chart to less than or equal to the 3rd percentile. Subsequent growth velocity is normal. Bone age is delayed. These

---

CASE STUDY 1: *RESOLUTION*

Previous growth data for the boy are plotted on the growth chart shown in (Fig. 13-8). His height has always been below the 3rd percentile. His growth velocity is normal, indicating that no pathologic process is present. If a bone age had been done, it would have been equal to his chronologic age. This child has genetic short stature. A mid-parental height range calculation indicates that his expected adult height is

$$([61 \text{ inches} + 5″] + 65.5″) ÷ 2 = 65.8″ ± 2″$$

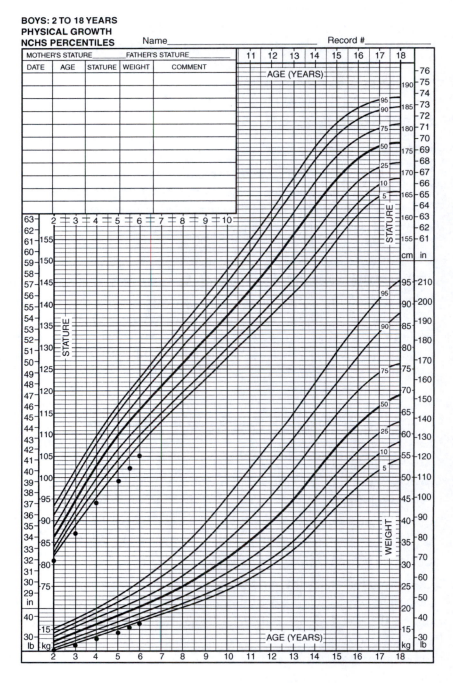

Fig. 13-8. Case Study 1 Growth Chart

NCHS = National Center for Health Statistics.

children enter puberty later than their peers, so they grow for a longer period of time. During puberty the growth spurt is normal, and their final adult height is within the normal range (Fig. 13.9). There is usually a history of a family member having been a "late bloomer." These children may have more psychological problems during adolescence than children with genetic short stature because they are both short and sexually immature for their age.

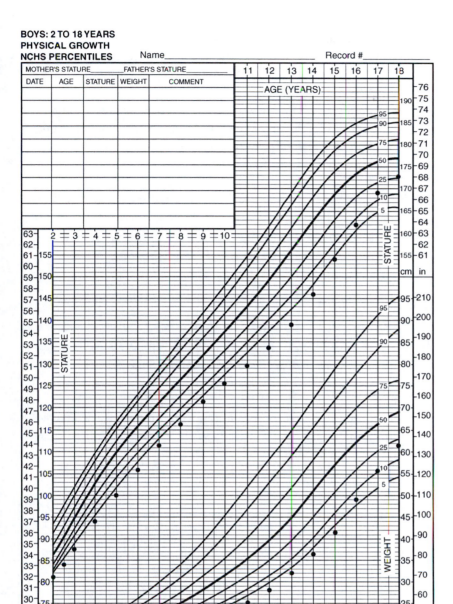

Fig. 13-9. Growth Chart of Patient with Constitutional Delay of Growth

Children typically are short and have delayed puberty. Final height is within the normal range. NCHS = National Center for Health Statistics.

NONENDOCRINE CAUSES

Chronic Disease

Any chronic disease or illness can interfere with normal growth. In some cases, linear growth failure is the initial manifestation or only manifestation of an underlying disorder. Examples of diseases that may be silent except for interfering with linear growth include inflammatory bowel disease, celiac sprue, renal insufficiency, and renal tubular acidosis.

Malnutrition

Nutritional deficiency is the most common cause for growth failure in the first 2 years of life. Poverty resulting in inadequate caloric intake is the most common cause of growth retardation worldwide.

If growth failure is due to malnutrition, the weight percentile decreases first. Linear growth is preserved initially but decreases as the chronicity and severity of malnutrition increases. Finally, the head circumference becomes affected.

Skeletal Dysplasia

Abnormal body proportions indicate that a skeletal dysplasia might be present. Over 100 different types of skeletal dysplasia have been identified. The most common are forms of achondroplasia.

Chromosomal Abnormalities and Syndromes

Many syndromes and chromosomal abnormalities are associated with short stature, including Down, Prader-Willi, Williams, Bloom, Russell-Silver, and Noonan syndromes.

CASE STUDY 2: INTRODUCTION AND RESOLUTION

Another 6-year-old boy is referred to the growth clinic for short stature. He has also been healthy. According to the mother, his birth history and development were normal, and his height was at the 50th percentile at 12 months of age, but he is now noticeably shorter than his peers. This child's recent growth data are not shown but look identical to those of the patient in case 1. Family history revealed that his mother is 5'3" tall and had late menarche at 17 years of age. His father is 5'9" and had onset of puberty at an "average" age. The physical examination is completely normal. A bone age x-ray reveals that his bone age is more than 2 SD below the mean for his chronologic age.

This child is shorter than his peers, but he appears healthy with no signs of systemic illness, hormone deficiency, or social deprivation. Although his height percentile shifted downward, his growth velocity is now normal for his delayed bone age. His family history indicates that his mother had constitutional delay of growth. It is likely that this child also has constitutional delay of growth. No treatment is needed. Counseling may be helpful later because of the expected delayed onset of sexual maturation compared with his peers.

Turner syndrome is an important cause of short stature in girls. Turner syndrome is due to a missing or abnormal X chromosome, which results in gonadal dysgenesis (ovaries are fibrous streaks) and ovarian failure (see Chapter 14). Because the phenotypic expression of Turner syndrome is extremely variable, a karyotype is required to make the diagnosis. The short stature of Turner syndrome is believed to be the result of haploinsufficiency of SHOX, a gene located on the short arm of the X chromosome.

Chromosome analysis is recommended for all girls with an abnormal growth velocity or height significantly below that expected for their families.

Intrauterine Growth Retardation

Intrauterine growth retardation is defined as a birth weight that is more than 2 SD below the mean adjusted for gestational age, race, and gender. Children with intrauterine growth retardation are a heterogeneous group with varied prognoses, depending on the cause and the time during gestation when the growth retardation occurred. Most "catch-up" growth, if any, takes place within the first 2 years after birth.

Psychosocial Dwarfism

Psychosocial dwarfism can be caused by emotional neglect (usually combined with poor nutrition) or by physical or psychological abuse. Children with psychosocial dwarfism have been shown to be GH deficient, but they have little response to treatment with GH. Their endocrine abnormalities usually disappear within a few days after they have been removed from a negative environment, and catch-up growth occurs.

ENDOCRINE CAUSES

Hypothyroidism

A decrease in linear growth is one of the most sensitive indicators of thyroid hormone deficiency in children. This may occur while other symptoms and signs of hypothyroidism are so subtle that they go unrecognized. If hypothyroidism develops after age 3, intellectual development is within normal limits. The most common cause of hypothyroidism in children is autoimmune thyroiditis (Hashimoto thyroiditis).

Thyroid function testing should be done in all children being evaluated for abnormal growth.

GH or IGF-I Deficiency

Congenital GH Deficiency. Congenital GH deficiency can be hereditary or can be due to structural abnormalities of the pituitary gland or other midline structures. Therefore, congenital GH deficiency can occur alone or in association with deficiencies of other pituitary hormones. Families with autosomal recessive, autosomal dominant, and X-linked GH deficiency have been found. Mutations in the pituitary transcription factors PIT-1 and PROP-1 typically result in combined pituitary hormone deficiencies. Examples of structural abnormalities include pituitary aplasia, pituitary hypoplasia, and septo-optic dysplasia. In some cases, the cause of congenital GH deficiency is unknown. Some of these cases might be due to deficiency of GHRH.

Children with congenital GH deficiency have normal length at birth. The growth rate slows during the first year of life and is quite apparent by the time a child is 2 years of age. Intellectual development is normal in children with isolated GH deficiency. They are at risk for hypoglycemia, especially during early infancy.

Acquired GH Deficiency. Acquired GH deficiency can cause growth failure at any age. Conditions that cause acquired GH deficiency include craniopharyngioma or other hypothalamic or pituitary tumors, cranial irradiation for brain tumors or leukemia, trauma, infection, autoimmune hypophysitis, and ischemia. Some cases are idiopathic.

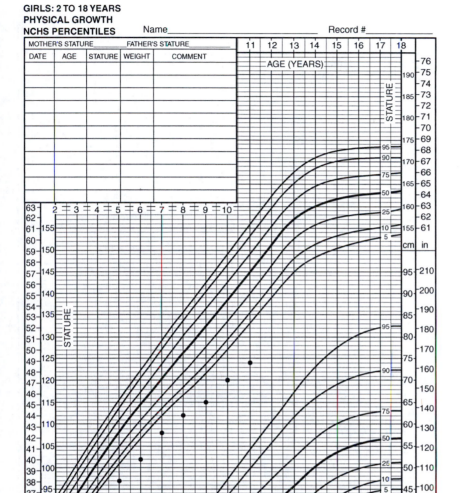

Fig. 13-10. Case Study 3 Growth Chart

NCHS = National Center for Health Statistics.

Resistance to GH. Complete insensitivity to GH results in Laron dwarfism. This severe form of dwarfism is caused by mutations in the GH receptor gene and is inherited as an autosomal recessive disorder. Partial GH insensitivity may be the cause of short stature in some children previously classified as having idiopathic short stature. Affected children have low levels of GHBP and IGF-I and high levels of GH, reflecting resistance to GH. These children do not respond to exogenous GH treatment with an increase in IGF-I.

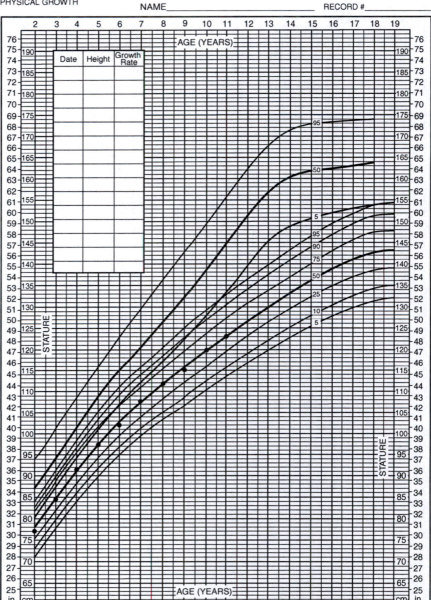

TURNER'S SYNDROME GIRLS: 2 TO 19 YEARS
PHYSICAL GROWTH
NAME_____ RECORD #_____

Fig. 13-11. Case Study 3 Growth Data Plotted on a Turner Syndrome Growth Chart

The chart shows the normal percentiles superimposed on the percentiles for girls with Turner syndrome. Although below the 5th percentile for the general population, this child is growing at the 50th percentile for girls with Turner syndrome.

IGF-I Deficiency. Pygmies have normal plasma GH and IGF-II levels, but they have a congenital inability to produce IGF-I. Growth failure due to a mutation in the IGF-1 gene has also been reported in association with prenatal growth retardation and abnormal neurologic development.

CASE STUDY 4: INTRODUCTION AND RESOLUTION

A 9-year-old boy was referred to the growth clinic for evaluation of dry skin and poor growth. He also had some problems with constipation. His parents mentioned that he was tired all the time, but they attributed his decreased energy to recent hot weather. Physical examination revealed an apathetic child with a slow pulse of 60 beats/min, blood pressure of 100/80 mm Hg, dry skin and hair, coarse features, an enlarged thyroid gland, and deep tendon reflexes with a delayed relaxation phase. His intelligence was normal for his age. Growth data obtained from his medical record are shown in Fig. 13-12.

This child's growth pattern could be the result of hypothyroidism or GH deficiency from a brain tumor. Laboratory studies revealed a thyroxine (T_4) level of 1.0 µg/dL (normal: 5.0–11.0 µg/dL) and a thyroid-stimulating hormone (TSH) level of 200 µU/L (normal: 0.4–5.0 µU/L), showing that he had primary hypothyroidism. Antimicrosomal and antithyroglobulin antibody titers were positive, indicating autoimmune thyroid disease. A bone age x-ray showed a delayed bone age.

He was treated with T_4 replacement, and normal growth resumed. If his initial thyroid tests had been normal, the next steps in his evaluation would have included GH stimulation testing and magnetic resonance imaging (MRI) of the brain to rule out a brain tumor.

Diagnosis and Treatment of GH Deficiency. Basal GH levels are low in normal children as well as in children with GH deficiency, so the diagnosis of GH deficiency depends on lack of GH response to provocative testing. At least 10% of normal children fail to respond to a single stimulus, so two methods must be used to confirm GH deficiency. Tests must be done when children are fasting because carbohydrate ingestion suppresses GH. Thyroid function testing should be done prior to testing for GH deficiency because hypothyroidism suppresses GH responsiveness. Hypothyroid children do not respond well to GH treatment. Children with psychosocial dwarfism have low GH levels that may not respond to provocative testing.

GH should rise during sleep and after 10 minutes of vigorous exercise. Pharmacologic stimuli for GH release include arginine, clonidine, levodopa, glucagon, GnRH, and enough insulin to cause acute hypoglycemia. Clonidine can cause hypotension and drowsiness, levodopa can cause nausea, and insulin can cause hypoglycemia, seizures, or coma. IGF-I levels cannot be used to make the diagnosis of GH deficiency because IGF-I is affected by nutrition, sex steroids, and psychosocial status.

Children who are GH deficient require treatment with synthetic human GH. Treatment with GH is currently approved for children

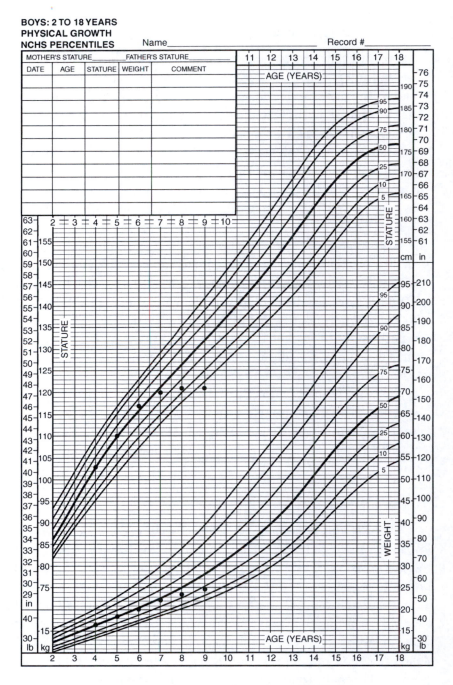

Fig. 13-12. Case Study 4 Growth Chart

NCHS = National Center for Health Statistics.

with confirmed GH deficiency and growth failure due to renal insufficiency, Turner syndrome, Prader-Willi syndrome, and intrauterine growth retardation (IUGR). GH treatment has also been approved by the Food and Drug Administration for children with idiopathic short stature, which commonly includes genetic short stature. Consideration for such treatment assumes careful exclusion of all other causes of short stature, along with close monitoring of height velocity and estimation of final adult height by a pediatric endocrinologist. GH should be limited to children who are more than 2.25 SD below the mean in height and, based on their bone age and height velocity, are unlikely to catch up in height. The predicted adult heights of children considered for treatment should be less than 63 inches for boys and less than 59 inches for girls. The expected increase in final adult height above the untreated predicted adult height is between 1.5 and 3 inches.

Glucocorticoid Excess. Glucocorticoid excess causes linear growth retardation in children. This may occur before other signs of hypercortisolism such as central obesity, muscle weakness, hypertension and glucose intolerance become apparent (see Chapter 5). Cushing disease and other causes of endogenous hypercortisolism do occur in children, but they are rare. Glucocorticoid excess in children is usually iatrogenic, since exogenous glucocorticoids are used to treat many conditions. The growth data plotted in Fig. 13-14 are those of a 14-year-old girl who had an adrenocorticotropic hormone-producing pituitary adenoma (Cushing disease).

Marked increase in weight associated with severe slowing of linear growth is characteristic of **Cushing syndrome** and **Cushing disease.**

Tall Stature

NORMAL VARIANT

Genetic Tall Stature

CASE STUDY 5: *INTRODUCTION AND RESOLUTION*

A 15-month-old girl was referred to the growth clinic for abnormal growth. Although her initial height and growth rate were within the normal range, she had been "falling off" her growth chart since she was approximately 9 months of age (Fig. 13-13). She was born at term, and development has been normal. She had problems with hypoglycemia in the newborn period but otherwise had been healthy. There was no family history of a growth disorder. The physical examination revealed a petite but otherwise normal child. A complete blood count, sedimentation rate, urinalysis, and serum chemistry screening were within normal limits. Her thyroid tests were also within normal limits. A karyotype was normal. Bone age was delayed.

There was no indication of another systemic illness, malnutrition, or parental neglect. Her growth chart was compatible with a diagnosis of congenital GH deficiency. Because of continued abnormal growth velocity, this child underwent provocative testing. Test results confirmed classic GH deficiency and she has been started on GH therapy.

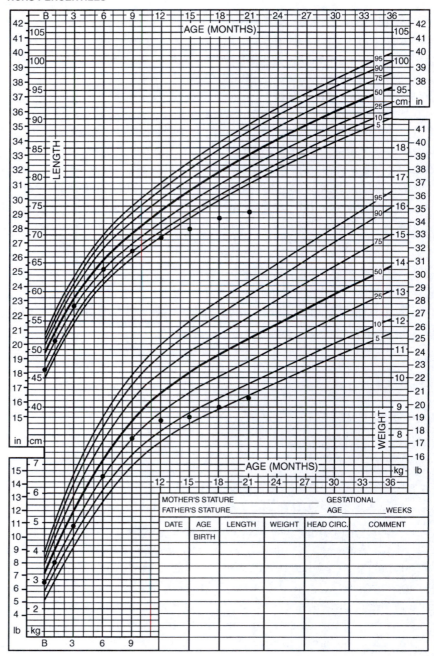

Fig. 13-13. Case Study 5 Growth Chart

NCHS = National Center for Health Statistics.

This represents a variation of normal growth in which height and weight are consistently above the 95th percentile. Growth velocity and bone age are normal, and there is a family history of tall stature. These individuals may achieve a final height at or above that of the general population, but their height is appropriate for their family.

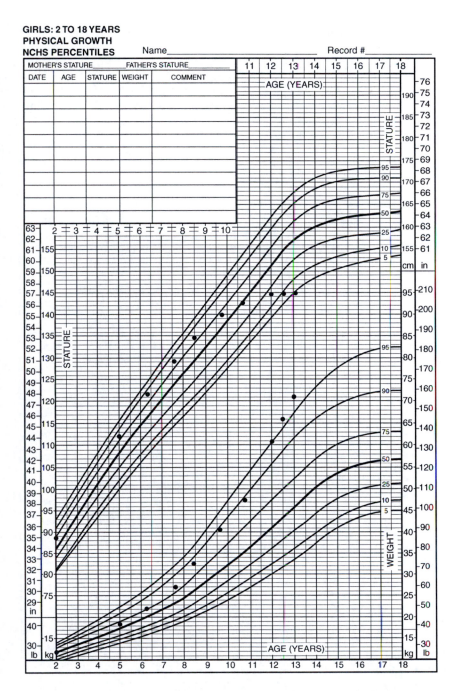

Fig. 13-14. Growth Chart of Patient with Cushing Syndrome

Note the acceleration in weight coinciding with linear growth failure. NCHS = National Center for Health Statistics.

NONENDOCRINE CAUSES

Syndromes/Chromosomal Abnormalities

Soto Syndrome. Children with Soto syndrome (also known as cerebral gigantism) have an acceleration of growth during the first few years of life, characteristic facial features, and developmental delay. The diagnosis is made by clinical criteria. The genetic defect causing Soto syndrome has been localized to a mutation on chromosome 5.

Klinefelter Syndrome. This syndrome is seen in males with a 47,XXY karyotype (see Chapter 14). Most patients are diagnosed when they present with delayed puberty and hypogonadism. They often have gynecomastia.

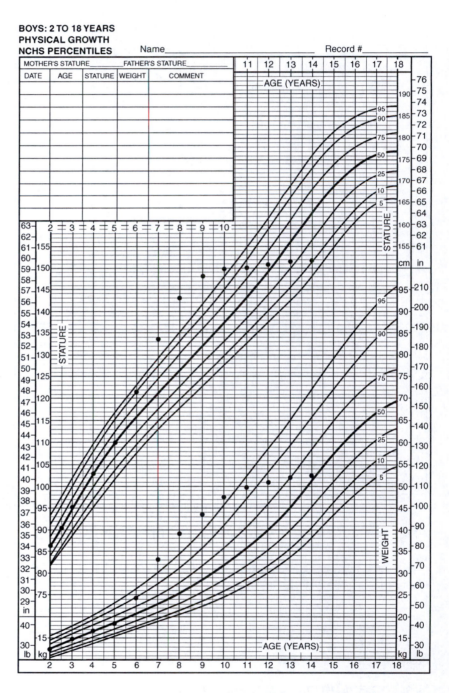

Fig. 13-15. Growth Chart of Patient with Precocious Puberty

This chart shows the initial height acceleration followed by premature cessation of growth. NCHS = National Center for Health Statistics.

Marfan Syndrome. This autosomal dominant disorder is caused by mutations in the gene coding for fibrillin, a constituent of connective tissue. Typical findings include tall stature, arachnodactyly (long fingers and toes), and eye, cardiac, and skeletal abnormalities.

Homocystinuria. This is an autosomal recessive disorder that is phenotypically similar to Marfan syndrome. This condition is caused by deficiency of the enzyme cystathionine ß-synthetase, which is important in the metabolism of amino acids. Mental retardation, seizures, and vascular thrombosis are common.

ENDOCRINE CAUSES

GH Excess

GH excess may be due to a GH-secreting pituitary adenoma, GHRH excess, or a decrease in somatostatin. These are rare causes of tall stature and growth acceleration in children. In adults, growth hormone excess causes acromegaly (see Chapter 2).

Precocious Puberty

Precocious puberty is present if signs of secondary sexual development appear before 8 years of age in girls and before 9 years of age in boys. Precocious puberty is an important cause of accelerated growth and tall stature in children. Bone age is advanced beyond chronologic age. Causes of precocious puberty are discussed in Chapter 14.

Paradoxically, untreated precocious puberty may ultimately result in short stature. Premature closure of the epiphyseal growth plates results from premature exposure to gonadal steroids. This is seen in the growth chart in Fig. 13-15, showing data from a patient with onset of precocious puberty at the age of 5 years.

REVIEW QUESTIONS

Directions: For each of the following questions, choose the *one best* answer.

1 An 8-year-old-boy is referred to the growth clinic for evaluation of obesity. Despite the fact that he "hardly eats anything," his weight has gone from the 75th to well above the 95th percentile during the last 4 to 5 years. Height has gone from the 75th to the 90th percentile. Developmental history is normal. According to the mother, several relatives on the paternal side are also "on the big side." What is the most likely diagnosis?

A Hypothyroidism
B Prader-Willi syndrome
C Exogenous obesity
D Growth hormone excess
E Normal variant

2 A 14-year-old boy presents with complaints of short stature and pubertal delay. He has otherwise been healthy but states that he is the smallest in his class and is being teased at school. His mother is 5′6″ tall and his father is 6″2″. His father reports that he grew 4 inches while he was in the military. On physical examination, the child is found to be well below the 5th percentile in height but is otherwise normal. Signs that puberty is just starting are noted. The most appropriate initial diagnostic test or tests would be

A bone age x-ray
B luteinizing hormone and testosterone measurements
C a karyotype
D a head magnetic resonance imaging (MRI) scan
E provocative growth hormone testing

3 An 18-month-old girl is referred to the growth clinic for growth failure. Her height has fallen from the 50th percentile at birth to the 10th percentile. Weight has decreased from the 50th percentile to below the 5th percentile. The child has otherwise been well. She lives at home with her mother, four siblings (ages 2 months–7 years), her mother's boyfriend, and his two children. The most likely etiology for this child's failure to thrive is

A growth hormone deficiency
B insulin deficiency
C thyroid hormone deficiency
D nutritional inadequacy
E congenital infection

4 A 10-year-old girl comes to an endocrinologist's office for evaluation of short stature. Her mother reports that she has always been small, but the difference from her peers has increased during the last several years. She has otherwise been well except for frequent ear infections. Her parents are of average height. A review of her growth chart reveals that her height has fallen from the 25th percentile to below the 5th percentile during the last few years. Weight has remained in the 25th percentile. Thyroid function tests, a complete blood count, sedimentation rate, urinalysis, serum electrolytes, and routine chemistries are normal. Her local physician has done a bone age x-ray, which is normal. Which of the following is the most essential next step in her evaluation?

A Analysis of her caloric intake
B Magnetic resonance imaging of the head
C A karyotype
D A stool sample for fecal fat
E A skeletal survey

5 A 7-year-old boy is referred to the growth clinic because of concerns about growth. He has been following the curve at approximately the 5th percentile. His mother's height is 5'1" and his father's height is 5'6". His parents are interested in treatment with growth hormone (GH). Which would be the most appropriate management for this child?

A Schedule the patient for GH stimulation testing now

B Schedule GH testing if the child is still at the 5th percentile in a year

C Prescribe growth hormone at this time

D Reassure the parents that the child is normal

E Schedule other testing first before considering the use of GH

6 An 11-year-old girl presents with slow growth. Review of previous records shows that her height has fallen from the 75th percentile to the 25th percentile during the last 2 years and that she has not grown at all during the past 6 months. Weight has remained at the 50th percentile. She has otherwise been well, although her parents report that she has decreased energy and problems with constipation. They also report that she insists on wearing a sweatshirt even on a hot summer day. The most likely cause of this child's growth failure is

A congenital growth hormone deficiency

B Cushing disease

C constitutional delay

D hypothyroidism

E psychosocial deprivation

References

Cohen LE, Radovick S: Molecular basis of combined pituitary hormone deficiencies. *Endocr Rev* 23:431–442, 2002.

Eugster EA, Pescovitz OH: Gigantism. *J Clin Endocrinol Metab* 84: 4379–4384, 1999.

Finkelstein BS, Silvers JB, Marrero U: Insurance coverage, physician recommendations and access to emerging treatments; Growth hormone therapy for childhood short stature. *JAMA* 270: 663–668, 1998.

Firth SM, Baxter RC: Cellular actions of the insulin-like growth factor binding proteins. *Endocr Rev* 23 :824–854, 2002.

Ong K, Kratzsch J, Kiess W: Size at birth and cord blood levels of insulin, insulin-like growth factor (IGF-1), IGF-11, IGF binding protein-1 (IGFBP-1), IGFBP-3 and the soluble IGF-II/mannose-6-phosphate receptor in term human infants. *J Clin Endocrinol Metab* 85: 4266–4269, 2000.

Robson H, Siebler T, Shalet SM, et al: Interactions between GH, IGF-1, Glucocorticoids, and thyroid hormones during skeletal growth. *Pediatr Res* 52(2): 137–147, 2002.

Tillmann V, Thalange NK, Foster PJ, et al: The relationship between stature, growth, and short-term changes in height and weight in normal prepubertal children. *Pediatr Res* 44: 882–886, 1998.

Vance ML, Mauras N: Growth hormone therapy in adults and children. *New Eng J Med* 341: 1206–1215, 1999.

14

Sexual Determination, Sexual Differentiation, and Puberty

Erica A. Eugster, M.D., and Antoinette M. Moran, M.D.

■ CHAPTER OUTLINE ■

■ LEARNING OBJECTIVES ■

At the completion of this chapter, the student will:
1. be aware of the determinants of genetic sex.
2. understand major features of male and female gonad and internal and external genitalia development.
3. be aware of gender identity, gender role, and sexual orientation.
4. recognize the causes and approach to therapy of ambiguous genitalia.
5. recognize the events of normal puberty in girls and boys.
6. understand the causes and approaches to therapy of precocious puberty.
7. understand the causes and approaches to therapy of delayed puberty.

Introduction

The sexual makeup of an individual is complex and is ultimately the result of a number of processes, including determination of genetic sex, development of the gonads, differentiation of internal and external sexual structures, establishment of gender role and gender identity, and postnatal pubertal development. Each of these processes takes place in a unique time frame during the evolution from fertilized ovum to complete sexual maturation. Successful completion of each stage is dependent on numerous factors, both endocrine and nonendocrine.

Determination of Genetic Sex

The chromosomal sex of the zygote is established with the fertilization of a normal ovum by an X or Y chromosome-bearing sperm at the moment of conception. Although conception usually takes place uneventfully, genetic accidents sometimes occur.

ABNORMALITIES OF SEX CHROMOSOMES

Abnormalities of the sex chromosomes occur at an approximate rate of 1 in 500 births. These abnormalities can occur in every cell or in a mosaic distribution. Sex chromosome abnormalities are usually sporadic events, and the phenotypes are typically milder than those observed with abnormalities of autosomal chromosomes. Either the number or the structure of the sex chromosomes may be affected.

Numerical Abnormalities

Abnormalities in the number of chromosomes (either sex or autosomal chromosomes) is termed *aneuploidy*. Examples of sex chromosome aneuploidy include Klinefelter syndrome (47, XXY karyotype) and Turner syndrome (45,X).

Structural Abnormalities

The most common structural abnormality of the sex chromosomes is duplication of the long arm of the X chromosome, with loss of all or part of the short arm. This type of chromosome is termed *isochromosome*.

Mosaicism refers to the presence of two or more different cell lines (e.g., 46,XX and 45,X) in the same individual.

Development and Differentiation of Sexual Structures

Until approximately 6 weeks fetal age, the gonads of males and females are morphologically indistinguishable and can differentiate into either ovaries or testes. The primordial germ cells migrate from the yolk sac to the developing gonad in the urogenital ridge at about 4 weeks fetal age.

TESTES

In the presence of a Y chromosome, the gonads differentiate into testes. This process is dependent on the existence of a gene known to be critical for male sexual differentiation that has been given the name *SRY*, or sex-determining region of Y. The *SRY* gene is located on the short arm of Y, near the pseudoautosomal region (Fig. 14-1). The pseudoautosomal regions of X and Y are the portions of the sex chromosomes that pair with each other during male meiosis and, in this way, behave much like a pair of autosomes (hence the term, pseudoautosomal). Genetic material may be exchanged between these portions of X and Y during meiosis. In addition to *SRY*, several other autosomal and/or X-linked genes are involved in sexual differentiation. Genes involved in gonadal differentiation act in a highly time-specific and dosage-specific manner. Thus, the phenotype resulting from duplication of a gene is vastly different from that resulting from a deletion or mutation within the same gene. In addition to *SRY*,

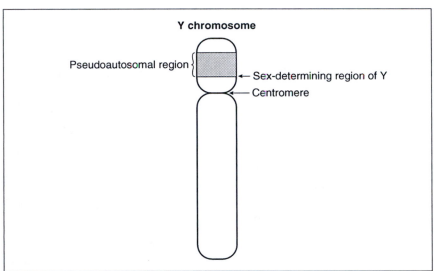

Fig. 14-1. Location of Pseudoautosomal Region and Sex-Determining Region of Y Chromosome

genes known to be essential for early gonadal development and normal male sexual differentiation include *SF-1*, *DAX-1*, *WT-1*, and *SOX-9*. Several of these are transcription factors that also play a role in the development of extragonadal tissues such as the adrenals (*SF-1*, *DAX-1*), the kidneys (*WT-1*), and the hypothalamic-pituitary axis (*DAX-1*).

46,XY females may result from point mutations within SRY. **46,XX males** may result from the translocation of SRY onto an X chromosome during male meiosis.

Normal male sexual differentiation is also dependent on two hormones secreted by the testes, müllerian-inhibiting substance (MIS), which is also called anti-müllerian hormone (AMH), and testosterone. MIS is secreted by the Sertoli cells, and testosterone is secreted by the Leydig cells of the testes. Testosterone secretion, which begins at about 9 weeks fetal age, results from stimulation of the testes by placental human chorionic gonadotropin (HCG) during the critical period of male sexual differentiation.

During later fetal and postnatal life, the testes are stimulated primarily by pituitary luteinizing hormone (LH). However, LH levels are low during early fetal development. Because HCG is structurally similar to LH, it is able to bind to LH receptors and stimulate the testes.

Spermatogenesis

Primordial germ cells destined to become spermatogonia are found within the developing seminiferous tubules early in testicular development. After several mitoses, they become quiescent until the pubertal period, when cell division again occurs, giving rise to primary spermatocytes.

OVARIES

The genes that actively promote ovarian development have only recently begun to be recognized. Thus far, the genes *DAX-1* and *WNT-4* have been shown to exert a critical influence on ovarian differentiation. Both are important in the early stages of gonad development in both males and females, but they become differentially expressed in the developing ovary. Germ cells must be present for ovarian differentiation. Once ovarian differentiation has occurred, two normal X chromosomes are required to maintain the normal ovarian life span. Girls with Turner syndrome have ovaries that appear histologically normal early in gestation. However, there is an accelerated rate of germ cell loss with subsequent fibrosis of ovarian stroma, leading to streak ovaries by the time the child is born or at a later point in postnatal life.

The classic concept of **female by default** has come under scrutiny because of the discovery of a gene on the short arm of the human X chromosome that, when duplicated, results in a male-to-female sex reversal, even in the presence of a functional *SRY* gene. Female sexual differentiation may be a more active process than previously believed.

During early development of the ovary, primary germ cells undergo active mitoses, giving rise to oogonia. The oogonia then enter meiotic division, becoming oocytes. Many oocytes degenerate during fetal life, but those that survive are arrested in the first meiotic division until ovulation occurs.

Karyotype 45,X

Turner syndrome
Accelerated germ cell loss
Early ovarian fibrosis
Streak gonads
Short stature

GENITAL DUCTS

By the seventh week of fetal life, both male (wolffian) and female (müllerian) ducts are present, derived from the mesonephros. During the third fetal month, either the wolffian or the müllerian ducts become fully formed, while the opposite structures degenerate (Fig. 14-2). The hormonal milieu plays the decisive role in determining which elements go on to differentiate, and which involute.

Testosterone, produced by the fetal testes, causes the wolffian ducts to complete their development, leading to formation of the epididymis, vas deferens, and seminiferous tubules. MIS, also produced by the fetal testes, causes degeneration of the müllerian structures.

In the absence of a functioning testes, the müllerian ducts differentiate, leading to the development of the uterus and fallopian tubes. This process is not dependent on the presence of an ovary; *therefore, it is the presence or absence of functioning testes that determines whether male or female internal structures develop.*

Development of the **wolffian structures** requires a high local concentration of testosterone. If only one functioning testis is present, male differentiation occurs on only one side and female internal structures develop on the other side. MIS also acts locally and unilaterally.

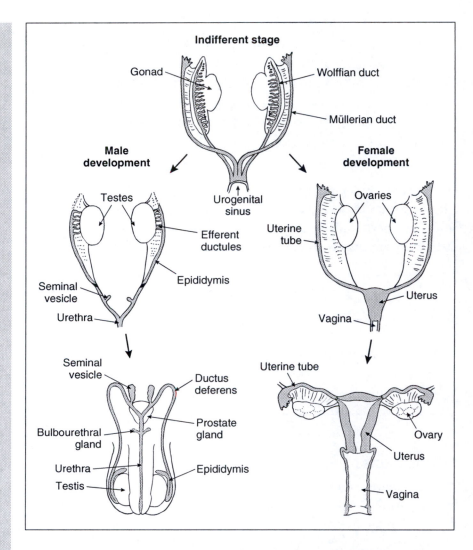

Fig. 14-2. Differentiation of the Müllerian and Wolffian Ducts Leading to Formation of Internal Structures

EXTERNAL GENITALIA

At 8 weeks fetal life, the external genitalia of males and females are identical and can differentiate in the direction of either sex. Homologous structures are shown in Fig. 14-3. Development of male external genitalia (and prostate) requires the presence of *dihydrotestosterone (DHT)* during 8 to 12 weeks of fetal life. DHT is formed from testosterone intracellularly by the action of the enzyme 5α-reductase. DHT binds to the androgen receptor with greater affinity than testosterone does. In the absence of DHT, female external genitalia develop.

In the female fetus, the vagina develops from the urogenital sinus. When normal müllerian structures are present, a septum develops that pushes the vaginal introitus posteriorly, creating a separate external opening. In the male, the prostate gland is derived from the urogenital sinus (Fig. 14-4). After the 12th fetal week, external genital formation is complete. Sexual determination and differentiation is summarized in Fig. 14-5.

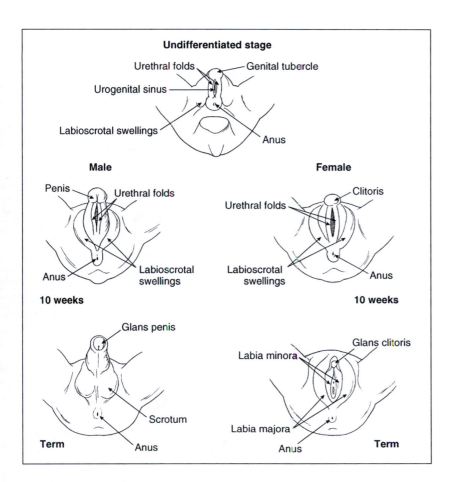

Fig. 14-3. Differentiation of the External Genitalia Showing Homologous Structures in the Male and Female

After the 12th week of gestation, abnormalities in the hormonal environment can affect the size of the clitoris and phallus, but not their morphologic structure.

Psychosexual Differentiation

In the area of psychosexual differentiation, the nature vs. nurture debate is far from resolved. There are three main concepts that define psychosexual development: gender identity, gender role, and sexual orientation.

Gender identity refers to the subjective sense of being "male" or "female," which is usually solidified between the ages of 2 to 2 1/2. With time, gender identity becomes basic to all other aspects of personal identity. Factors influencing the formation of gender identity are complex and poorly understood, but include both biologic and environmental forces.

Gender role refers to objective behaviors within a given social group, which are assigned to either male or female members of the species. Differences in the behavior of boys and girls from early infancy have been observed, although such observations are influenced substantially

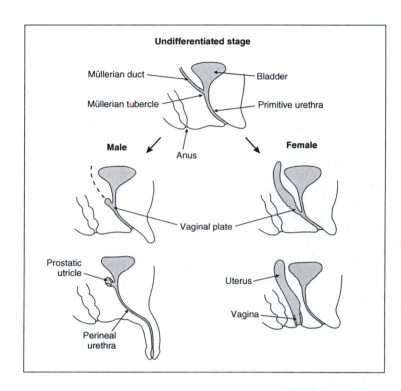

Fig. 14-4. Differentiation of the Urogenital Sinus

(*Source:* Reprinted with permission from Lifshitz, *Pediatric Endocrinology*, 3rd ed. New York, NY: Marcel Dekker, 1996 p 285.)

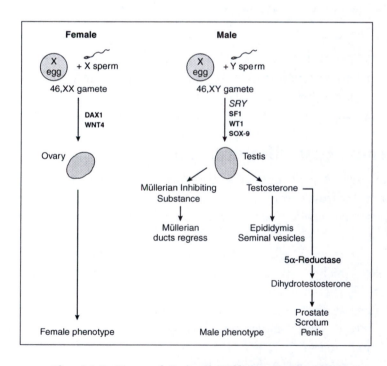

Fig. 14-5. Normal Sexual Differentiation from Fertilization to Formation of External Genitalia

SRY = sex-determining region of Y.

by observer bias based on sex stereotypes. There is evidence that gender role behaviors may be influenced by prenatal hormones, but these behaviors can also be learned. They are mediated initially by parents or other care-givers and later by same sex peer groups.

Some researchers have found structural differences in certain areas of the brain in men and women. This has led to speculation about the role of the brain in human psychosexual differentiation.

Sexual orientation refers to an individual's sexual attraction to the opposite or same sex and usually develops after puberty.

Fifty percent concordance for homosexuality among identical twins, as well as a higher than expected incidence of homosexuality in women with prenatal androgen exposure, indicates the contribution of both genetic and environmental factors in the development of sexual orientation.

Ambiguous Genitalia

The birth of an infant with ambiguous genitalia is considered both a medical emergency, because potentially life-threatening conditions are part of the differential diagnosis, and a psychological emergency, because of the need for an unequivocal sex assignment as soon as possible. Sex assignment cannot be made before all necessary information has been collected and analyzed. There are four general categories of ambiguous genitalia: virilization of the XX female, undervirilization of the XY male, gonadal differentiation disorders, and anatomic or syndromic abnormalities. Conditions in which ambiguous genitalia occur are often referred to as "intersex disorders."

VIRILIZATION OF THE XX FEMALE INFANT

Exposure of the female fetus to androgens prior to the 12th fetal week results in labial fusion, clitoral hypertrophy, and sometimes even formation of a male urethra. After the 12th fetal week, exposure to androgens causes only clitoral hypertrophy. There are three general categories of disorders that cause virilization of the XX female.

Causes of Virilization of an X,X Female
Congenital adrenal hyperplasia
Excess maternal or placental androgens
Idiopathic or teratogenic factors

Congenital Adrenal Hyperplasia (CAH)

CAH is the most common cause of ambiguous genitalia in female infants. This autosomal recessive disorder is caused by the deficiency of an enzyme involved in adrenal steroidogenesis.

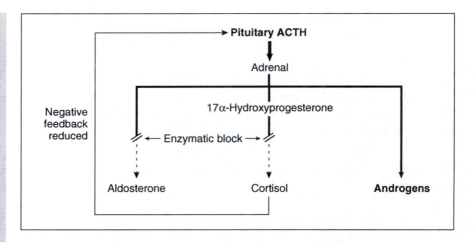

Fig. 14-6. Pathophysiology of Congenital Adrenal Hyperplasia (CAH)

This figure shows a block at the level of the 21-hydroxylase enzyme with accumulation of cortisol precursor 17-OH progesterone and increased production of adrenal androgens. The decreased production of cortisol leads to continued stimulation of the adrenals by pituitary adrenocorticotropic hormone (ACTH).

The enzyme block is within the synthetic pathway of cortisol. If the defect is severe, synthesis of aldosterone is also affected. Low cortisol levels cause a rise in pituitary ACTH levels, producing hyperstimulation of the fetal adrenals. There is buildup of steroid precursors that are shunted into the androgen synthetic pathway, resulting in adrenal androgen excess (Fig. 14-6). A defect in the enzyme 21-hydroxylase is the most common enzyme defect causing CAH.

The diagnosis of **21-hydroxylase deficiency** is made by finding an elevated level of plasma 17-hydroxyprogesterone, the substrate for the defective enzyme in the synthetic pathway of cortisol.

Approximately two-thirds of individuals with 21-hydroxylase deficiency have a defect in both cortisol and aldosterone synthesis, resulting in both virilization and salt-wasting. The other one-third have a defect only in cortisol production, resulting in virilization.

If synthesis of **aldosterone** is blocked, patients with **CAH** are at risk for a "salt-wasting crisis," characterized by electrolyte abnormalities, dehydration, and shock. This usually occurs within the first 5 to 10 days of life. In many states all newborns are screened for 21-hydroxylase deficiency.

Girls with CAH have a normal 46,XX karyotype and normal internal reproductive organs, although their external structures are virilized. In contrast, boys with 21-hydroxylase deficiency appear normal at birth. Levels of androgens from the testes are very high in utero, so an extra contribution from the adrenals has no phenotypic consequences. Boys may present in the newborn period if they are salt wasters, or later in life with precocious puberty (see Precocious Puberty).

Treatment of CAH involves glucocorticoid replacement and mineralocorticoid replacement, if indicated. Historically, feminizing genital surgery has been performed early in life in virilized girls with CAH. This practice has recently been challenged. Some advocate delaying genital surgery until the patient is able to participate in the decision of when or whether to have surgery performed. The psychological effects of delaying genital surgery in virilized girls with CAH are unknown.

Maternal or Placental Androgens

Maternal or placental androgens may also cause virilization of a female fetus. Sources include maternal virilizing tumors of adrenals or ovaries, maternal CAH, ingestion of androgens or progestins, or abnormal placental enzyme activity (rare). In all of these cases, the mother is virilized.

Idiopathic or Teratogenic Virilization

Virilization of the XX female fetus can also be *idiopathic* or *teratogenic*. In idiopathic cases the etiology of the virilization is not identified. Teratogenic virilization implies a specific exposure.

UNDERVIRILIZATION OF THE XY MALE INFANT

Conditions giving rise to undervirilization of the male infant result in a spectrum of phenotypic findings, ranging from normal female genitalia to various degrees of ambiguous genitalia. The phenotype depends on the severity of the defect and the time during which the defect occurs. Several general categories of disorders cause undervirilization of the male infant.

Causes of Undervirilization of an X,Y Male

Deficient enzyme for testosterone synthesis
Deficient 5α-reductase for DHT synthesis
Abnormal androgen receptors (androgen resistance)
    Complete (testicular feminization)
    Partial
Testicular regression
Maternal drug ingestion

Defect in the Pathway of Testosterone Synthesis

Deficiency of an enzyme needed for the synthesis of testosterone can be present in the adrenals and testes, or in the testes alone. Patients with adrenal enzyme deficiencies may also be at risk for salt-wasting.

Patients with 5α-reductase deficiency cannot convert testosterone to DHT. Since the development of normal male external genitalia is dependent on DHT, these patients have female or ambiguous external genitalia. Their internal reproductive structures develop normally since these structures are dependent only on the presence of testosterone. At puberty, receptor-affinity relationships change. The external structures are responsive to the high level of testosterone, leading to partial virilization of external genitalia. In some cultures in which the incidence of 5α-reductase deficiency is quite high, complete reversal of sex assignment at puberty is an accepted and well-recognized phenomenon called "guevedoce," which means "penis at 12."

Androgen Resistance

Androgen resistance is another cause of undervirilization of male infants. End organ resistance to androgens, which can be complete or partial, is caused by abnormalities in the number or function of androgen receptors. These abnormalities are due to mutations in genes on the X chromosome coding for the androgen receptor or mutations that cause postreceptor defects.

Complete androgen resistance due to a severe abnormality or absence of the androgen receptor results in *testicular feminization syndrome*. Testes are present and testosterone is produced, but the tissues are unable to respond. The genotype is 46,XY but the external genitalia are unambiguously female. There are no wolffian structures because tissues cannot recognize testosterone. There are no müllerian structures because testes produce MIS normally. The external genitalia are female.

At puberty, when testosterone increases, follicle-stimulating hormone (FSH) and LH levels remain high because the pituitary lacks testosterone receptors and cannot respond to negative feedback. Constant FSH and LH stimulation results in high levels of testosterone, which is converted to estrogen in peripheral tissues. Breast development occurs in response to estrogen stimulation. Patients present with primary amenorrhea because the vagina ends in a blind pouch. They have little or no pubic hair and no acne because both require effective androgens for development.

The testes are intra-abdominal and must be removed after puberty has been completed, because intra-abdominal testes are at high risk for malignancy. Estrogen replacement therapy is given after the testes are removed.

Partial androgen resistance resulting in variable degrees of genital ambiguity accounts for most cases of ambiguous genitalia in boys. The pattern of inheritance in many kindreds is consistent with an X-linked recessive trait with variable penetrance. Wolffian duct structures are poorly developed.

FSH, LH, testosterone, and estrogen levels are all high in **testicular feminization syndrome.** FSH and LH are high because the pituitary lacks receptors to recognize testosterone and cannot respond to negative feedback. Continual stimulation of the testes by high levels of LH results in high levels of testosterone, which are converted to estrogen in peripheral tissues.

LH Resistance

LH resistance is caused by a loss-of-function mutation in the LH receptor. Boys with this abnormality have Leydig cell hypoplasia and present with a spectrum of undervirilization ranging from female external genitalia to a normal male phenotype with micropenis.

Testicular Regression

Testicular regression, also known as "vanishing testes" refers to a 46,XY male infant with absence of identifiable gonads. The underlying defect is unknown but can result in varying degrees of genital ambiguity or micropenis, depending on the timing of the regression.

Maternal Drug Ingestion

Maternal drug ingestion can interfere with normal male sexual differentiation. Estrogens, progestins, and spironolactone are examples of drugs ingested by the mother that can result in undervirilization of a male fetus.

GONADAL DIFFERENTIATION DISORDERS

In disorders of gonadal differentiation, both male and female elements are present. Individuals with *true hermaphroditism* have both ovarian and testicular tissue. The genitalia may be male, female, or ambiguous. The most common finding is an ovary on one side of the abdomen, and a testes on the other, although both may be combined as an ovotestes. The most common karyotype is 46,XX.

In contrast, *mixed gonadal dysgenesis* is a disorder that is associated with mosaicism of 2 or more cell lines with different karyotypes, one of which includes a Y or portions of a Y chromosome. A wide range of phenotypes has been described. Various combinations of dysgenetic testes, ovotestes, or streak ovaries are present, as well as a rudimentary uterus and at least one oviduct. Approximately one third of these patients have stigmata of Turner syndrome (see Turner syndrome).

ANATOMIC AND SYNDROMIC CAUSES

Anatomic causes of ambiguous genitalia include morphologic defects, which often occur in association with other congenital anomalies of the hindgut such as imperforate anus or renal agenesis. In rare cases ambiguous genitalia can be due to mechanical disruption such as that caused by a hemangioma or amniotic band. A number of *chromosomal abnormalities and syndromes,* including trisomies 13 and 18, and CHARGE, Robinow, Smith-Lemli-Opitz, and Vacterl syndromes, are associated with ambiguous genitalia.

MANAGEMENT OF INFANTS WITH AMBIGUOUS GENITALIA

There is an ongoing international debate regarding the clinical management and rationale for sex assignment in "intersex" infants. This was precipitated by the emergence of highly vocal patient groups along with the recognition that psychosexual outcome data in intersex individuals is sorely lacking. While there is little consensus, current existing strategies attempt to incorporate multiple factors in determining sex-of-rearing. These include sexual and reproductive potential, prenatal androgen exposure, cultural and societal mores, and the limited follow-up information that is available in specific intersex populations.

Micropenis

Micropenis is the condition in which unambiguously male genitalia are abnormally small. The length of the phallus is at least 2.5 SD below the mean for age. From the 6th to the 12th fetal week, HCG from the placenta stimulates production of testosterone from the fetal testes. Testosterone is converted to DHT, which stimulates differentiation of the external genitalia. After the 12th fetal week, LH from the fetal pituitary stimulates the testes to produce testosterone. A defect anywhere along the fetal hypothalamic-pituitary-gonadal axis or a defect in peripheral androgen action can result in failure of the phallus to grow. Some cases of micropenis are classified as *idiopathic.*

Micropenis is defined as a phallic length that is 2.5 SD below the mean for age. In a term newborn, a phallus less than or equal to 2 cm is considered a micropenis.

Gonadotropin deficiency due to a pituitary defect is the most common cause of micropenis. LH deficiency can be isolated or can be associated with deficiencies in other pituitary hormones. Isolated gonadotropin deficiency can also be due to a hypothalamic defect resulting in failure of gonadotropin-releasing hormone (GnRH) secretion.

Primary hypogonadism can lead to micropenis if the testes cannot secrete enough testosterone for normal genital development. This can occur in boys with Klinefelter syndrome (47,XXY) and with other causes of primary testicular failure such as "vanishing testes."

Mild *partial androgen resistance* can cause micropenis. *Syndromes and chromosomal disorders* with micropenis as an associated feature include Noonan, Prader-Willi, and various trisomies.

Newborn children with micropenis must be examined carefully for signs of multiple pituitary hormone deficiencies. If they are present, these infants are at risk for hypoglycemia due to growth hormone (GH) and ACTH deficiencies, hypothyroidism due to thyroid-stimulating hormone (TSH) deficiency, and adrenal insufficiency due to lack of ACTH. A karyotype may be necessary to rule out Klinefelter syndrome. Children with micropenis due to inadequate testosterone production usually respond well to a trial of testosterone therapy. Alternatively, an HCG stimulation test can give important information regarding testicular function and end-organ responsiveness.

The newborn with a micropenis must be monitored closely for signs of other pituitary hormone deficiencies. Hypoglycemia may develop due to ACTH deficiency, growth hormone deficiency, or both.

Adrenarche

Adrenarche refers to the rise in serum androgens resulting from the increased production of weak androgens (dehydroepiandrosterone [DHEA], dehydroepiandrosterone sulfate [DHEAS], and androstenedione) from the adrenal glands. Adrenarche normally begins at the age of 6 or 7 years. This process is independent of *gonadarche*, which refers to the activation of the hypothalamic-pituitary-gonadal axis with increased production of sex steroids from the gonads at the onset of "central" puberty. The levels of adrenal androgens continue to rise but are usually not high enough to cause physical changes until the age of puberty.

Puberty

The onset of puberty marks the beginning of a complex process that results in complete sexual maturation. This process includes growth and development of primary sexual characteristics (genitalia and gonads), development of secondary sexual characteristics, psychological

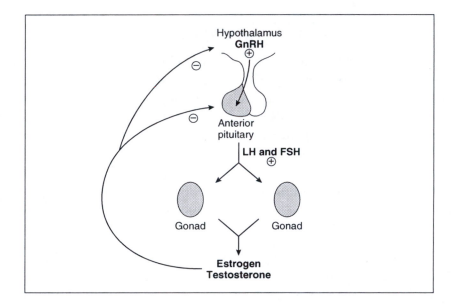

Fig. 14-7. Hypothalamic-Pituitary-Gonadal Axis

This figure shows feedback relationships at the level of the pituitary and hypothalamus. GnRH = gonadotropin-releasing hormone; LH = luteinizing hormone; FSH = follicle-stimulating hormone.

changes, and the acquisition of fertility. These events are brought about by gonadal production of sex steroids resulting from the activation of the hypothalamic-pituitary-gonadal axis (Fig. 14-7).

HYPOTHALAMIC-PITUITARY-GONADAL AXIS AND SEX STEROIDS

Puberty can be thought of as part of the continuum of gonadal development. Hypothalamic-pituitary activity is high during fetal life, becomes relatively quiescent during childhood, and then becomes high again at puberty.

Episodic release of GnRH from hypothalamic neurons known as the GnRH pulse generator stimulates intermittent release of *gonadotropins LH and FSH* from the pituitary. Prior to puberty, infrequent low-amplitude pulses of LH and FSH occur. Puberty is heralded by a dramatic increase in the amplitude and frequency of LH pulses, occurring first during sleep and later throughout the day. Patterns of gonadotropin secretion from infancy through puberty are shown in Fig. 14-8. FSH and LH stimulate the gonads to produce estrogen and androgens such as testosterone.

The physical changes of puberty are caused by estrogens and androgens, both of which are present in male and female individuals. *Estrogen* is produced by the ovaries in females and by peripheral conversion of androgens in both sexes. Estrogen causes breast enlargement, maturation of the vaginal mucosa, growth acceleration, and advancement of skeletal maturation. *Androgens* are produced by the adrenals, by the testes (males), and by the ovaries (females).

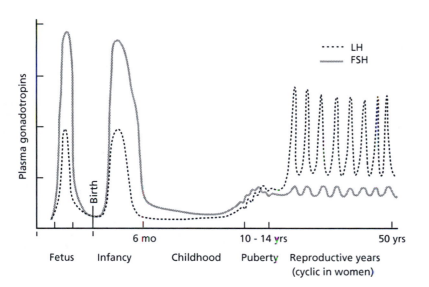

Fig. 14-8. Levels of Luteinizing Hormone and Follicle-Stimulating Hormone at different Ages.

Androgens cause acne; axillary, pubic, and facial hair growth; body odor; voice changes; growth acceleration; and skeletal maturation.

Androgens and estrogens cause skeletal maturation, but estrogen is essential for complete epiphyseal fusion. This was demonstrated recently in a 28-year-old man with complete absence of estrogen receptors. He was 6'11" tall and still growing.

STAGES OF PUBERTY

Breast development, genital changes in boys, and pubic hair growth during puberty are staged according to the system derived by Dr. James Tanner (called Tanner staging). Tanner stage I represents the prepubertal stage, and Tanner stage V represents full sexual maturation.

Pubertal Changes in Girls

The first visible sign of puberty in 70% of girls is breast budding, known as *thelarche*. Appearance of pubic hair, known as *pubarche*, occurs first in 30% of girls. Whichever of these occurs first, the other usually follows within 6 months. The first physical change of puberty in girls is actually enlargement of the ovaries, but this is observable only by ultrasound.

The normal age range for the onset of puberty in girls is 8 to 13 years. There are ethnic variations, with this range being shifted downward approximately 6 months in girls of African American or Hispanic descent.

Table 14-1. Onset of the Events of Puberty

Puberty in Girls*	AVERAGE AGE OF ONSET	AGE RANGE
Breast budding	11 years	8–13 years
Pubic hair appears	11 years	8–14 years
Growth spurt	11 years	9.5–14.5 years
Menarche	12.8 years	10–16.5 years
Puberty in Boys		
Testes enlarge	12 years	9–14 years
Pubic hair appears	12.2 years	10–15 years
Penile enlargement	13 years	11–14.5 years
Growth spurt	13 years	10.5–16 years

*The first event of puberty in girls is ovarian enlargement, but this can be detected only by ultrasound.

Notes

Additional events during puberty include the pubertal growth spurt and *menarche*, or the first menstrual period. Menarche, the final milestone of puberty in girls, marks the point at which growth is almost complete. The timing of these events is shown in Table 14-1.

Menarche usually occurs 2 to 2.5 years after the onset of breast development. The average age of menarche in the United States is 12.8 years.

Pubertal Changes in Boys

The first sign of puberty in boys is testicular enlargement. The timing and sequence of pubertal events in boys is shown in Table 14-1. *Pubertal gynecomastia* (excessive growth of male breast tissue) is due to an imbalance in the relative amounts of androgens and estrogens. Increased conversion of androgen to estrogen in fat cells during puberty temporarily lowers the testosterone to estrogen ratio expected in male individuals. Individual differences in sensitivity to normal levels of estrogen may also play a role. In most cases, gynecomastia resolves spontaneously within 1 to 2 years. However, if pubertal gynecomastia is persistent and cosmetically unacceptable, surgical removal of the breast tissue is possible.

The age range of onset of puberty in boys is 9 to 14 years. The **pubertal growth spurt** is due to the combined effects of sex steroids and growth hormone. In boys, this begins later, lasts longer, and reaches a higher amplitude than the pubertal growth spurt in girls. As a result, men are taller on average than women.

Pathologic causes of gynecomastia include hypogonadism (another cause of a lower than normal testosterone:estrogen ratio), drug ingestion (marijuana, ketoconazole, estrogens), and very rare estrogen-producing tumors of the testes or adrenals.

Gynecomastia occurs in nearly 90% of normal boys during puberty.

Precocious Puberty

Precocious puberty is premature sexual development, which occurs at an age more than 2.5 SD below the mean age of puberty. Premature increases in estrogen and androgens cause acceleration of growth in the short term but ultimately compromise final adult height due to premature closure of the epiphyseal growth plates (see Chapter 13). Assessments of growth velocity and skeletal maturation are an important part of the evaluation of children with precocious puberty.

Precocious puberty is defined as the onset of pubertal development in girls before age 8 and in boys before age 9.

BENIGN VARIANTS

Premature Thelarche

Premature thelarche is a condition of isolated breast development in a girl with no other signs of puberty. Growth velocity and bone age are normal, and the onset of puberty occurs at a normal age. No treatment is needed and there are no sequelae. The breast tissue may resolve, persist, or enlarge but does not usually surpass Tanner stage-III development. Asymmetric breast development is not a cause for concern; it is quite common for breasts to develop at different rates.

Follow-up is essential for a child with premature thelarche. This could also represent the beginning of true precocious puberty.

Premature Pubarche or Adrenarche

This refers to isolated pubic hair development in boys and girls. Body odor, axillary hair, and mild acne may also be present. Growth velocity is normal. Bone age is often mildly advanced but is usually within 2 SD of the mean. These children have mildly elevated levels of adrenal androgens, which do not interfere with the onset of normal puberty or with normal growth. Girls with premature pubarche are at increased risk for insulin resistance, the development of polycystic ovarian syndrome, and type II diabetes as adults (see Chapter 12). The terms pubarche and adrenarche are often used interchangeably, but *adrenarche* refers to the biochemical changes in adrenal androgen levels; *pubarche* refers to the physical changes caused by these androgens.

Causes of Precocious Puberty

Benign Variants
Premature thelarche
Premature pubarche

Central Precocious Puberty
Idiopathic
Congenital CNS abnormality
CNS trauma, infection, or ischemia
CNS tumor

Peripheral Precocious Puberty
CAH
Androgen or estrogen ingestion
Adrenal or gonadal tumor
G-protein abnormality
Ovarian cysts

CENTRAL PRECOCIOUS PUBERTY

This refers to puberty occurring via activation of the hypothalamic-pituitary-gonadal axis at a younger than normal age. In childhood the pituitary is unresponsive to GnRH. Once central puberty has been activated, the pituitary responds to GnRH by secreting gonadotropins (Fig. 14-9), and the gonads enlarge in response to LH and FSH stimulation. Random levels of LH and FSH are not helpful in making the diagnosis of central precocious puberty, since baseline values are indistinguishable in the prepubertal and pubertal state. The diagnosis of central precocious puberty can be made if administration of an exogenous GnRH analog results in a brisk rise in pituitary gonadotropins (a positive GnRH stimulation test).

Central precocious puberty can be caused by congenital central nervous system (CNS) abnormalities such as septo-optic dysplasia, hypothalamic hamartoma, and neurofibromatosis, or by acquired CNS insults such as infection, ischemia, trauma, and neoplasm. However, in 90% of cases of central precocious puberty in girls, the etiology of premature activation of the hypothalamic-pituitary-gonadal axis is unknown. In boys with central precocious puberty, approximately 50% of cases are idiopathic. Children with central precocious puberty are treated with a long-acting GnRH analog, which down-regulates GnRH receptors so that they no longer respond to GnRH pulses.

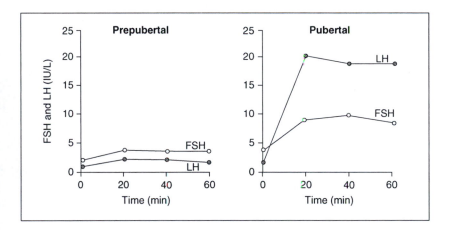

Fig. 14-9. Gonadotropin-Releasing Hormone (GnRH) Stimulation Test

Luteinizing hormone (LH) and follicle-stimulating hormone (FSH) are measured sequentially after administration of intravenous GnRH. In the prepubertal child, there is no significant response to the GnRH analog. A pubertal response is characterized by a brisk rise in gonadotropins with a predominance of LH.

Central precocious puberty is confirmed if a GnRH stimulation test elicits a brisk rise in pituitary gonadotropins with LH predominance. Central precocious puberty is treated with long-acting **GnRH analog therapy** in the form of intramuscular or subcutaneous injections. Sustained high concentrations of GnRH lead to down-regulation of pituitary GnRH receptors and subsequent suppression of the pituitary-gonadal axis.

Peripheral Precocious Puberty

Peripheral precocious puberty is initiated by a process outside the central hypothalamic-pituitary-gonadal axis that results in either endogenous or exogenous androgen/estrogen exposure. Since the central axis is still immature, gonadotropin levels are low and do not respond to GnRH stimulation.

In **peripheral precocious puberty,** a GnRH stimulation test elicits no increase in FSH and LH, indicating that the hypothalamic-pituitary-gonadal axis is still immature.

Congenital Adrenal Hyperplasia (CAH)

CAH is an important cause of ambiguous genitalia, but CAH can also present as precocious puberty in girls and boys. The type of presentation depends on the severity of the enzyme block. Since the adrenals produce androgens but not estrogen, premature breast development does not occur in girls with peripheral precocious puberty due to CAH.

CAH that is due to 21-hydroxylase deficiency is the most common cause of postnatal virilization in boys and girls.

Exogenous Causes

Ingestion of androgens or estrogen found in birth control pills or contaminated meat also causes peripheral precocious puberty. Ingestion of estrogen results in breast development, whereas ingestion of androgens causes body hair and other signs of abnormal virilization.

Tumors

Adrenal, testicular, or ovarian tumors that produce androgen or estrogen are rare causes of peripheral precocious puberty in children. Tumors producing HCG can also cause precocious puberty because HCG is structurally similar to LH and stimulates the testes to produce testosterone.

Gain-of-Function Mutations

FSH and LH act via cell surface receptors on the gonads, resulting in activation of G-rpotein-induced formation of cyclic adenosine monophosphate (cAMP). Peripheral precocious puberty may be caused by mutations in the gene coding for the G-protein stimulatory subunit (Gs_α) resulting in constitutive activation of G-protein-driven formation of cAMP. Gonadal cells behave as though they are constantly stimulated with FSH and LH and continue to produce estrogen and testosterone even though the gonadotropin receptors are not occupied. This is the etiology of McCune-Albright syndrome, which is characterized by the classic triad of precocious puberty, polyostotic fibrous dysplasia of bone, and café au lait spots. Familial male precocious puberty (also known as testotoxicosis) is caused by an activating mutation in the LH receptor and is inherited in an autosomal dominant pattern.

Ovarian Cysts

Functional ovarian cysts can produce estrogen, causing acute onset of breast enlargement in girls. The cysts resolve spontaneously, often resulting in withdrawal bleeding from the estrogen-stimulated endometrium, after which the breast tissue regresses. The diagnosis is made by ultrasound, and no treatment is necessary.

Delayed Puberty

Delayed puberty is defined as the failure of progression of puberty or the absence of any signs of puberty in a girl by age 13 or in a boy by age 14.

BENIGN VARIANT

Constitutional Delay of Growth and Puberty

This is characterized by a slow rate of growth during the first few years of life, delayed skeletal maturation (bone age is less than chronologic age), and delayed puberty. There is usually a family history of delayed growth. Puberty begins late, but because these children grow for a longer period of time than their peers, final adult height is normal (see Chapter 13).

PATHOLOGIC CAUSES

Pathologic causes of delayed puberty include defects in the hypothalamic-pituitary-gonadal axis at any level and end-organ resistance to gonadal hormones. Delayed puberty can also be seen in the context of *any* significant chronic disease or illness.

Gonadotropin Deficiency

This is the result of inadequate hypothalamic GnRH or inadequate pituitary LH and FSH. Hypothalamic causes of delayed puberty include Kallman syndrome, a condition originating from a deletion of the KAL gene, which encodes for the protein anosmin and is known to be involved in neuronal migration. This disorder is characterized by hypogonadotropic hypogonadism and a deficient or absent sense of smell (hyposmia or anosmia). Gonadotropin deficiency may also arise from mutations in the GnRH receptor gene. Prader-Willi and Lawrence-Moon-Biedl syndromes are also associated with hypogonadotropic hypogonadism. Patients with anorexia nervosa, whose weight is markedly below normal, have disturbances in the GnRH pulse generator. In some cases gonadotropin deficiency is idiopathic.

If **delayed puberty** is due to a **hypothalamic or pituitary disorder**, LH and FSH levels are low. Testosterone and estrogen levels also are low.

Gonadal Failure

Gonadal failure in females is most often caused by Turner syndrome (karyotype 45,X). The incidence of Turner syndrome is approximately 1 in 2000 live female births. Approximately 30% of those affected are mosaics. This disorder is characterized by ovarian dysgenesis, short stature (see Chapter 13), and a spectrum of physical stigmata including low posterior hairline, high-arched palate, webbed neck, shield-shaped chest, coarctation of the aorta, hyperconvex fingernails, cubitus valgus (increased carrying angle), and lymphedema. Most patients have normal intelligence but have difficulty with math, especially spatial relationships. Since many girls with Turner syndrome lack some or most of the phenotypic features, the diagnosis must be made by chromosomal analysis.

Gonadal failure also occurs in boys with Klinefelter syndrome (karyotype 47,XXY), which is characterized by seminiferous tubule dysplasia and varying degrees of testicular failure. The incidence of Klinefelter syndrome is 1 in 400. Boys usually present at puberty with gynecomastia and small testes due to lack of seminiferous tubules. Many are infertile from their first presentation; others become infertile in early adulthood due to premature testicular failure. Phenotypic features, which include decreased body hair, decreased muscle mass, and female-type subcutaneous fat distribution, vary widely, and a chromosomal analysis is required to make the diagnosis. Causes of acquired gonadal failure include infection (tuberculosis), irradiation, trauma, and torsion.

If **delayed puberty** is caused by **gonadal failure**, LH and FSH levels are high due to lack of pituitary suppression by testosterone or estrogen.

End Organ Resistance

Delayed puberty due to end-organ resistance to gonadal hormones occurs in patients with complete androgen resistance, or testicular feminization syndrome. These phenotypic females typically present at puberty with primary amenorrhea.

CASE STUDY: *RESOLUTION*

Anna had symptoms and signs of true (central) precocious puberty in which both estrogens and androgens are produced. If she had benign premature thelarche, she would have exhibited no signs of puberty except breast enlargement, and her growth velocity would have been normal. If she had benign premature pubarche due to adrenal androgens, she would not have breast development, and her growth velocity would have been normal.

To confirm central precocious puberty, a GnRH stimulation test was performed. Anna was given a bolus of an exogenous GnRH analog. This provoked a brisk rise in pituitary gonadotropins as shown in Fig. 14-9. This rise was due to premature maturation of her hypothalamic-pituitary-ovarian axis. A magnetic resonance imaging (MRI) scan of her head was normal, indicating that her central precocious puberty was not caused by a tumor or other CNS abnormality. Central precocious puberty in girls is usually idiopathic.

Anna was started on monthly injections of a potent long-acting GnRH analog to down-regulate pituitary GnRH receptors. Within 6 months, the progression of her puberty had stabilized, her growth velocity had slowed, and the rapid increase in her bone age also decreased. She and her family were given counseling because children with precocious puberty may be teased by or feel uncomfortable with other children. Also, since these children do not have the social maturity to match their physical maturity, they may encounter unrealistic expectations from adults.

If Anna were left untreated, her growth chart would look very much like that shown in Chapter 13, Figure 13-15. She would be tall initially due to her early estrogen-induced growth spurt, but she would be short as an adult due to premature closure of her epiphyses.

REVIEW QUESTIONS

Directions: For each of the following questions, choose the *one best* answer.

1 An endocrinologist is called to evaluate a newborn with ambiguous genitalia. On exam, gonads are palpable in the scrotum. The genitalia are ambiguous and include a phallic-like structure measuring approximately 1 cm. The parents are very concerned about the sex assignment. The endocrinologist should tell them that

A since the phallic structure is very small, the sex assignment will be female

B since the infant has testes, the sex assignment will be male

C the sex assignment will depend on what the chromosomes are

D multiple factors need to be taken into consideration in determining the sex assignment.

E the child should be allowed to choose his or her own sex at puberty

2 One week later, another child is born with ambiguous genitalia. The mother had amniocentesis done, so it is known that the infant's karyotype is 46,XX. No gonads are palpable. The external genitalia include a phallic-like structure measuring approximately 1 cm. An ultrasound done shortly after birth reveals a normal uterus, fallopian tubes, and ovaries. The most likely cause for this infant's ambiguous genitalia is

A complete estrogen resistance

B mixed gonadal dysgenesis

C 21-hydroxylase deficiency

D paternal androgen-secreting tumor

3 A mother is concerned because her 13-year-old daughter is only 4'9" tall. Her daughter is otherwise healthy and has been menstruating regularly for the last 1 1/2 years. The mother wants to know if this child will grow taller. What is the most accurate response?

A The child will grow, but may need treatment with growth hormone to help her

B While *most* girls have their pubertal growth spurt before menarche, a few have it after menarche

C The child will grow, but only if she is given medication to stop her menses

D During the 2 years after menarche, the child should grow approximately the same amount as she grew in the 2 years before menarche

E Menarche represents the end-point of puberty in girls and, therefore, the child does not have any significant growth potential left

4 A 7-year-old boy comes to clinic because he recently has developed pubic hair. The parents also report an adult body odor, which started about 1 month before the clinic visit. The child has otherwise been healthy. On examination, Tanner stage II pubic hair and axillary odor are noted. The testes are 2 cc (normal: prepubertal size 1–3 cc), and the phallus is Tanner stage I. The examination is otherwise normal. Review of previous growth charts reveals that the child has been growing normally at about the 75th percentile. Bone age x-ray is normal (within 2 SD of the mean). Based on this information, the most likely diagnosis is

A benign premature thelarche

B congenital adrenal hyperplasia

C central precocious puberty

D benign premature pubarche (adrenarche)

E ingestion of anabolic steroids

5 A 17-year-old girl comes to the clinic because of primary amenorrhea. Breast development started several years ago but she has had no menses. She has otherwise been well. On exam, height is above the 95th percentile. Breasts are Tanner stage V, but there is no pubic or axillary hair. The endocrinologist attempts a pelvic exam but is unable to visualize the cervix. These findings are most consistent with which of the following syndromes?

A Turner syndrome

B Kallman syndrome

C Testicular feminization syndrome

D Klinefelter syndrome

E Prader-Willi syndrome

6 The mother of a 3-year-old girl has noticed gradual enlargement of the girl's right breast followed shortly by enlargement of the left breast during the last few months. The child has otherwise been healthy. No one in the home is on birth control pills. Examination reveals height and weight to be at the 50th percentile (where they were 1 year ago), Tanner stage II breast development with no axillary hair or odor, and Tanner stage I pubic hair. Her records show that her growth velocity is normal. A bone age x-ray is also normal (i.e., equal to chronologic age). What is the most likely cause of this child's breast development?

A Premature thelarche
B Premature pubarche
C Congenital adrenal hyperplasia
D McCune-Albright syndrome
E Central precocious puberty

7 A 6-year-old boy is referred for evaluation of pubic hair, which his father first noticed about 6 months ago. It has increased in amount since then. He also thinks his child's penis has gotten bigger and states, "He is growing like a weed." His son has otherwise been healthy. Examination reveals height and weight above the 95th percentile, and Tanner stage III pubic hair and genital development. The testes are 3 cc (normal prepubertal size: 1–3 cc). A bone age is read as 12 years. Laboratory tests include a serum 17-hydroxyprogesterone level of 3900 ng/dL (normal 3–90 ng/dL). This child has

A idiopathic central precocious puberty
B congenital adrenal hyperplasia
C premature pubarche
D McCune Albright syndrome
E familial testotoxicosis

8 A 14-year-old girl has not yet had menses. She developed pubic hair at approximately 12 years but has had no breast development. She has always been short but has otherwise been healthy. On examination, height and weight are below the 5th percentile. Other findings include Tanner stage I breasts, Tanner stage III pubic hair, low-posterior hairline, a webbed neck, and cubitus valgus (increased carrying angle). Chromosome analysis reveals a 45,X karyotype. Her hormone profile is most likely to be

A low follicle stimulating hormone (FSH), low luteinizing hormone (LH), and low estrogen
B normal FSH, normal LH, and low estrogen
C high FSH, high LH, and high estrogen
D high FSH, high LH, and low estrogen

References

Achermann JC, Ito M, Hindmarsh PC, et al: A mutation in the gene encoding steroidogenic factor-1 causes XY sex reversal and adrenal failure in humans. *Nat Genet* 22: 125–126, 1999.

Fenton C, Tang M, Poth M: Review of precocious puberty parts 1 and II: Gonadotropin-dependent precocious puberty: gonadotropin-independent precocious puberty. *The Endocrinol* 10: 107–112, 397–402, 2000.

Kulin H: Delayed puberty. *J Clin Endocrinol Metab* 81(10): 3460–3464, 1996.

Stein MT, Dandberg DE, Mazur T, et al: A newborn infant with a disorder of sexual differentiation. *J Dev Behav Pediatr* 24: 115–119, 2003.

Tilmann C, Capel B: Cellular and molecular pathways regulating mammalian sex determination. *Recent Prog Horn Res* 57: 1–18, 2002.

Vanio S, Heikkila M, Kispert A, et al: Female development in mammals is regulated by Wnt-4 signaling. *Nature* 397: 405–409, 1999.

Zucker KJ: Intersexuality and gender identity differentiation. *J Pediatr Adolesc Gynecol* 15: 3–13, 2002.

Notes

15

Endocrinology of Pregnancy and Lactation

Virginia R. Lupo, M.D.

■ CHAPTER OUTLINE ■

■ LEARNING OBJECTIVES ■

At the completion of this chapter, the student will:
1. recognize the hormonal milieu necessary to maintain early pregnancy.
2. understand the role of human chorionic gonadotropin.
3. recognize the major peptide hormones of the placenta.
4. recognize the role of steroid hormones in the physiologic changes of pregnancy.
5. be aware of the hormone changes after delivery.
6. understand the anatomy of the breast and neural and hormonal control of lactation.
7. be aware of the relationship between lactation and contraception.
8. be aware of the normal changes in glucose metabolism and the complications of diabetes in pregnancy.
9. be aware of the complications of thyroid disease and pregnancy.

CASE STUDY: *INTRODUCTION*

A 28-year-old woman came to the company health service for a physical examination, as she had just started her new job as a computer programmer. She had had one normal pregnancy and was breast-feeding her 6-month-old infant. Menses had not yet recurred. She used oral contraceptives in the past, but since her child was born she has used a diaphragm for contraception. Recently she has experienced frequent nausea and increased fatigue, which she attributes to the stress of her new job. Her past medical history was unremarkable except for an appendectomy at age 7. She has a sister with hypothyroidism and two grandmothers who have type 2 diabetes mellitus.

Physical examination revealed a modestly obese woman with mild acne. She had lost 5 lb since her examination 3 months ago. Her blood pressure was within normal limits. Her resting heart rate (HR) was 88 beats/min (past HR: 76 beats/min). Her eye examination was unremarkable. Her thyroid gland was slightly enlarged but not changed from her last examination. Her urine human chorionic gonadotropin (HCG) level was high.

Hormonal Events of Early Pregnancy

Fertilization of the egg by the sperm occurs in the fallopian tube within 48 hours of ovulation. Tubal peristalsis propels the zygote into the endometrial cavity. The endometrium is primed to receive a fertilized egg by the estrogen already secreted during the first half of the menstrual cycle (see Chapter 12). As soon as ovulation occurs, the remaining granulosa cells in the follicle that has released the egg begin producing progesterone in large quantities. Progesterone deposits appear yellow, and after ovulation the follicle is called a corpus luteum ("yellow body"). Progesterone stabilizes the endometrium in preparation for implantation, which occurs 6 to 7 days after conception, when the embryo is at the blastocyst stage.

For most pregnancies, the date of conception is not known. By convention "weeks of gestation" or "gestational age" is dated from the first day of the last menstrual period.

If implantation does not occur, the corpus luteum makes progesterone for approximately 10 days after ovulation. Progesterone feedback inhibits luteinizing hormone (LH) production by the pituitary gland. This results in menses, because without LH the corpus luteum fails. However, if implantation does occur, the developing embryo begins making HCG within 24 hours. HCG is a peptide hormone that mimics the effect of LH. HCG combines with LH–HCG receptors and stimulates the corpus luteum to continue producing progesterone; thus the endometrial lining is maintained and menses do not occur. Ablation of the corpus luteum at this time causes loss of the pregnancy because there is no other adequate source of progesterone. By approximately 9 weeks after conception (approximately 11 weeks gestation), the rudimentary placenta is able to synthesize enough progesterone to support the pregnancy, and the corpus luteum involutes.

Hormones of the Placenta

The placenta is an active metabolic factory, producing peptide hormones, steroid hormones, and many releasing and inhibiting factors for these hormones. The role of many of these hormones in pregnancy is not well understood.

POLYPEPTIDE HORMONES

Polypeptide hormones are made entirely within the placenta. They are too large to cross the placental barrier into the fetus, so they are found only in the maternal circulation. Their impact on maternal metabolism is uncertain. Several cytokines and growth factors are also produced by the placenta and may act locally. Polypeptide-releasing hormones synthesized by the placenta include gonadotropin-releasing hormone (GnRH), thyrotropin-releasing hormone (TRH), and corticotropin-releasing hormone (CRH). Pituitary-like products from the placenta include placental lactogen (similar to prolactin [PRL]), HCG (similar to LH), chorionic thyrotropin (similar to thyroid-stimulating hormone [TSH]), and chorionic adrenocorticotropin (similar to adrenocorticotropic hormone [ACTH]).

HUMAN CHORIONIC GONADOTROPIN (HCG)

HCG is produced by placental tissue and rare germ cell tumors and is virtually undetectable in the maternal circulation before pregnancy. HCG is a glycoprotein with two subunits: the α-chain is common to HCG, LH, follicle-stimulating hormone (FSH), and TSH; the β-chain has some homology to the LH β-chain but is unique to HCG. In the past, pregnancy tests identified the entire HCG molecule. When other hormones with the common α-subunit were present in high concentrations, cross-reactivity occurred and resulted in false-positive pregnancy tests. Now pregnancy tests measure only the β-subunit of HCG, eliminating false-positive results. Home urine pregnancy tests use a monoclonal antibody specific for the β-subunit of HCG and give highly accurate results within a few minutes. Quantitative measurement of serum HCG is used primarily to distinguish between a viable pregnancy and an ectopic pregnancy or a miscarriage. Serum and urine tests can be positive by 9 days after conception unless the urine is very dilute.

The HCG level doubles every 48 hours during the first few weeks of pregnancy, rising to a peak at 10 weeks of gestation (Fig. 15-1). After

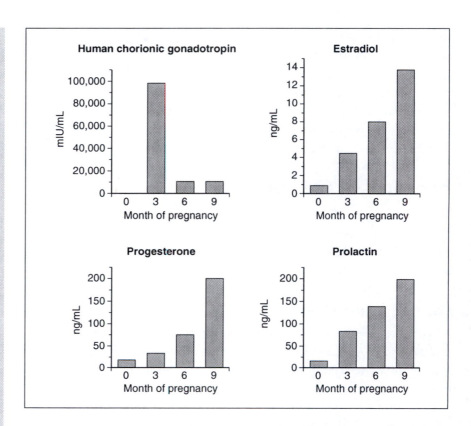

Fig. 15-1. Plasma Levels of Human Chorionic Gonadotropin, Estrogen, Progesterone, and Prolactin before and during Pregnancy

Since prepregnancy levels of estrogen and progesterone fluctuate throughout the menstrual cycle, values shown are at the upper limits of the normal ranges in nonpregnant women.

10 weeks the HCG level decreases but remains above the nonpregnant level until delivery.

> Specific biochemical identification of the pregnant state requires measurement of human chorionic gonadotropin (HCG), which is present only during pregnancy. Pregnancy tests measure HCG, a placental hormone, which is detectable in serum and urine as early as 9 days after conception.

An abnormal rise in HCG early in gestation indicates a nonviable pregnancy. A very high HCG level indicates a trophoblastic tumor such as a hydatidiform mole or a choriocarcinoma.

HUMAN PLACENTAL LACTOGEN (HPL)

As pregnancy progresses, exponential growth of the placenta results in an exponential increase in the placental polypeptide hormone HPL. This is a single polypeptide chain of 191 amino acids, sometimes

CASE STUDY: *CONTINUED*

The patient's high urine HCG level indicated that she was pregnant again. Her nausea, fatigue, and mild tachycardia might be due to pregnancy, but because of her family history of thyroid disease, thyroid function tests were obtained. She had an elevated total thyroxine (T_4) level with a normal free T_4. Her TSH level was within normal limits. Her fasting plasma glucose level was lower than a previous nonpregnant level.

As her pregnancy progressed, the patient's acne resolved, but she complained of chronic sinus drainage and constipation. During her second trimester, her fasting plasma glucose was higher than expected, and an oral glucose tolerance test revealed a blood glucose level more than two standard deviations (SD) above the mean for her stage of pregnancy.

referred to as human chorionic somatomammotropin (HCS), which has some structural homology to pituitary growth hormone. Placental growth, fetal growth, and HPL levels all increase exponentially in the third trimester of pregnancy (see Fig. 15-1). The role of HPL during pregnancy is uncertain, but HPL does stimulate maternal lipolysis, making more fatty acids available for fuel during periods of fasting. HPL is thought to contribute to the increase in maternal insulin resistance that occurs as pregnancy progresses.

STEROID HORMONES

The placenta is unable to synthesize steroid hormones de novo. Cholesterol precursors from the maternal compartment are required for placental synthesis of progesterone. Placental estrogen synthesis also requires cholesterol precursors from the maternal compartment, but these must be further metabolized by the fetal adrenal and fetal liver. Most estrogens are actually metabolites of androgens, which require fetal and placental steps in their synthesis. When the precursors do become available, the syncytiotrophoblast has extraordinary ability to complete estrogen and progesterone synthesis and to secrete the hormones into the maternal and fetal circulations.

> Placenta steroid synthesis requires cholesterol precursors from the maternal compartment. Placenta estrogen synthesis also requires processing by the fetal adrenal and fetal liver.

Maternal estradiol levels increase markedly during pregnancy (see Fig. 15-1) as do the levels of estrone and estriol. Since estrogen

Table 15-1. Effects of Increased Estrogen During Pregnancy

Increased hepatic protein synthesis	Increased uterine blood flow
Peripheral vasodilatation	Increased blood volume
Increased heart rate	Physiologic anemia
Increased stroke volume	Increased coagulation factors
Increased cardiac output	Increased renal perfusion and creatinine clearance

Notes

synthesis requires synergy between the fetus and the placenta, estrogen levels were once thought to reflect the metabolic integrity of the placenta, and serial estrogen levels were used to assess fetal well-being. Now more direct measures of fetal well-being are used. Maternal progesterone levels also increase dramatically during pregnancy (see Fig. 15-1). Placental estrogen and progesterone have profound effects on the mother, but their roles in the development of the fetus are still not well defined.

Estrogen

Major physiologic effects of increased estrogen are listed in Table 15-1. Hepatic synthesis of most proteis, including thyroid hormone–binding globulin and cortisol-binding globulin, is increased, but serum transaminase levels are not elevated.

Estrogen is a profound vasodilator. Blood flow to the uterus increases due to the estrogen-induced decrease in uteroplacental resistance. Peripheral vasodilatation requires an increase in cardiac output; both stroke volume and heart rate rise, and cardiac output increases up to 50%. Women with lesions restricting cardiac output may suffer worsening of their heart disease. Peripheral blood pressure falls initially due to the vasodilatation, but eventually returns to prepregnancy levels. Blood vessels are less sensitive to angiotensin during pregnancy, probably due to a change at the angiotensin receptor level.

Estrogen-induced vasodilatation is responsible for the following:

- Increased sinus congestion
- Increased epistaxis (nosebleeds)
- Bleeding gums
- Better healing of acne and chronic ulcerations
- Sensation of warmth

Plasma volume increases more than red blood cell (RBC) mass, and a physiologic anemia occurs routinely in pregnant women. Coagulation factors and venous thromboembolic disease increase. This problem persists until estrogen levels fall postpartum. One third of thromboses occur in the postpartum period.

Table 15-2. Effects of Increased Progesterone during Pregnancy

Increased minute ventilation	Decreased intestinal motility
Compensated respiratory alkalosis	Urinary collecting system stasis
Smooth muscle relaxation	Decreased uterine contractions
Lower esophageal sphincter relaxation	

The increase in venous thromboembolic disease during pregnancy is due to the following:

- Increased coagulation factors
- Stasis
- Vessel wall damage

Renal perfusion increases. Creatinine clearance increases by 50%; serum creatinine and blood urea nitrogen (BUN) levels fall. The glomeruli cannot reabsorb all the glucose filtered, so many pregnant women have glucosuria even with normal plasma glucose levels.

Progesterone

Major physiologic effects of increased progesterone are listed in Table 15-2. Progesterone acts upon the central respiratory centers to produce a sense of air hunger. Tidal volume increases, resulting in a respiratory alkalosis that is compensated by increased bicarbonate excretion. Minute ventilation also increases, but there is no change in respiratory rate. The expiratory reserve is decreased by elevation of the diaphragm as the uterus enlarges.

Progesterone is responsible for smooth muscle relaxation during pregnancy. Relaxation of the lower esophageal sphincter can result in reflux esophagitis. Gastric emptying is delayed. Decreased intestinal motility causes constipation in many women. Increased stasis in the ureters and urethra contributes to the increase in urinary tract infections during pregnancy.

Progesterone-induced smooth muscle relaxation causes:
- Increased esophageal reflux and esophagitis
- Delayed gastric emptying
- Constipation
- Urinary tract stasis and infections

Other Hormonal and Metabolic Alterations during Pregnancy

The metabolic and hormonal adaptations to pregnancy are extensive (Table 15-3). Pituitary production of GnRH, LH, and FSH remains

Table 15-3. Major Maternal Hormonal and Metabolic Changes during Pregnancy

Higher estrogen	Increased total and free cortisol
Higher progesterone	Increased calcium absorption; normal ionized calcium
Low LH and FSH	Lower fasting glucose; increased postprandial glucose
Increasing prolactin	Higher postprandial insulin; increased insulin resistance
High total T_4; normal free T_4 and TSH	

Note. LH = luteinizing hormone; FSH = follicle-stimulating hormone; T4 = thyroxine; TSH = thyroid-stimulating hormone.

suppressed by the high circulating levels of estrogen and progesterone until delivery. Pituitary size increases, primarily due to the estrogen-induced stimulation of lactotrophs, which produce PRL.

Renal clearance of iodide is increased during pregnancy. Mild thyroid enlargement is common during pregnancy, especially in areas of iodine deficiency. The concentrations of total T_4 and total T_3 increase as a result of the estrogen-induced increase in thyroid-binding globulin (TBG) [see Chapter 4], but free thyroid hormone concentrations and TSH are normal. Maternal TSH does not cross the placenta. Only minute amounts of maternal T_4 and T_3 cross the placenta, but they are sufficient for a fetus without a thyroid gland to develop normally until after delivery.

Total plasma cortisol increases due to the estrogen-induced increase in cortisol-binding globulin. Plasma free cortisol is also higher during pregnancy, but pregnant women do not develop signs of cortisol excess. The diurnal variation of cortisol levels is maintained.

Calcium (Ca^{2+}) is needed for the fetal skeleton, especially in the third trimester. Maternal parathyroid glands become hyperplastic, and Ca^{2+} absorption efficiency increases. Ionized Ca^{2+} remains normal.

Fetal nutritional requirements alter maternal fuel metabolism. Fasting glucose levels decrease because glucose is transported across the placenta to the fetus by facilitated diffusion, and amino acids actively transported to the fetus are not available for maternal gluconeogenesis. Lipolysis and ketogenesis increase, and fasting ketone and free fatty acid levels are higher. Fatty acids do not cross the placenta. Maternal insulin is bound and degraded by the placenta and does not cross into the fetal compartment. The fetus depends on its own insulin for glucose disposal; fetal insulin is produced by 12 weeks gestation.

There is a shift in maternal carbohydrate metabolism after meals, especially as pregnancy advances from the second into the third trimester. Postmeal glucose levels are higher than in nonpregnant women, even though postprandial insulin secretion increases. This insulin resistance has been attributed to higher levels of HPL, progesterone, and cortisol. Lipolysis is suppressed after meals despite the insulin resistance. Triglyceride synthesis increases due to the high estrogen levels.

Endocrine Changes at Parturition

Levels of placental hormones fall precipitously after the placenta is delivered. The plasma half-lives of the placental hormones determine how quickly they disappear from the maternal circulation. Some women are sensitive enough to the rapid fall in estrogen levels that they perceive hot flashes similar to those which occur after menopause. The decrease in circulating estrogen quickly returns peripheral vascular resistance to its nonpregnant levels. The diminished smooth muscle tone of pregnancy resolves as progesterone levels fall. In nonlactating women the estrogen and progesterone are back to prepregnancy levels by 6 week' postpartum. At this time the increased risk of thromboembolism from estrogen-induced hepatic synthesis of coagulation factors is over, the renal collecting system is back to normal, and the risk of urinary tract infection is back to the prepregnancy level.

In lactating women, estrogen levels are suppressed for months by increased PRL secretion (see Role of Prolactin). Bone loss occurs as a result of this hypoestrogenism, but this is promptly reversed after lactation ceases.

The insulin resistance induced by pregnancy resolves very rapidly after delivery.

Diabetes Mellitus and Pregnancy

In women who have diabetes *before* pregnancy, control of blood glucose early in gestation influences the occurrence of congenital malformations. Glucose is transported across the placenta by means of facilitated diffusion, so maternal hyperglycemia exposes the fetus to hyperglycemia. Poor diabetes control at conception is highly correlated with increases in fetal heart and neural tube defects, spontaneous abortion, and premature deliveries. Infants of poorly controlled diabetic mothers are also at risk for death at term. The mechanisms are not known.

In women who have diabetes *before* pregnancy, the degree of control of blood glucose at conception and during the first few weeks of gestation influences the occurrence of congenital malformations in the fetus.

Some women develop diabetes *during* pregnancy because they cannot increase insulin secretion enough to counteract the physiologic increase in insulin resistance. Prospective screening with an oral glucose challenge test in midpregnancy may reveal maternal glucose levels more than 2 standard deviations higher than expected. This is called *gestational* diabetes. Because gestational diabetes develops after organogenesis has occurred, the risk of congenital malformations is not increased.

When maternal hyperglycemia results in fetal hyperglycemia, the fetus secretes more insulin. Insulin is a major growth factor for the fetus, and fetuses of diabetic mothers are more likely to be large *(macrosomia)* as a result of the hyperinsulinemia and the increased fuel supply. Macrosomia increases the risk for birth trauma, especially shoulder dystocia, and the need for cesarean section.

Fetuses of diabetic mothers are often larger than those of nondiabetic mothers **(macrosomia)**. Macrosomia is due to the excessive fuel (glucose) supplied to the fetus and to fetal hyperinsulinemia.

Gestational diabetes develops in the second half of pregnancy. Because it occurs after fetal organogenesis, the risk for congenital malformations is not increased.

Most women with gestational diabetes are treated with changes in diet alone, but sometimes insulin therapy is necessary. If so, large doses of insulin may be required to overcome the insulin resistance. All pregnant women with diabetes need careful blood glucose monitoring to avoid fasting hypoglycemia as well as hyperglycemia.

Women with diabetes need very careful glucose monitoring during pregnancy to avoid the complications of hyperglycemia, hypoglycemia, and ketosis.

After delivery of the infant, maternal insulin requirements plummet because the factors produced by the placenta that cause insulin resistance are no longer present. Gestational diabetes resolves as the insulin resistance resolves, unless pregnancy has unmasked underlying diabetes that was unrecognized previously. Approximately 40% of women with gestational diabetes will develop diabetes within 10 to 15 years. The risk of subsequent diabetes increases if women are obese or have a family history of diabetes.

Exposure of the infant to hyperglycemia stops abruptly at delivery, but fetal hyperinsulinemia is still present. Therefore, newborns of diabetic mothers must be watched for the development of hypoglycemia. Infants of diabetic mothers are also more likely to have polycythemia, hyperbilirubinemia, and hypocalcemia, the causes of which are uncertain. Lactation is not contraindicated for women with diabetes.

Newborns of diabetic mothers are at risk for hypoglycemia.

Thyroid Disorders and Pregnancy

Some of the symptoms of pregnancy mimic those of hyperthyroidism: nausea, a sensation of warmth due to vasodilatation, tachycardia, and increased cardiac output. Thyroid function testing and pregnancy testing are required to make the correct diagnosis.

Hyperthyroidism causes menstrual irregularity and infertility, but this is not universal, and hyperthyroid women can become pregnant. Maternal hyperthyroidism is most often due to Graves disease, with thyroid-stimulating immunoglobulins (TSI) causing stimulation of the thyroid gland (see Chapter 4). TSI can cross the placenta into the fetal compartment and stimulate the fetal thyroid gland. This results in fetal tachycardia, hypermetabolism, and fetal growth restriction. Since hyperthyroidism can be life-threatening for both mother and fetus, hyperthyroidism must be treated during pregnancy. However, the antithyroid medications used to treat maternal hyperthyroidism do cross the placenta into the fetal compartment and can cause fetal hypothyroidism. The minimum dose required to bring the mother's thyroid function tests into the upper limit of the normal range should be given. Inadvertent administration of radioactive iodine to a pregnant woman can result in destruction of the fetal thyroid gland. Since untreated hypothyroidism in the newborn period causes irreversible brain damage, many states perform routine heel-stick capillary screening for hypothyroidism after birth.

CASE STUDY: *CONTINUED*

The patient's thyroid function tests were typical for a pregnant woman. Total T_4 levels were increased due to the estrogen-induced increase in TBG (see Chapter 4) but her normal free T_4 and TSH indicated that she was euthyroid. The improvement in her acne and her increased sinus drainage were consequences of estrogen-induced vasodilation, and the constipation was caused by progesterone-induced smooth muscle relaxation.

Initially, her fasting plasma glucose level was lower than before her pregnancy, an expected adaptation to the nutritional requirements of the fetus. However, by midpregnancy she had developed gestational diabetes. After this diagnosis was made, she watched her caloric intake carefully, and her glucose control was excellent. She delivered a 9 lb girl 2 weeks before her due date. Her constipation and excessive sinus drainage resolved after delivery. Within a week after delivery, her plasma glucose levels were similar to those prior to her pregnancy. Her constipation and excessive sinus drainage resolved after delivery. She decided to breastfeed this baby also.

Maternal hypothyroidism has no impact on the fetal thyroid axis unless the hypothyroidism is due to previously treated Graves disease and antibodies still remain in the maternal circulation. Thyroid hormone replacement for the mother crosses the placenta in such small amounts that fetal thyroid hormone levels are not increased. Several studies have shown that requirements for thyroid hormone replacement increase during pregnancy. The high estrogen levels stimulate hepatic synthesis of thyroid binding globulin. More T_4 is bound and less free T_4 is available. Thyroid function tests should be followed carefully.

The Breast and Lactation

ANATOMY OF THE BREAST

The breast is composed of clusters of secretory alveoli (lobules), which empty into intralobular ducts. These empty into larger collecting ducts that converge under the nipple (Fig. 15-2). The alveoli are lined by cuboidal epithelial cells, which produce milk after pregnancy. The alveoli are surrounded by myoepithelial cells, and the contraction of these muscle cells causes ejection of milk in the alveoli into the ducts.

Many systemic hormones act jointly to produce breast enlargement and priming for lactation during pregnancy. Estrogen, progesterone, PRL, growth hormone, insulin, cortisol, epithelial growth factor, and probably parathyroid hormone–related peptide are required.

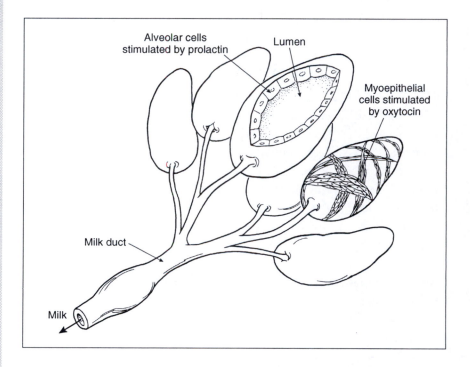

Fig. 15-2. Anatomy of the Breast

A cluster of alveoli showing alveolar and myoepithelial cells.

New alveoli and ducts are formed, and alveolar cells proliferate. Estrogen and PRL stimulate accumulation of adipose tissue, which results in breast enlargement. Each breast enlarges by approximately 0.5 kg during pregnancy. By the second trimester the breasts are developed enough for milk production, if premature birth makes this necessary.

ROLE OF PROLACTIN (PRL)

PRL is the main hormonal support of lactation, although insulin and cortisol are also required. PRL is a polypeptide consisting of 198 amino acids held together by three disulfide bonds. PRL is made in the lactotroph cells of the anterior pituitary and binds to membrane receptors on breast alveolar cells. In nonpregnant women PRL secretion is kept tonically suppressed by dopamine from the hypothalamus. The rise in PRL during pregnancy is due to the high levels of estrogen. Estrogen stimulates lactotroph hyperplasia and PRL gene expression in the pituitary. Estrogen also inhibits dopamine release and decreases pituitary dopamine receptors.

In the nonpregnant state, the lactotrophs make up 10% to 25% of the pituitary, and PRL production is tonically suppressed by dopamine. During pregnancy, PRL levels rise as much as twenty- to fortyfold and up to 70% of the gland is involved in synthesis of PRL.

Although PRL levels rise early and dramatically under the influence of estrogen (see Fig. 15-1), milk production does not occur during pregnancy. Estrogen blocks terminal differentiation of alveolar epithelium, and progesterone blocks the onset of milk production. At term, with delivery of the placenta, estrogen and progesterone levels fall dramatically and lactation can begin.

During pregnancy, milk production is suppressed by estrogen and progesterone.

Suckling on the nipple is the main regulator of PRL secretion during lactation. Suckling activates sensory receptors and transmission of impulses via thoracic nerves T4, T5, and T6 to the spinal cord and hypothalamus. Dopamine secretion is suppressed. This results in release of stored PRL from the anterior pituitary (Fig. 15-3). The PRL level can increase ten- to twentyfold. PRL increases gene expression of milk proteins; stimulates synthesis of lactose, the main sugar in milk; and increases milk yield. PRL released during suckling stimulates milk production from the breast for 3 to 4 hours, allowing alveolar cells to replenish the milk supply.

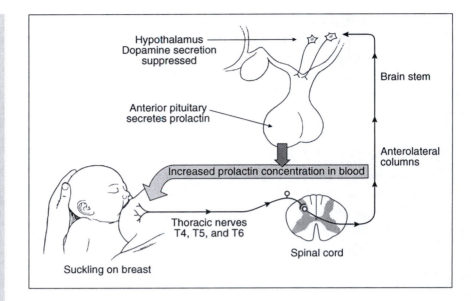

Fig. 15-3. Neural Repsonses to Suckling Resulting in Prolactin Secretion from the Pituitary Gland

Over time, PRL levels fall even in women who continue to breast-feed. Nevertheless, a rise in PRL still occurs with each episode of breast-feeding. Even 6 months after delivery, PRL levels are higher than nonpregnant levels and increase twofold with suckling.

PRL is also found in ovarian follicle fluid, in the lining of the pregnant uterus, and in amniotic fluid. In other species PRL plays a role in osmotic regulation. Some studies suggest that the very high PRL concentration in amniotic fluid helps maintain fetal water balance until squamous epithelium develops and fetal skin becomes impermeable to water.

ROLE OF OXYTOCIN

Suckling on the areola stimulates afferent nerves running with thoracic nerves T4, T5, and T6, and impulses are transmitted to the spinal cord and hypothalamus. Oxytocin, a peptide produced in the supraoptic and paraventricular nuclei of the hypothalamus, is then released into the circulation from the posterior pituitary (see Chapter 3). Oxytocin stimulates contraction of the myoepithelial cells surrounding the breast alveoli, causing milk to be expressed into the nipple.

Milk release from the breast is due primarily to suckling-induced release of the hormone oxytocin.

The infant's tongue strokes the nipple from back to front, stripping the milk out of the nipple. Initially the oxytocin level is elevated only during actual breast-feeding. However, after women have been breast-feeding for a time, central nervous system (CNS) effects can also cause oxytocin secretion. Hearing a baby cry can be sufficient stimulation for oxytocin release.

Oxytocin receptors are also found in the uterus. Oxytocin increases the frequency and strength of uterine contractions. Estrogen potentiates the action of oxytocin by altering membrane potentials of uterine smooth muscle cells. The uterus is especially sensitive to oxytocin at the end of pregnancy, when the estrogen levels are very high. Dilation of the uterus, cervix, and vagina during delivery also stimulates oxytocin secretion. In the postpartum period, a woman who is breast-feeding may experience uterine contractions. Oxytocin-induced muscle contraction helps the uterus return to its normal size and reduces postpartum bleeding.

COMPOSITION OF BREAST MILK

The fluid produced during the first 2 to 3 days postpartum is colostrum, a thick mixture composed of desquamated epithelial cells, lymphocytes, and transudate. Milk production usually begins within 3 days of delivery. Breast milk is the ideal energy source for the growing newborn. It is digestible, sterile, and always the correct temperature. IgA is present in colostrum and breast milk and helps to protect the infant's mucosal surfaces from infection. Immunocompetent cells are also present in breast milk and help boost neonatal immunologic defenses.

The content and composition of breast milk adapt to changing conditions. For example, the milk from the breast at the end of a session of suckling has a higher fat content than the earlier milk. This may trigger satiety in the infant when the majority of the milk has been extracted from that feeding. Preterm milk contains more protein, lower lactose, and more essential long-chain fatty acids than term milk, making it ideal for preterm infants needing more brain growth than term infants.

Breast milk provides 20 kcal/oz, which is the caloric equivalent of whole cow milk (see Table 15-4). Breast-fed infants are less likely to become obese than formula-fed infants, perhaps due to the increased

Table 15-4. Comparison of Human Milk and Cow Milk

	HUMAN MILK	COW MILK
Caloric content (Kcal/L)	750	700
Fat (g/100 g milk)	4.5	3.8
Lactose (g/100 mL)	140	110
Protein (g/100 mL)	1.0	3.3
Casein (g/100 mL)	0.4	2.7
Whey:casein ratio	70:30	30:70
Cholesterol (mg/L)	139	110
Sodium (mEq/L)	7.8	22
Potassium (mEq/L)	14	36
Calcium (mg/100 mL)	34	120
Phosphorous (mg/100 mL)	15	90
Iron (mg/L)	0.3	0.5

work of suckling from the breast. Approximately half the calories in mature milk come from fat. The fat content gradually increases for approximately 3 months after delivery. Breast milk contains fatty acids that are essential for myelin production and brain maturation. PRL stimulates breast lipoprotein lipase, which makes fatty acids more available for milk production.

The main proteins of human milk and cow milk are different. Human milk contains less casein and more whey. Casein is the mixture of cheese-generating proteins in milk that precipitate when milk is acidified to pH 4.0. The remaining supernatant is whey. Whey proteins contain more essential amino acids and are easier for the infant's immature gastrointestinal tract to digest than casein.

The main sugar of milk is lactose, a combination of glucose and galactose, which provides approximately 42% of the calories of mature milk. Lactose accounts for 70% of the osmolality of human milk, which has a low sodium (Na^+) content. PRL stimulates resorption of Na^+ from human milk and thus protects the infant from hypernatremia.

Iron is available in very small amounts in breast milk, but its bioavailability is so great that levels are as high in nursing infants as in infants fed iron-fortified formula.

Breast-fed infants have fewer gastrointestinal illnesses, food allergies, and ear infections in the first year of life.

Maternal nutrition during lactation should include 1500 mg calcium daily from dairy products or other foods or supplements. Maternal iron supplementation is often required during breast-feeding, although adequate dietary intake is possible with attention to iron-rich foods. Drugs taken by the mother are transported into breast milk mainly by passive diffusion, but lipid solubility, ionization, and protein binding affect the concentration in breast milk. Lactic acid, which accumulates after heavy exercise, and alcohol are also transported into breast milk. Many women note aversion of the newborn to breast-feeding after maternal alcohol ingestion or vigorous exercise. Nicotine decreases milk production.

SUSTAINING LACTATION

Milk yield is mainly determined by infant demand. There is a synergism between breastfeeding and milk production that allows increased milk production as the infant grows. The more an infant suckles, the more milk a woman produces. Milk volume reaches a maximum of 800 to 1200 mL/day, after 6 to 7 months of lactation. Maintenance of ongoing milk production *(galactopoiesis)* is maximal if milk is emptied completely from the breast. Supplementation of breast-feeding with

Table 15-5. Barriers to Lactation

MATERNAL	NEONATAL
Cultural	Marked prematurity
Infection	Hypotonia
Medications	Ventilator support
	Congenital malformations

formula or food can decrease the infant's sucking frequency and intensity very quickly. This diminishes milk supply and results in greater hunger for exogenous nutritional sources by the infant. Only with long-standing breast-feeding can milk production be maintained even if feedings are decreased to only once or twice a day. Breast-feeding can be maintained for several years after birth. Occasionally, women breast-feed through a subsequent pregnancy, although this is uncommon in the United States.

Despite the advantages of breast-feeding for the infant, many women in the United States choose not to do this. Barriers to lactation are listed in Table 15-5. Motivation to breast-feed is culturally influenced to a large extent. Maternal infections and medications may also limit lactation. Human immunodeficiency virus (HIV) is transmitted in breast milk, and in the United States nursing is not recommended for HIV positive women. The World Health Organization does not discourage breast-feeding among HIV positive women when infants are more likely to die of malnutrition or diarrheal disease if they are not nursing, than of HIV if they are nursing. Maternal hepatitis B (HBV) infection is not a contraindication to breast-feeding, as long as the newborn receives passive prophylaxis for HBV shortly after delivery and begins the primary immunization series against the virus while in the hospital.

Breast-feeding is contraindicated in women taking cocaine or methadone, which are transferred into breast milk. Tetracyclines can cause staining of baby teeth and permanent teeth. Quinolone antibiotics can cause disordered growth of the cartilagenous epiphyses during the first year of life.

Infant barriers to suckling include marked prematurity, hypotonia, congenital malformations such as facial clefts, and need for ventilator support.

Decreased suckling during weaning results in decreased PRL and accumulation of local inhibitors of galactopoesis. Postlactation involution of the breast is mostly due to the decrease in PRL. Alveoli, ducts, and adipose tissue regress to approximately the prepregnancy state.

If a woman does not breast-feed, PRL levels begin to fall soon after delivery. Pharmacologic suppression of lactation with bromocriptine, a dopamine agonist that blocks PRL release, is no longer approved by the Food and Drug Administration because of the side effects (hypertension, seizures, strokes, and nausea). Failure to complete a full 2-week course of the drug can result in rebound breast engorgement. When women do not wish to breast-feed, ice packs and firm support of the breasts are used for the discomfort of breast engorgement. Breast stimulation should be avoided. The pressure stasis of not breast-feeding causes prompt cessation of new milk production. Estrogen can be used to suppress engorgement and lactation. The mechanism of this inhibition is uncertain.

LACTATION AND CONTRACEPTION

Breast-feeding is a low estrogen state. The high PRL level suppresses pulsatile GnRH secretion, so FSH and LH levels are tonically reduced to the low-normal range. Estrogen production is decreased and ovulation is suppressed. Lactation is an effective contraceptive from the standpoint of large populations where breast-feeding is common. However, in a given individual return of ovulatory function is unpredictable, and lactation is not a dependable method of contraception. As breast-feeding frequency wanes, baseline PRL levels fall. Eventually only a small peak is seen with each breast-feeding episode. Ovulation may occur and will precede the return of menses. In general, the period of anovulation during nursing lasts longer when maternal nutrition is poor.

Hormonal contraception during lactation is highly effective, but estrogen-containing pills can decrease milk production and should not be prescribed until several months after breast-feeding is well established. A progesterone-only contraceptive is a good choice while breast-feeding. Progesterone inhibits the initiation of milk production in the postpartum period, but progesterone does not interfere with the maintenance of lactation once it has been established. Barrier methods of contraception such as diaphragms or condoms do not interfere with breast-feeding, but they are less effective than hormonal contraception.

CASE STUDY: *RESOLUTION*

The patient breastfed her daughter for 6 months and experienced amenorrhea during that time. Since she became pregnant while breast-feeding her first child and using a barrier method of contraception, she decided to use a progesterone-only contraceptive while breast-feeding her second child. Her risk for developing diabetes in the future is increased because she is moderately obese and has a family history of diabetes. After she finished breast-feeding her daughter, she was given a modest weight reduction diet. Her exercise level increased as she coped with the demands of her job and two small children.

REVIEW QUESTIONS

Directions: For each of the following questions, choose the *one best* answer.

1 A 34-year-old woman's last menstrual period began 9 weeks ago. She is fatigued and nauseated, and she has lost 3 pounds in the past few weeks. The first step in her evaluation should consist of

A urine human chorionic gonadotropin
B thyroid-stimulating hormone (TSH) and free thyroxine
C oral glucose tolerance test
D follicle-stimulating hormone (FSH)

2 A 26-year-old woman's last menstrual period was 6 weeks ago, and pregnancy has been confirmed. At this time the necessary uterine environment to sustain pregnancy is maintained by

A maternal gonadotropin-releasing hormone (GnRH)
B human chorionic gonadotropin (HCG) from the endometrium
C progesterone from the corpus luteum
D luteinizing hormone (LH) from the developing fetal pituitary

3 A 36-year-old woman who is 7 months pregnant complains of heartburn, palpitations, rhinitis, and always feeling too warm. Which of the following conditions is due to the effects of progesterone during her pregnancy?

A Increased reflux esophagitis
B Peripheral vasodilation
C Increased cardiac output
D Heat intolerance

4 A 22-year-old woman volunteers for a study of hormonal adaptation during the third trimester of pregnancy. She previously has been well except for mild hypothyroidism, which was treated with thyroid-hormone replacement. If her pregnancy is progressing normally, the physician would be most likely to expect which of the following?

A Increased fasting plasma glucose and decreased postprandial glucose and insulin levels
B Decreased thyroid size and a decreased requirement for thyroid hormone replacement
C Increasing prolactin levels and postpeak human chorionic gonadotropin (HCG) levels
D Decreasing levels of estrogen and progesterone
E Decreased total and free cortisol levels

5 A woman wishes to breast-feed her infant. Forty-eight hours after delivery, she still has no milk production. Her infant has lost 5% of his initial birth weight. She is reassured when told that infants often lose up to 10% of their body weight before milk production begins. The cause of her inability to lactate at this time is most likely to be

A low estrogen and progesterone levels after delivery of the placenta
B residual inhibition of prolactin (PRL) action by estrogen and progesterone
C a low prolactin level due to postpartum pituitary infarction
D a low oxytocin level due to excessive suckling

6 After a normal pregnancy and delivery, a young woman is trying to decide whether or not to breast-feed her infant. Her physician would be most likely to tell her that compared to cow milk, breast milk

A is more likely to cause autoimmunity due to transmission of maternal IgG
B is less likely to cause infant obesity because it is lower in calories
C is less likely to cause hypernatremia but is likely to cause iron deficiency
D contains mostly carbohydrate in the form of sucrose
E contains more easily digestible whey than casein

7 A 38-year-old previously healthy woman had a blood glucose level more than 2 standard deviations above the expected mean after an oral glucose tolerance test at 28-weeks' gestation. If she has gestational diabetes, her infant is most at risk for

A cardiac malformations
B incomplete closure of the neural tube
C low birth weight
D shoulder dystocia
E postpartum hyperglycemia

References

Ben-Jonathan N, Hnasko R: Dopamine as a prolactin (PRL) inhibitor. *Endocrine Rev* 22: 724–763, 2001.

Challis JRG, Matthews SG, Gibb W, et al: Endocrine and paracrine regulation of birth at term and preterm. *Endocrine Rev* 21: 514–550, 2000.

Freed GL, Clark SJ, Sorenson J, et al: National assessment of physicians' breast-feeding knowledge, attitudes, training and experience. *JAMA* 273: 472–476, 1995.

Garner P: Type I diabetes and pregnancy. *Lancet* 346: 157–161, 1995.

Glinoer D: The regulation of thyroid function in pregnancy: pathways of endocrine adaptation from physiology to pathology. *Endocrine Rev* 18: 404–433, 1997.

Jovanovic L: Medical emergencies in the patient with diabetes during pregnancy. *Endocrinol Metab Clin N Am* 29: 771–787, 2000.

Kjos SL, Buchanan TA: Gestational diabetes mellitus. *N Engl J Med* 341: 1749–1756, 1999.

Kovacs CS, Kronenberg HM: Maternal-fetal calcium and bone metabolism during pregnancy, puerperium, and lactation. *Endocrine Rev* 18: 832–872, 1997.

Kovacs CS: Calcium and bone metabolism in pregnancy. *J Clin Endocrinol Metab* 86: 2344–2348, 2001.

Smallridge RC, Ladenson PW: Hypothyroidism in pregnancy: consequences to neonatal health. *J Clin Endocrinol Metab* 86: 2349–2353, 2001.

Answers and Explanations

Chapter 1

1. **The answer is E.** Many peptide hormones (first messengers) produce their effects by interacting with cell membrane receptors coupled to GTP-binding proteins. This generates second messengers such as cyclic adenosine monophosphate (cAMP), which activates kinases and alters cell phosphorylation. The more prolonged the second messenger response, the longer the effects of the hormone persist. Peptide hormones cannot be taken orally because they are digested by acid in the stomach and peptidases in the intestine. Most peptide hormones are not attached to binding proteins in plasma. Inactivating the receptor G-protein would abolish the hormone response. Peptide hormones interact with receptors in the cell membrane. They do not enter the nucleus and do not interact directly with DNA.

2. **The answer is D.** Without the stabilizing effect of carrier proteins, small steroid hormones could be filtered through the kidney more easily and lost in urine. All other conditions listed would likely increase steroid hormone action.

3–5. **The answers are: 3-D, 4-A, 5-B.** (3-D) As the result of the congenital defect, gland X produces too little of hormone A. Without the stimulus of target hormone A, target tissue Y cannot produce hormone B. (4-A) Overproduction of hormone A results in excessive stimulation of target hormone Y, which then overproduces hormone B. (5-B) Tissue Y does not produce hormone B because it cannot respond to hormone A. The endocrine system is designed to maintain homeostasis. Therefore, lack of hormone B signals gland X to produce excess hormone A in an attempt to overcome the defect.

Chapter 2

1. **The answer is A.** Dopamine produced by the hypothalamus normally inhibits PRL secretion. If the pituitary stalk was severed during the accident so that the portal circulation from the hypothalamus to the pituitary was interrupted, dopamine could not reach the pituitary gland. Phenothiazines cause hyperprolactinemia because they *inhibit* dopamine. GnRH does not stimulate PRL secretion. Hypothyroidism is associated with high PRL. When thyroid hormone levels are low, absence of negative feedback causes the hypothalamus to increase thyrotropin-releasing hormone (TRH) production. High concentrations of TRH stimulate prolactin production; normal TRH concentrations do not. A TSH-producing pituitary tumor would result in hyperthyroidism, and the high levels of thyroid hormones would suppress TRH.

    This woman might have a large PRL-producing tumor. Since she is a postmenopausal woman, she would not have early warning signs of excess PRL production (amenorrhea, galactorrhea, infertility), which might have brought her to medical attention earlier.

2. **The answer is B.** Absence of negative feedback due to low thyroid hormone levels should stimulate the pituitary to produce TSH. Since she is a postmenopausal woman, her ovaries do not produce enough

estrogen and progesterone to suppress the hypothalamus and pituitary. FSH and LH levels are high in postmenopausal women.

3. **The answer is C.** The patient's GH level was not suppressed to less than 1 ng/mL after a glucose load. This is the gold standard for the diagnosis of acromegaly. Patients with acromegaly have increased lipolysis, increased hepatic glucose production (gluconeogenesis), and decreased insulin action (insulin resistance) due to their high GH levels. This combination can produce hyperglycemia and diabetes mellitus. GH stimulates protein synthesis, which is necessary for longitudinal growth in children and tissue proliferation in adults. IGF-1 is increased by high GH.

4. **The answer is A.** The optic chiasm is located superiorly to the sella. In most people it is directly over the pituitary gland and is separated from the pituitary only by the thin fold of dura called the diaphragm sella. A large tumor can cause the pituitary gland to expand upward until it impinges on the optic chiasm. The major sign of such compression is bitemporal hemianopsia. The cranial nerves affected by pituitary or hypothalamic tumors are III, IV, V, and VI. Pituitary tumors cause headaches by stretching the dura, not shrinking it. Cushing disease is due to adrenocorticotropic hormone (ACTH)-producing tumors, not craniopharyngiomas. If the pituitary stalk is damaged, dopamine from the hypothalamus cannot reach the pituitary to inhibit PRL secretion, and PRL secretion increases.

5. **The answer is C.** The 10-year-old child is at risk for panhypopituitarism. If this has developed, the cortisol response to stress would be decreased due to low adrenocorticotropic hormone (ACTH). Sexual maturation and the normal growth spurt during puberty would not occur due to low levels of luteinizing hormone (LH), follicle-stimulating hormone (FSH), gonadal hormones, growth hormone (GH), insulin-like growth factor-1 (IGF-1), thyroid-stimulating hormone (TDSH), and thyroid hormones. A goiter would not develop without TSH to stimulate growth of thyroid tissue.

Chapter 3

1. **The answer is D.** Osmoreceptors in the hypothalamus are exquisitely sensitive to cellular dehydration, which occurs when extracellular osmolality becomes greater than intracellular osmolality and water exits from cells. Baroreceptors are sensitive to volume depletion. Both stimuli elicit ADH release. Low osmolality suppresses ADH secretion. Thirst is stimulated by hypovolemia and angiotensin II. ADH increases translocation of water channels to the surface of the collecting duct lumen and stimulates water flow from the collecting duct to the interstitium.

2. **The answer is C.** Transient DI following pituitary surgery occurs in up to 10% of cases. Her thirst mechanism is intact, as she is drinking large amounts of water. In the setting of recent pituitary surgery, sudden onset of central DI is much more likely than nephrogenic DI. SIADH and excess intravenous fluids do not cause thirst.

3. **The answer is D.** She has central DI. Since she cannot secrete ADH, she is unable to concentrate her urine, and urine osmolality is lower than plasma osmolality. Her kidneys should respond to exogenous ADH, which is given as part of the water deprivation test, and the treatment of choice is a long-acting ADH agonist. Primary polydipsia results in a hypotonic state, so plasma osmolality would be low.

4. **The answer is C.** The syndrome of inappropriate ADH is common in hospitalized postoperative patients. Continued infusion of hypotonic solution with concomitant ADH release from the posterior pituitary results in inappropriate free water retention. The ADH release is likely stimulated by physiologic stressors including postoperative pain and the opiate analgesic. The test of choice would be urine osmolality. Urine osmolality should be inappropriately high (inappropriate concentration of urine in the setting of dilute plasma osmolality) in this patient. There is no evidence for any of the other choices.

5. **The answer is B.** Pathologic water drinkers have hypotonic plasma and are volume replete, so ADH should be suppressed. In patients with nephrogenic DI, urine cannot be concentrated, and plasma osmolality rises. ADH is secreted in response to hypertonicity, but the renal collecting duct cannot respond. Hypovolemia from any cause stimulates ADH secretion. ADH would be inappropriately high

if the patient had an ectopic tumor secreting ADH, because secretion by ectopic tumors is not suppressed when normal osmolality and plasma volume have been achieved.

Chapter 4

1. **The answer is B.** FT_4 and T_3 are elevated in hyperthyroidism. Graves disease is characterized by hyperfunction of the thyroid gland due to autoantibodies (thyroid stimulating immunoglobulins) stimulating the TSH receptor. This leads to a high radioactive iodine uptake. The TSH level should be suppressed (low), since the pituitary and hypothalamus respond to feedback inhibition by the high FT_4 and high T_3.

2. **The answer is E.** Her symptoms and signs and the low FT_4 indicate hypothyroidism. The high TSH indicates normal pituitary response to primary hypothyroidism. If she had secondary hypothyroidism, the TSH level would be low or low-normal. If she had hypothyroidism due to autoimmune destruction (chronic lymphocytic thyroiditis), the high TSH stimulation might have caused a goiter. The absence of a goiter suggests destruction of the thyroid by radioiodine. Development of hypothyroidism often occurs after radioactive iodine treatment of Graves disease, which takes advantage of the unique ability of the thyroid gland to trap and concentrate iodine. The hypothyroidism may take years to develop, so ongoing follow-up is needed. Since the hypothyroidism can be easily treated with replacement T_4, the benefits of treatment with radioiodine outweigh the risks on persistent hyperthyroidism. The ophthalmopathy associated with Graves disease can progress even if the hyperthyroidism is treated successfully. However, her physical examination revealed no abnormal eye findings.

3. **The answer is A.** If T_4 and T_3 cannot be hydrolyzed from the thyroglobulin molecule, the thyroid gland will be unable to release the thyroid hormones into the circulation, and thyroid hormone levels in the serum will be low. In response, the pituitary should increase the synthesis and secretion of TSH, leading to a high serum TSH concentration. Feedback inhibition is based on the amount of thyroid hormone reaching the pituitary and hypothalamus, not the amount of thyroid hormone in the thyroid gland. If T_4 cannot be released from the thyroid gland, the serum T_3 level is likely to be low because most of the serum T_3 comes from peripheral deiodination of T_4.

4. **The answer is B.** She has symptoms and signs of hypothyroidism. This cannot be primary thyroid disease because the TSH level would be elevated in response to a primary thyroid problem. The data are compatible with secondary (pituitary) disease with low TSH resulting in low FT_4. If she had pituitary disease with low or low-normal TSH, she would not have a goiter. If she had tertiary (hypothalamic) disease causing hypothyroidism, the TRH level and T_3 would be low. (Serum TRH level cannot be measured, as TRH is found primarily in the hypothalamic-pituitary portal system [see Chapter 2]). Excess thyroxine ingestion would result in suppressed TSH and high FT_4 and thyrotoxicosis, not hypothyroidism.

5. **The answer is C.** He has symptoms and signs of hyperthyroidism. The proptosis and diplopia indicate that this is due to Graves disease. Thyrotoxicosis from any cause increases sensitivity to circulating epinephrine. This results in increased contraction of palpebral muscles of the eyelid, lid lag, and stare, and increased (not decreased) cardiac contractility and heart rate. Thyroid hormones also have direct effects upon the heart. Thyrotoxicosis from any cause results in an increase in metabolic rate; heat production; and fat, protein, and bone turnover; with net catabolism resulting in weight loss because the caloric intake does not keep up. The proptosis and diplopia are the result of Graves ophthalmopathy, in which the extraocular muscles are infiltrated with lymphocytes and mucopolysaccharides, not malignant cells.

6. **The answer is B.** The findings (older age, enlarged irregular thyroid gland, and gradually developing hyperthyroidism) are often associated with a multinodular goiter. This is not an autoimmune disorder, so a strong family history would not be expected. Thyroid cancer tissue does not produce thyroid hormones efficiently, so hyperthyroidism is rare unless the tumor burden is very large. His slow, mild

clinical course does not suggest this. The clinical course and physical findings are more compatible with multinodular goiter than thyroiditis. Because the entire gland is irregular, more than one nodule is probably present.

Chapter 5

1. **The answer is C.** Cortisol is called a glucocorticoid because it increases gluconeogenesis. Cortisol decreases glucose uptake by muscle and adipose tissue by increasing resistance to insulin. The net result is to make more glucose available to non–insulin-requiring tissues such as the brain. Cortisol decreases CRH and ACTH secretion by negative feedback inhibition. Cortisol decreases inflammation, the major reason for pharmacologic administration of cortisol or one of its analogs, and retards wound healing.

2. **The answer is B.** The combination of fatigue, vomiting, weight loss, postural hypotension, and abnormal Na^+ and K^+ levels suggests the possibility of adrenal insufficiency. The problem is likely to be primary adrenal insufficiency, since Na^+ and K^+ are regulated primarily by the renin-angiotensin system. The patch of depigmented skin is probably vitiligo, an autoimmune condition caused by antibodies to skin cells that produce melanin pigment. The presence of vitiligo suggests that autoimmune adrenalitis is the cause of the adrenal failure. The diagnosis is best established by demonstrating an inadequate cortisol response following ACTH administration. The dexamethasone suppression tests and the midnight plasma cortisol are used to diagnose cortisol excess (Cushing syndrome). Aldosterone suppression tests are used in the evaluation of hyperaldosteronism.

3. **The answer is D.** The combination of hypertension, obesity, hirsutism, ecchymoses, and abdominal striae strongly suggest the possibility of Cushing syndrome. A good screening test for Cushing syndrome is the 1 mg (overnight) dexamethasone suppression test. Normally, dexamethasone would suppress pituitary ACTH secretion, thereby causing suppression of plasma cortisol. However, in Cushing syndrome, ACTH and cortisol do not suppress normally following dexamethasone administration. Other screening tests for Cushing syndrome include measurement of urine free cortisol, midnight plasma cortisol, and bedtime salivary cortisol. The CRH stimulation test and the high-dose dexamethasone tests are used to determine the source of ACTH once the diagnosis of ACTH-dependent Cushing syndrome has been made.

4. **The answer is A.** Pituitary tumors that produce ACTH are not completely autonomous. Although ACTH and therefore cortisol production do not suppress normally after low-dose dexamethasone, they are suppressed by administration of high-dose dexamethasone. Levels increase in response to CRH. Ectopic ACTH production by a lung carcinoma is less likely to decrease in response to high-dose dexamethasone or increase in response to CRH. Cortisol production by adrenal adenomas and carcinomas is not ACTH dependent and is unaffected by CRH or dexamethasone administration. Surreptitious prednisone ingestion would suppress ACTH by negative feedback. Plasma cortisol would be low and would not change in response to CRH or dexamethasone.

5. **The answer is E.** Prednisone administration would suppress CRH and ACTH secretion and thereby plasma cortisol and urine free cortisol excretion.

6. **The answer is C.** The finding of hypertension in association with low serum K^+ suggests the possibility of primary hyperaldosteronism. Hyperaldosteronism decreases urinary sodium (Na^+) excretion and causes sodium retention and volume expansion, and plasma renin activity is suppressed. Measurement of plasma ACTH, cortisol, 17-hydroxyprogesterone, or 11-deoxycortisol would not help determine the cause of his hypertension.

Chapter 6

1. **The correct answer is C.** In response to stress, catechol-induced oxygen consumption increases, and catecholamines stimulate both fat and glycogen catabolism to provide fuel.

2. **The correct answer is B.** Increased blood flow to muscles and less to viscera would theoretically aid the man's escape in this "flight or fight" situation.

3. **The correct answer is C.** The patient presents with classic symptoms of catecholamine excess characteristic of pheochromocytoma: paroxysmal hypertension, palpitations, headache, and sweating. The diagnosis of pheochromocytoma is based upon the measurement of elevated catecholamines or their metabolites in the urine. Since catecholamine secretion by these tumors can be episodic, a 24-hour urine specimen that integrates catecholamine production over a 24-hour period is a better diagnostic test than a single plasma catecholamine measurement. Measurement of plasma free metanephrines is also useful. In patients who have multiple endocrine neoplasia 2B, pheochromocytoma is associated with medullary carcinoma of the thyroid, which arises from parafollicular cells, not thyroid follicle cells, Parafollicular cells do not take up iodine. Patients with a pheochromocytoma should have α-adrenergic blockade before β-adrenergic blockade because unopposed α-adrenergic secretion can worsen vasoconstriction and volume depletion. Her anxiety is one of the symptoms of pheochromocytoma; diagnosis and treatment should be directed toward the underlying tumor.

4. **The correct answer is A.** The family history of this woman suggests multiple endocrine neoplasia 2A. If this is correct, her father's thyroid cancer was a medullary carcinoma of the thyroid, which produced calcitonin. Her aunt's history of hypercalcemia suggests hyperparathyroidism, and her hypertension might be due to a pheochromocytoma. Excess epinephrine secretion by a pheochromocytoma stimulates gluconeogenesis and glycogenolysis and can result in hyperglycemia.

5. **The correct answer is B.** The next step in the management of this woman is to localize the pheochromocytoma, not to search for a calcitonin-producing tumor or parathyroid hyperplasia, which are the other components of MEN-2A. The consequences of untreated pheochromocytoma are more life threatening, and the stress of anesthesia could precipitate a pheochromocytoma paroxysm. A careful history and physical examination may yield important clues as to the location of a pheochromocytoma. For example, postmicturition hypertension can be the result of a tumor in the wall of the urinary bladder. Approximately 90% of pheochromocytomas are located in the adrenal glands, and MRI and CT scans are useful for localizing the tumor. Because pheochromocytomas have a characteristic hyperintense image on T_2-weighted scans, MRI is preferable but is more expensive. Scanning with ^{131}I-metaiodobenzylguanidine is less widely available, but it reveals 80% to 95% of pheochromocytomas and can be particularly useful with familial pheochromocytomas, where bilateral and extra-adrenal involvement are more common.

6. **The answer is D.** After removal of the tumor, the sudden loss of excessive α-adrenergic-induced vasoconstriction results in vasodilatation and hypotension, which can be treated with fluids. Further volume depletion with a diuretic would only exacerbate the hypotension. This woman should be offered genetic counseling, as it is likely that she has familial MEN-2A. She should have 24-hour urine metanephrine levels measured 2 weeks postoperatively to assess whether she has residual tumor. To check for recurrence or new tumors, 24-hour urine measurements should be done annually for at least 10 years. It would be appropriate to test her for medullary carcinoma of the thyroid, which produces calcitonin.

Chapter 7

1. **The answer is C.** Ms. R. is a thin, postmenopausal woman with a family history of osteoporosis. She gets little exercise because of her asthma, and her dietary intake of calcium is low. Her bone mass is low. A first-degree relative (her sister) has breast cancer, so estrogen therapy is not an option. Thyroxine stimulates bone turnover, and excess thyroxine increases bone loss in postmenopausal women. Calcium suppresses PTH and suppresses bone resorption, Ms. R. should increase her calcium intake. Bisphosphonates and calcitonin suppress osteoclast activity and decrease bone resorption, which will diminish additional bone loss. Bisphosphonates are more effective than calcitonin.

2. **The answer is C.** Glucocorticoid therapy causes bone loss by inhibiting bone formation. Urine calcium loss also increases.

3. **The answer is D.** Mr. T. has familial hypocalciuric hypercalcemia (FHH), an autosomal dominant disorder caused by a defective calcium sensor protein. His parathyroid cells do not decrease PTH secretion until serum calcium is higher than normal. Most patients with FHH are asymptomatic except for newborns homozygous for the abnormal calcium sensor protein gene.

4. **The answer is E.** This man is most likely to have hypercalcemia of malignancy due to tumor production of PTHrP. It is very rare for a solid tissue malignancy to produce enough PTH to cause hypercalcemia. The diagnosis could be confirmed by measuring PTH, which should be suppressed by the hypercalcemia. (Measurement of PTHrP is more difficult and is usually not available.) Excess endogenous $1,25(OH)_2D$ is produced primarily by lymphomas and granulomatous diseases. Calcitonin is produced by medullary carcinoma of the thyroid, but patients with this malignancy are not hypercalcemic, perhaps due to down-regulation of receptors in the face of such high concentrations of calcitonin.

5. **The answer is A.** This 66-year-old patient has classic symptoms and signs of long-standing primary hyperparathyroidism. The 74-year-old woman has osteomalacia. This most likely is due to vitamin D deficiency, which results in hypocalcemia and a compensatory increase in PTH. The 32-year-old man has renal failure resulting in hyperphosphatemia and low activation of vitamin 25(OH)D. These result is hypocalcemia, which elicits an increase in PTH. The 27-year-old woman has pseudohypoparathyroidism (the classic form also known as Albright's hereditary osteodystrophy). This patient is resistant to PTH because a defective $G_{S\alpha}$ protein results in decreased formation of cAMP after PTH interacts with its receptor. Resistance to several hormones may be present if the defect in G-protein is widespread.

6. **The answer is F.** The 82-years-old woman has classic signs of hypocalcemia and osteomalacia due to $1,25(OH)_2D$ deficiency. She has been confined indoors, and her diet is poor. Decreased calcium absorption results in high PTH. Phosphorous is low partly due to low absorption and partly due to action of PTH on the kidneys.

7. **The answer is E.** The 45-year-old man has symptoms and signs of hypocalcemia, which are most likely due to inadvertent destruction of the parathyroid glands during thyroid surgery. Low PTH results in hypocalcemia and hyperphosphatemia. The hypocalcemia is partly due to decreased bone resorption and renal calcium retention and partly due to low 1α-hydroxylase activity and decreased activation of vitamin D in the absence of normal PTH.

8. **The answer is A.** The clinical picture of the 65-year-old woman is most likely the result of vitamin D excess due to years of taking multiple vitamin pills containing vitamin D. Both phosphorous and calcium would be high, and PTH would be suppressed by the hypercalcemia. The long history of symptoms makes hypercalcemia due to malignancy unlikely.

9. **The answer is F.** The 3-year-old girl represents the classic picture of rickets due to vitamin D deficiency in childhood.

Chapter 8

1. **The answer is B.** The 58-year-old man is likely to have type 2 DM because he is an overweight adult with increased serum glucose in the absence of ketonuria. His age, size, and lack of ketonuria make type 1 DM unlikely. Diabetes insipidus results from an inadequate quantity or inadequate effect of antidiuretic hormone (see Chapter 3). It causes dehydration due to the inability to concentrate urine, but it does not cause glucosuria. A simple urinary tract infection may cause polyuria but should not cause weight loss or glucosuria.

2. **The answer is A.** Patients with type 2 diabetes mellitus (type 2 DM) have insulin resistance. Their beta-cell capacity for insulin secretion is sufficient to prevent ketoacidosis but not sufficient to prevent hyperglycemia. Type 2 DM is not an autoimmune disorder and is not HLA-associated.

3. **The answer is B.** Normalizing glucose concentrations has been shown to slow the rate of development and perhaps prevent the microvascular complications of diabetes. Blood pressure control is also very important in slowing the rate of development of retinopathy, nephropathy, and the macrovascular complications of diabetes. Annual monitoring of blood pressure may not be enough, and fundus examinations should be done annually. Modest alcohol consumption is not necessarily contraindicated, but the calories and any accompanying carbohydrate should be taken into account. Regular exercise is excellent but may have to be modified if the patient develops significant retinopathy, neuropathy, or coronary or peripheral vascular disease. Patients who develop peripheral neuropathy or have impaired blood flow to their feet should examine their feet daily. Increasing his hepatic glucose output on an ongoing basis would increase his hyperglycemia. A better way to avoid hypoglycemia would be to match his insulin needs carefully with his carbohydrate intake and his exercise.

4. **The answer is C.** The patient is no longer able to recognize hypoglycemia before he develops neuroglycopenic symptoms because his ability to secrete catecholamines is gone or severely impaired. He is also unable to secrete glucagon in response to hypoglycemia. Increased cortisol and growth hormone are appropriate responses to hypoglycemia and would not cause his symptoms. Frustration would not account for his loss of adrenergic symptoms and signs in response to hypoglycemia.

5. **The answer is B.** The 30-year-old Native American man illustrates a classic presentation of type 2 DM, which is prevalent among Native American populations. Patients with type 2 DM are often asymptomatic, and their diabetes is often discovered as part of another investigation. Obesity and a family history of type 2 DM are common in patients with type 2 DM.

6. **The answer is A.** The 25-year-old woman has classic symptoms of severe hyperglycemia. Low C-peptide indicates insulin deficiency consistent with type 1 DM. Weight loss, polyphagia, polyuria, and polydipsia all occur with hyperglycemia.

7. **The answer is A.** The 12-year-old boy has severe type 1 DM and is presenting with diabetic ketoacidosis. The presence of ketones indicates that he needs insulin. His orthostatic blood pressure changes and lightheadedness indicate that he has severe volume depletion.

8. **The answer is D.** High glucose in the face of considerable insulin secretion, as indicated by the high-normal level of C-peptide in the 65-year-old woman, illustrates insulin resistance. Her obesity makes her insulin resistant. She has abnormal glucose tolerance and is at high risk for type 2 DM. The cause of her fatigue is uncertain.

9. **The answer is D.** The 34-year-old day-care worker has signs and symptoms of autonomic neuropathy (delayed gastric emptying, orthostatic hypotension) and peripheral neuropathy (loss of deep tendon reflexes, loss of light touch sensation) in her feet.

10. **The answer is D.** The 72-year-old retired electrician has symptoms (abnormal sensation, particularly at night) and signs (absent vibration and pinprick sensation in legs) of peripheral diabetic neuropathy.

11. **The answer is A.** The 23-year-old librarian has retinopathy. The findings on fundoscopic examination are classic for background retinopathy.

12. **The answer is C.** The urinary albumin excretion rate of the 28-year-old medical student is elevated, indicating that she has diabetic nephropathy. Her hypertension may be due to the renal complications of diabetes.

13. **The answer is B.** The 58-year-old basketball coach has peripheral vascular disease as indicated by exercise-induced leg pain (claudication) and decreased pulses in his legs. His neurologic examination is normal, so he does not have clinical evidence of severe neuropathy. He should be tested for pinprick and vibratory sensation, which are more sensitive indicators of developing neuropathy than abnormal light touch.

Chapter 9

1. **The answer is B.** Both cholesterol and triglyceride levels are high. A high triglyceride level indicates high VLDL or chylomicrons. Since the triglyceride level is below 400 mg/dL, chylomicrons are not present. The ratio of triglyceride to cholesterol in VLDL is approximately 5 to 1, so VLDL cholesterol can be calculated by dividing the triglyceride level by 5.

$$VLDL = TG \div 5 = 210 \text{ mg/dL} \div 5 = 42 \text{ mg/dL (optimal: } \leq 30 \text{ mg/dL)}$$

   The Friedwald formula can be used to calculate the LDL level.

$$LDL = \text{total cholesterol} - (VLDL + HDL) = 255 \text{ mg/dL} - (42 \text{ mg/dL} + 58 \text{ mg/dL})$$
$$= 155 \text{ mg/dL (optimal} \leq 130 \text{ mg/dL)}$$

2. **The answer is D.** Glucocorticosteroids cause insulin resistance, which can result in increased VLDL and LDL production. It is impossible to know if this is a secondary disorder only or a combined primary and secondary disorder because no family history concerning lipid levels is available. After the glucocorticoid is discontinued, a lipid profile should be repeated to determine whether a primary hyperlipidemia is present. At this point, since the patient is young and has no known atherosclerosis risk factors, drug treatment should not be initiated.

3. **The answer is B.** Since the patient's sister had triglyceride elevation with normal cholesterol, his father had both cholesterol and triglyceride elevations, and the patient has isolated hypercholesterolemia, distracters A, C, and D are incorrect. Secondary causes are not likely given his normal laboratory tests and no intake of drugs affecting lipids. Different members of a family with familial combined hyperlipidemia can present with isolated cholesterol elevation, isolated triglyceride elevation, or a combination of the two.

4. **The answer is C.** Pancreatitis in a child who also has eruptive xanthomas is likely to be due to inability to clear chylomicrons after eating a fatty meal. Deficiency of lipoprotein lipase (LpL) or its cofactor apo C-II can cause chylomicronemia in a child. None of the other disorders listed result in chylomicronemia.

5. **The answer is E.** An adult patient with plasma triglycerides above 1000 mg/dL and a creamy layer on top of refrigerated plasma has elevated chylomicrons and VLDL due to combined overproduction and clearance defects. A secondary cause of hyperlipidemia like poorly controlled diabetes, which affects both production and clearance of VLDL, and an underlying primary disorder like familial hypertriglyceridemia or familial combined hyperlipidemia, which causes overproduction of VLDL, are usually present. Chylomicrons and VLDL are cleared by the same pathway, so both increase when VLDL production exceeds clearance capacity.

6. **The answer is C.** The NCEP-III guidelines recommend a lipid profile every 5 years in everyone beginning at age 20. This is particularly true for this patient, who has a family history of hyperlipidemia and a low HDL level. Individuals should be fasting for 12 to 14 hours before a fasting lipid profile is obtained to be sure that chylomicrons have been cleared. The Friedwald formula for calculating LDL is not valid if chylomicrons are present. There is not enough information to assess the severity of her mother's disorder. The estrogen in oral contraceptives increases HDL cholesterol but also causes increased VLDL production and turnover. If this patient has a defect in VLDL clearance, she could develop marked hypertriglyceridemia.

   In a patient who is not fasting, total atherogenic cholesterol in apo B–containing particles (VLDL + remnants + LDL) can be assessed by calculating the non-HDL cholesterol level. Her non-HDL level = 198 mg/dL − 32 mg/dL = 166 mg/dL. The desirable non-HDL level for primary prevention is ≤160 mg/dL.

7. **The answer is A.** Distracters B and C are excluded because her cholesterol level is normal. The patient is taking no medications, and her laboratory profile shows no secondary cause for hypertriglyceridemia. Since her triglyceride level is <400 mg/dL, chylomicrons are not present.

With so little family history available, it is impossible to tell whether this patient has familial hypertriglyceridemia or familial combined hyperlipidemia. It might be helpful to obtain an apo B level, since there is one apo B per lipoprotein particle. If she has familial hypertriglyceridemia, she should have a normal number of large, triglyceride-laden particles, and her apo B level should be normal. If she has familial combined hyperlipidemia, she should have a high number of smaller, more atherogenic particles containing triglyceride, and her apo B level should be high.

If the physician prescribes an estrogen-containing oral contraceptive, the patient should have another fasting lipid profile to be sure that she does not develop marked hypertriglyceridemia. Lifestyle modifications are very important for treatment of hypertriglyceridemia. She should be placed on a low-fat diet that includes more slowly digested carbohydrates (e.g., legumes, whole grain products, nuts) than sugars and rapidly digested starches (e.g., potato, white bread, rice, pasta). She should restrict her alcohol intake and should exercise for 30 minutes daily, if possible.

Chapter 10

1. **The answer is B.** This man and his identical twin have morbid obesity. Comorbidities such as diabetes increase the risk that his obesity will have major medical consequences. Since the man is young, the cumulative risk posed by his obesity is increased. The other individuals would benefit from weight loss, but they have mild to moderate obesity or less severe central obesity (indicated by waist circumference) which is associated with less risk of major complications.

2. **The answer is C.** This patient's high waist circumference indicates that she has severe central obesity, and women with central or android obesity experience a significantly increased health risk. High leptin levels are seen in obesity but have no known effect on risk. High adiponectin levels are associated with decreased insulin resistance, inflammation, and atherosclerosis. A family history of obesity provides information on the cause of obesity, not the level of risk.

3. **The answer is C.** Diet and exercise changes are the cause of all weight loss, even when they are supported by drugs or surgical therapy. No diet can increase metabolic rate in a way that will produce weight loss, and if the effects of seratonin were suppressed, appetite would be likely to increase. No medical treatment program can claim such a high percentage of weight loss in so many people over a sustained period. Mean weight reduction in responders to current pharmacologic therapy is 10% of body weight. There is no current method of changing fat distribution short of making major changes in the gonadal hormone milieu (i.e., substituting estrogen for androgens).

4. **The answer is D.** Orlistat is described correctly and has been shown to cause weight loss when used appropriately. Sibutramine is an anorectic agent that suppresses appetite by blocking presynaptic re-uptake of seratonin and norepinephrine. It is associated with hypertension. Phentermine is an attenuated amphetamine that reduces appetite by acting at norepinephrine synapses in the brain. Phentermine has a low potential for abuse. Thyroid hormone does increase energy expenditure, but the high dose of thyroid hormone required for weight loss increases cardiac output, reduces muscle mass, and increases bone turnover and loss of bone density, especially in postmenopausal women.

5. **The answer is A.** In most humans, a complex, polygenic contribution of inheritance to obesity is likely. Estimates of the number of genes involved range from 10 to 40. Mutations in the leptin receptor could cause obesity, but monogenic obesity in humans is rare. Since NPY stimulates feeding behavior, loss of the NPY gene would not result in obesity. Hypothyroidism does not cause obesity. Weight gain associated with hypothyroidism is primarily due to accumulation of mucopolysaccharides, not adipose tissue. This patient has central obesity and hypertension, but these are common conditions, and familial Cushing syndrome due to a gene mutation or a familial autoimmune disorder is very rare.

Chapter 11

1. **The answer is D.** Klinefelter syndrome is a chromosomal disorder resulting in premature testicular failure. The hypothalamic and pituitary responses to low testosterone are normal, so laboratory testing reveals high gonadotropin levels. In each of the other disorders, LH and FSH levels would be low because of a defect at the hypothalamic or pituitary level. Congenital hypogonadotropic hypogonadism coupled with anosmia (a defective sense of smell) is an X-linked disorder known as Kallman syndrome.

2. **The answer is D.** With all axis hormones low, it is important to look for a hypothalamic or pituitary cause of hypogonadism. Finasteride is a 5α-reductase inhibitor that blocks dihydrotestosterone synthesis in androgen target tissues. It would not interfere with hormones of the hypothalamic-pituitary-gonadal (HPG) axis. Mumps orchitis in adults causes premature testicular failure and low testosterone, but pituitary gonadotropins would be high. Androgen receptor blockade would result in high follicle-stimulating hormone (FSH), luteinizing hormone (LH), and testosterone because the pituitary would not recognize testosterone, and feedback inhibition would not occur. Sertoli cell damage would result in lack of inhibin B, and FSH levels would be high.

3. **The answer is A.** Pulsatile release of GnRH is critical. A long-acting agonist of GnRH would down-regulate the system. LH and FSH levels would be suppressed, resulting in low testosterone. This is the basis of GnRH agonist treatment for prostate cancer.

4. **The answer is B.** When all axis hormone levels are high, target tissues, including the regulatory areas in the hypothalamus and pituitary, are not getting an adequate androgen signal. Androgen receptor blockade would be a way to acquire such a condition. The study subjects developed gynecomastia because they had high levels of testosterone that could be converted to estrogen by aromatase in peripheral tissues. Patients with testicular feminization who have deficient or defective androgen receptors due to a genetic defect have a similar hormone profile and have a female phenotype, including breast development.

5. **The answer is C.** In malnutrition or severe illness, the input from the central nervous system down-regulates the entire axis by suppressing normal pulses of GnRH from the hypothalamus.

6. **The answer is E.** Since dihydrotestosterone is necessary for normal development of male external genitalia, 5α-reductase deficiency results in an apparently female infant. At the time of puberty, GnRH, FSH, and LH pulses increase and testosterone levels increase markedly. Testosterone interacts with androgen receptors resulting in masculinization. Since testosterone exerts normal feedback on the hypothalamus and pituitary, FSH and LH levels are normal.

    In men aromatase deficiency results in low estrogen, tall stature due to failure of the epiphyses to close, and osteoporosis. Estrogen-receptor deficiency presents the same way because tissues cannot recognize estrogen that is present. However, the HPG axis and masculinization are normal. Anosmin deficiency results in abnormal migration of olfactory and GnRH neurons and hypogonadotropic hypogonadism (all hormones of the HPG axis are low) [Kallman syndrome]. Inhibin B deficiency results in high FSH and abnormal control of spermatogenesis.

Chapter 12

1. **The answer is D.** If a young woman is in the late proliferative phase of her menstrual cycle, ovulation will occur very soon. A well-developed dominant follicle that is producing estrogen is required for the LH surge, which precedes ovulation.

2. **The answer is C.** Early in pregnancy, the endometrium cannot support ongoing development of the fetus unless corpus luteum progesterone production is sustained. During the first trimester, the corpus luteum is maintained by HCG produced in the placenta. After that, the placenta produces enough progesterone, and the corpus luteum is no longer necessary.

3. **The answer is D.** If the uterus is present, the outflow tract is patent, and no bleeding follows a progesterone challenge, it is certain that there is not enough estrogen to prepare the endometrium for progesterone action. From the information given, it is not possible to tell whether the problem is at the level of the hypothalamus, the pituitary gland, or the ovaries. The negative pregnancy test indicates that this woman's HCG level is not high.

4. **The answer is B.** Jennifer L. has clinical and laboratory evidence for pituitary failure. The vaginal dryness and nonferning cervical mucous indicate estrogen deficiency, which is confirmed by laboratory testing. The accompanying low or low-normal FSH and LH levels show that the problem is in the pituitary or hypothalamus, not the ovaries. Her fatigue and frequent flu-like illnesses suggest cortisol deficiency. Her fatigue, dry skin, and low-normal TSH in the presence of a low thyroid hormone level indicate secondary hypothyroidism. GnRH failure due to stress is not accompanied by evidence of cortisol deficiency. CAH is unlikely. Her testosterone level is low, she has no signs of virilization, and even late-onset CAH is unlikely at 32 years of age. Amenorrhea due to Turner syndrome or XO/XX mosaicism is the result of ovarian failure and is accompanied by high FSH and LH levels.

5. **The answer is A.** The history of irregular menses, acne, hirsutism, a high-normal LH level, and a low-normal FSH level are compatible with PCOS. The long duration of her irregular bleeding, lack of severe virilization, and a free testosterone level that is not markedly elevated indicate that she does not have an adrenal or ovarian tumor. The normal DHEAS level suggests that the androgen excess is not solely of adrenal origin. The normal 17α-hydroxyprogesterone level makes CAH unlikely. Testicular feminization results in primary amenorrhea because no ovaries and uterus are present.

6. **The answer is E.** Women with PCOS have increased insulin resistance, not decreased insulin resistance. Women with PCOS are not always obese, and progesterone does not cause morbid obesity. Chronic estrogen and androgen secretion protects women with PCOS from loss of bone mass. Women with PCOS are usually anovulatory; they do not have increased ovulation frequency. Chronic estrogen production that is unopposed by cyclic progesterone results in endometrial hyperplasia.

7. **The answer is A.** Ms. Z.'s history is compatible with normal menopause, which is associated with marked depletion of ovarian follicles and low estrogen and progesterone production. The normal compensatory increase in FSH and LH requires GnRH stimulation.

8. **The answer is B.** Atrophic urethritis, vaginal atrophy, higher LDL cholesterol, lower HDL cholesterol, hot flashes, and sleep disturbance are consequences of estrogen deficiency, not estrogen replacement. After menopause ovarian follicles are depleted, and it is not possible to restore fertility with hormone therapy.

Chapter 13

1. **The answer is C.** The fact that this child's linear growth has been normal indicates that his obesity is not due to organic pathology. The presence of a positive family history is also consistent with a diagnosis of exogenous obesity. No routine testing is indicated in such cases. A long-term, structured program of regular exercise combined with dietary intervention is the only effective therapy. Currently there is no approved pharmacologic treatment for obesity in children.

2. **The answer is A.** The finding of a delayed bone age would be consistent with a diagnosis of constitutional delay of growth and puberty. This should be suspected on the basis of the patient's presentation and family history. For most patients, reassurance and follow-up are all that are indicated. Some patients receive a short course of testosterone to allow them to develop the physical changes of puberty if they are experiencing significant psychological stress.

3. **The answer is D.** The weight percentile has decreased more than the height percentile, which is consistent with a nutritional basis for failure to thrive. Initial management should consist of a 5-day diet history analyzed for caloric intake. In the first years of life, the average daily caloric requirement in children is 1000 Kcal plus 100 Kcal per year of life.

4. **The answer is C.** All girls with unexplained slow growth should have a karyotype to rule out Turner syndrome. There is no evidence for malnutrition or malabsorption. There is no evidence for a bone disease or skeletal dysplasia. She has had abnormal growth with no other clinical signs of pituitary disease for several years, and her thyroid tests are normal. It is more important to rule out Turner syndrome, especially in view of the history of ear infections, than to rule out a slow-growing pituitary tumor at this time.

5. **The answer is D.** This child has been consistently in the 5th percentile, so his growth velocity is normal. He has genetic short stature, which is a normal variant. No testing or treatment is indicated. GH treatment has been approved for boys with idiopathic or genetic short stature with predicted adult height under 5′3″. A midparental height range calculation for this child indicates that his minimum predicted height is 5′4″. He does not meet the criteria for GH treatment. As the benefit of GH treatment in these children is modest (an additional 1–2 inches on average), there are ethical concerns about the use of GH.

6. **The answer is D.** This child has classic symptoms of hypothyroidism (fatigue, constipation, cold intolerance) along with dramatic failure of linear growth. Congenital growth hormone deficiency would have presented at an earlier age. She has no symptoms or signs of Cushing disease, and her weight has remained in the 50th percentile. Her growth chart data are not consistent with constitutional delay. There is no evidence of psychosocial deprivation.

Chapter 14

1. **The answer is D.** While the genotypic sex *is* most likely male (ovaries do not descend), sex assignment must be made on the basis of multiple factors and multidisciplinary input. Ideally, the management of an infant with ambiguous genitalia involves a team of specialists with expertise in both biological and psychological aspects of intersex disorders. While decisions regarding genital surgery may be deferred, there is universal agreement on the need for a sex-assignment in the immediate newborn period.

2. **The answer is C.** The most common cause of ambiguous genitalia in a female is congenital adrenal hyperplasia (CAH) caused by 21-hydroxylase deficiency. Mixed gonadal dysgenesis is associated with mosaicism and the presence of both male and female internal structures. Estrogen resistance and paternal tumor are not causes of ambiguous genitalia.

3. **The answer is E.** Menarche is the final milestone of puberty in girls. Most girls do not gain more than an additional 1–2 inches in height after menarche. By 1 1/2 years postmenarche, linear growth is essentially complete. Once the epiphyseal growth plates are fused, there is no way to increase stature. Unfortunately, it is too late to do anything about this child's short stature.

4. **The answer is D.** Isolated pubic hair and body odor with prepubertal testes and phallus and a normal growth velocity and bone age are consistent with premature pubarche (adrenarche). However, follow-up is essential to be sure that his condition remains stable.

5. **The answer is C.** Complete androgen resistance, or testicular feminization syndrome, is due to absence of functional testosterone receptors, resulting in a phenotypic female with normal breast development but a paucity of body hair (which requires androgen action). The testes are intra-abdominal. Müllerian structures are absent because the testes produce müllerian inhibiting substance (MIS). Wolffian structures do not develop because testosterone receptors are absent. The vagina ends in a blind pouch. The other syndromes listed can present with delayed puberty, but they are not consistent with the findings in this patient.

6. **The answer is A.** This child has isolated breast development. She has no pubic hair, no signs of virilization, and no other signs of puberty. Her growth velocity and her bone age are normal. She needs no treatment, but she does need follow-up to be sure that this is not the beginning of true puberty.

7. **The answer is B.** The physical findings and advanced bone age indicate that puberty is underway. The testes are small, indicating that they are not the source of the androgen and that this is a type of

peripheral precocious puberty. The high level of 17-hydroxyprogesterone confirms a block in cortisol synthesis and the diagnosis of CAH.

8. **The answer is D.** This girl has classic features of Turner syndrome, which is confirmed by the karyotype 45,X. Since her ovaries are fibrous streaks without follicle cells, she is unable to produce ovarian estrogen. Her pituitary gonadotropins are high due to lack of estrogen feedback. She has developed some pubic hair due to adrenal androgens.

Chapter 15

1. **The answer is A.** Pregnancy testing is mandatory in a premenopausal woman who presents with amenorrhea. Her complaints of fatigue, nausea, and weight loss are compatible with hyperthyroidism, but some symptoms and signs of pregnancy and hyperthyroidism are similar, and pregnancy should be excluded before ordering TSH and free T_4 levels to assess thyroid status. Fatigue and nausea can also be presenting signs of diabetes, but in the absence of polyuria and polydipsia or ketosis, a pregnancy test should be done first. An oral glucose tolerance test would not be the first step in an evaluation for diabetes in any case (see Chapter 8). Evaluation for ovarian failure with measurement of FSH is not indicated unless pregnancy has been excluded and there are other symptoms or signs of premature ovarian failure.

2. **The answer is C.** Early pregnancy is maintained by progesterone from the corpus luteum until the placenta can make enough progesterone to assume this function. Withdrawal of progesterone from the estrogen-primed endometrium would result in bleeding and miscarriage of the newly implanted blastocyst. HCG is made in the *trophoblast*, not the endometrium. HCG occupies the same corpus luteum receptors as LH and stimulates progesterone production. Maternal GnRH pulses are suppressed by negative feedback from the high progesterone levels during pregnancy. Maternal LH and FSH are also suppressed to the low-normal range during pregnancy. The fetal pituitary has not developed into a hormone-secreting gland early in pregnancy.

3. **The answer is A.** Progesterone has generalized effects on smooth muscle, decreasing its tone. Progesterone-induced relaxation of the lower esophageal sphincter is most likely responsible for the frequent complaints of heartburn during pregnancy. Progesterone effects on smooth muscle relaxation are also responsible for increased constipation, more frequent urinary tract infections, decreased gall bladder emptying, and increased gallstones. Estrogen causes marked peripheral vasodilation during pregnancy, which increases blood supply to the uterus. A compensatory increase in cardiac output occurs in response to decreased afterload. Facial acne and ulcerations are often improved by increased blood supply to the skin, which contributes to the feeling of warmth.

4. **The answer is C.** Fasting plasma glucose is lower during pregnancy due to transfer of glucose to the fetus, and postprandial glucose levels are higher due to postprandial insulin resistance. Hypothyroidism often worsens and requirements for thyroxine are higher during pregnancy. The thyroid gland is often mildly enlarged during pregnancy. Prolactin levels increase throughout pregnancy, but HCG levels peak during the first trimester. After the placenta matures, HCG no longer is required to sustain progesterone production. HCG levels then decline but remain above the prepregnancy level. Estrogen and progesterone levels are high until delivery of the placenta. Total plasma cortisol is high due to the estrogen-induced increase in cortisol-binding globulin. Plasma free cortisol is also increased, but pregnant women have no signs of cortisol excess.

5. **The correct answer is B.** This woman should be reassured that milk production is rarely seen prior to the third day after delivery. During pregnancy high levels of estrogen and progesterone inhibit PRL action on the breast. Estrogen and progesterone levels must drop, as they do after delivery, for milk production to occur. There is no indication that a severe postpartum pituitary hemorrhage has occurred. However, this would be a consideration if this woman continues to have no milk production,

Newborn suckling stimulates prolactin-induced milk production and milk letdown by the action of oxytocin on myoepithelial cells.

6. **The answer is E.** Whey is more digestible and contains more essential amino acids than casein, so the nutritional value of breast milk is higher. Breast milk is not more likely to transmit autoimmunity. The IgA transmitted in breast milk is protective. Breast milk and cow milk are equivalent in calories. Breast-fed infants may be less likely to be obese because they must do more work to suck milk from the breast than from a bottle. Breast milk is lower in both sodium and iron. The iron in breast milk is more available than the iron in cow milk. Most of the carbohydrate in milk is in the form of lactose.

7. **The answer is D.** Infants of diabetic mothers receive more glucose during pregnancy than infants of nondiabetic mothers. In response, these infants secrete more insulin, which is a major growth hormone for the fetus. Infants of diabetic mothers are more likely to be large (macrosomia) and to suffer shoulder dystocia and other trauma during delivery. Since gestational diabetes occurs after organogenesis is complete, the infants are not at increased risk for congenital malformations. After delivery, these infants are no longer receiving glucose via the placenta and must be watched for hypoglycemia until their higher insulin levels return to normal.

Index

Bitemporal hemianopsia, 27
Blastocyst, 364
Blood glucose concentration, regulation
  of, 164–169, 164f
  glucose transporters, 168–169, 169t
  pancreatic islet hormones, 165–168,
    166f, 166t, 167t, 168f
  pancreatic islet structure, 165–166,
    165f
Bloom syndrome, 320–321
Body fat, distribution of, 228
Body mass index (BMI), 227–228, 228t,
    229, 229f
Bone
  bone-forming units (BFUs), 149–150
  chondrocyte differentiation, 315, 315f
  diseases, metabolic, 148–159
  formation
    cortisol suppression of, 90–91
    vitamin D deficiency and, 145–146
  growth plate, 314f, 315, 315f, 316, 351
  hormone effects on, 151–152, 151t
  loss
    during lactation, 371
    postmenopausal, 296, 297
  mineralization disorder, 156–157. See
    also Osteomalacia
  osteoporotic, 153, 153f. See also
    Osteoporosis
  Paget disease of, 148, 158
  resorption
    in hyperparathyroidism, 138, 138f
    postmenopausal, 150
    PTH effect on, 130–131, 130f
  turnover/remodeling, 149–150, 149f
Bone age, as growth parameter, 307, 308f
Bone balance, and bone mass, 148–152
Bone mass
  changes with age, 151f
  determinants of, 151–152, 151t, 152t
  index (BMI), and obesity, 227–228,
    228t, 229f, 231t
  and metabolic bone diseases, 148–152
  postmenopausal, 296, 297
  regulators of, 150
Bone mineral density, in osteoporosis,
    153, 155
Brain centers, in obesity, 235–237, 237f
Brain development, and thyroid hormone
    deficiency, 60
Breast
  anatomy of, 374–375, 374f
  and lactation, 374–380. See also Breast
    milk; Lactation
  suckling on
    neural responses and oxytocin
      release, 376
    neural responses and prolactin
      secretion, 375–376, 376f
Breast cancer
  and HRT, 297
  hypercalcemia in, 140
  and oral contraceptives, 294
Breast-feeding, contraindications to, 379
Breast milk
  and breast anatomy, 374–375, 374f
  composition of, 377–378, 377t

production
  hormone levels and, 375
  maintenance of, 378–380
  release, oxytocin role in, 376
  yield/volume, 378
Bromocriptine, 379–380

Caffeine, in obesity treatment, 242
CAH. See Congenital adrenal hyperplasia
Calcitonin, 3t
  in calcium balance regulation,
    132–133
  in osteoporosis prevention/treatment,
    155, 156
  versus PTH, 132t
Calcium
  circulating levels in calcium disorders,
    139t
  daily intake, optimal, 127, 127t
  deficiency, and osteomalacia, 157
  dietary sources of, 126–127, 127t
  in lactating females, 127, 127t
  in osteoporosis prevention/
    treatment, 155
  in plasma
    decrease with age, 150
    feedback loops regulating, 131–132,
      131f
    levels of, 126t
  in pregnant females, 370, 370t
  reabsorption in kidney, 131
  supplements, 128t, 156
Calcium balance
  failure of calcium homeostasis,
    136–148
  feedback loops regulating,
    131–132, 131f
  hormonal regulators of, 129–136
  maintenance of, 128, 128f
Calcium homeostasis, 125–128
  failure of, 136–148. See also
    Hypercalcemia; Hypocalcemia
Calcium receptor mutations, 140–141
Calcium-regulating hormones, 3t,
    129–136. See also Calcium
    balance
  calcitonin, 132–133, 132t
  parathyroid hormone (PTH),
    129–132, 132t
  parathyroid hormone-related protein
    (PTHrP), 132
  vitamin D, 133–136, 133f, 134t, 135t
cAMP. See Cyclic adenosine
    monophosphate
Carbohydrate metabolism
  cortisol effect on, 90
  in pregnancy, 370
Carrier proteins, 58
Catecholamines, 110–121
  actions of, 114–115, 114t, 115t
  metabolism and disposal of,
    115, 116t
  paroxysmal release of, 120, 120t
  plasma levels of, 112, 112t
  receptor interaction, 113–117
  release of, 112–113
  synthesis of, 110–112, 111f

tumors secreting, 117–121. See also
    Pheochromocytoma
Cerebral gigantism, 329–330
Cerebrospinal fluid (CSF), and pituitary
    tumors, 27
Cervical mucus, ferning of, 274,
    274f, 275
CHARGE syndrome, 348
Children
  calcium, optimal daily intake,
    127, 127t
  chylomicronemia in, 213, 221
  growth. See also Growth
    cortisol inhibition of, 91
    rates, 311–312
    thyrotoxicosis and, 69
  hypothyroidism in, 74, 321
  LH/FSH levels in, 351f
  obesity in
    and diabetes mellitus, 174
    and growth, 305–306, 306t
  treatment of GH deficiency in,
    33–34
  vitamin D deficiency in, 145
Cholesterol. See also Hyperlipidemias;
    Lipids; Lipoproteins
  ACAT enzyme, 204, 204f
  cellular regulation of, 203–204, 204f
  cholesterol ester transfer protein
    (CETP), 205f, 206
  elevation in hyperlipidemia, combined
    with triglyceride elevation, 214
  function of, 197
  hypercholesterolemia, 206, 208–211,
    219–220, 219t
  LCAT enzyme, 205–206, 205f
  National Cholesterol Education
    Program III (NCEP-III)
    guidelines, 208
  reverse cholesterol pathway,
    204–206, 205f
Chorionic adrenocorticotropin, 365
Chorionic gonadotropin. See Human
    chorionic gonadotropin
Chorionic somatomammotropin
    (CS), 311
  human (human placental lactogen),
    365, 366–367
Chorionic thyrotropin, 365
Chromosomal abnormalities and
    syndromes
  and ambiguous genitalia, 348
  and hypercalcemia, 139
  and micropenis, 348
  and short stature, 320–321
  and tall stature, 329–331
Chronic lymphocytic thyroiditis, 66, 68t,
    73, 78, 321
Chylomicron remnants, 199–200,
    201t, 202
  remnant disease (familial
    dysbetalipoproteinemia), 214
Chylomicronemia syndrome, 207,
    213–214, 221
  in adults, 214
  in children, 213
  treatment of, 217, 221

pathogenesis of, 169–174
  abnormal insulin, 169–172
  insulin resistance, 171, 172f, 173, 177
and pregnancy, 371–373
primary versus secondary, 169, 170
treatment of, 175–179
type 1, 169–171
  age of onset, 170
  causes of, 169–170
  clinical features of, 170–171, 171t
  complications of
    acute, 179–180
    chronic, 182–188, 183f
    hypoglycemia, 189, 190
    ketoacidosis, 180, 181f
  pathophysiology of, 169–170
  prevalence of, 170
  treatment/management of, 175–177
    insulin-dosing regime, 177f
    insulin preparations, 176, 176t
  versus type 2 diabetes mellitus, 171t
type 2, 171–174
  age of onset, 173
  causes of, 172–173
  clinical features of, 173–174
  complications of
    acute, 179, 180–182
    chronic, 182–188, 183f
  MODY (maturity onset diabetes of the young), 172
  pathophysiology of, 171–173, 171t
    hyperglycemia, 171–172, 174, 177–179, 180–185
    insulin resistance, 171, 172f, 173, 177
    insulin secretion in, 171–172, 172f
    multiplier hypothesis, 172f
  prevalence of, 173
  prevention of, 174
  treatment/management of, 175–176, 177–179
    major drugs for, 179t
  versus type 1 diabetes mellitus, 171t
Diabetic nephropathy, 185–186
Diabetic neuropathy, 186, 186t
Diabetic retinopathy, 187
Diaphragm sella, 13f, 14, 27, 32
Diazoxide, and hirsutism, 289
Diet
  in diabetes mellitus management, 177–178
  as factor in obesity, 233–234
  in treatment of obesity, 238–241
Dihydrotestosterone (DHT), 3t, 247, 247t, 340, 342f
  and hirsutism, 289
  versus testosterone, 258
Diurnal rhythms, in hormone secretion, 7, 15, 19, 87, 94
Donahue syndrome, 310
Dopamine, 16t, 110, 111f
  inhibition of PRL synthesis and secretion, 25, 25f, 375
  inhibition of TSH secretion, 19
  normal plasma and urine values of, 116t
  receptors, 113–114

Dopamine agonists
  bromocriptine suppression of lactation, 379–380
  suppression of PRL secretion, 25
  in treatment of amenorrhea, 279
  in treatment of pituitary tumors, 29
Dopamine antagonists, increase of PRL levels by, 25
Down syndrome, 320–321
Dura, 13f, 14
Dwarfism, 16t
  GH resistance, 323
  psychosocial, 321
Dysbetalipoproteinemia, familial, 214
Dysgenesis, gonadal, 321, 347. See also Turner syndrome
Dysmenorrhea, 277

Ectopic pregnancy, 365
Elderly people, calcium requirements, 127, 127t
Empty sella syndrome, 32
End organ resistance, in delayed puberty, 358
Endocrinology
  defined, 2
  general concepts in, 2–8
Endometrium
  during normal menstrual cycle, 271f, 274t, 275–276
  maintenance during pregnancy, 364–365
  proliferative phase, 271f, 274t, 276
  secretory phase, 271f, 274t, 276
Environment
  as factor in obesity, 233–234
  in prenatal growth, 309, 309f
Ephedrine, in obesity treatment, 242
Epidermal growth factor (EGF), 311
Epinephrine, 3t, 110, 111f, 112
  actions of, 114, 114t, 115t
  normal plasma and urine values of, 116t
  upright posture and, 115
Epiphyseal growth plate, 314f, 315, 315f, 316
  fusion of, 351
Erythropoietin, in prenatal growth, 311
Estradiol, 3t. See also Estrogen
  activity of, 269
  in female reproduction, 268f
  secretion stimulated by LH and FSH, 21
  testosterone conversion to, 258, 258f, 259, 269, 269f
Estrogen, 16t
  actions of, 270, 270t, 368, 368t
  agonists (SERMs), 155, 156, 298
  binding to SHBG, 269
  in contraceptives, 291–293
  deficiency, 283
    and bone turnover, postmenopausal, 150
  depletion of in menopause
    early consequences of, 295–296, 295t
    long-term consequences of, 295t, 296

in epiphyseal growth plate fusion, 316
and epiphyseal growth plate fusion, 351
in female reproduction, 268f, 269–270, 271f, 273–276, 274t
and lactation, 26, 374–375, 380
and male maturation, 260
in osteoporosis prevention/treatment, 155–156
and ovulation, 274
phytoestrogens, 298
placental production of, 367, 368–369, 368t
plasma levels before and during pregnancy, 366f
and PRL levels, 26
in puberty, 316, 350–351, 350f
receptors, 156
  in men, 150, 259
  selective estrogen receptor modulators, 155, 156, 298
replacement
  for amenorrhea, 283
  therapy (ERT) for menopause, 296–297
secretion of, 269
synthesis and structure of, 269, 269f
treatment, and changes in TBG, 62, 62t
Exercise, in treatment of obesity, 238–241
External genitalia, development/ differentiation of, 341–342, 341f, 342f, 348
Ezetimbe, in treatment of hyperlipidemia, 219t, 220

Failure to thrive, 304–305, 306t
Fallopian tubes, development/ differentiation of, 339, 340f
Familial combined hyperlipidemia, 210–211, 212, 214, 220
Familial defective apo B, 209–210
Familial dysbetalipoproteinemia, 214
Familial hypercholesterolemia, 208–209
Familial hypertriglyceridemia, 212
Familial hypocalciuric hypercalcemia (FHH), 140–141
Familial pheochromocytoma, 118–119
Fat, 198. See also Lipids
  body distribution of, 228
  metabolism, cortisol effect on, 90
Fatty acids, 197. See also Lipids
Feedback loops, 7, 12–13, 17, 17f
  in growth hormone regulation, 23
  long loop, 17, 17f
  short loop, 17, 17f
Female by default, 339
Female reproduction, 266–298
  androgen excess, disorders of, 284–291
  hormonal contraception, 291–294
  hypothalamic hormone secretion in, 267–268, 268f
  hypothalamic-pituitary-ovarian hormone system, 267–270, 268f
  LH/FSH levels in reproductive years, 351f
  menopause, 294–298, 295t

Vitamin D (*Continued*)
regulators of, 136
resistance
as cause of hypocalcemia, 139t,
146–147
treatment of, 146–147
and rickets, 145, 146
supplements, 134, 135t
Vitiligo, 97
Von Hippel-Lindau (VHL) disease,
118, 119t

Water balance
disorders of, 44–49
diabetes insipidus, 44–47, 45t
hypertonic disorders, 44–47, 44t
hypotonic disorders, 47–49, 47t
maintenance of, 39–43
ADH action in, 40–42, 40f, 41f, 43f
osmoreceptors and baroreceptors,
40, 40f, 42–43

oxytocin and, 49
thirst in, 42–43, 43f
water repletion reaction, 39–40, 40f
Weight, as growth parameter, 304–306,
306t
Williams syndrome, 320–321
Wolffian duct/structures, 339, 340f

X chromosome
in genetic sex determination,
336–338, 342f
pseudoautosomal region of, 337
45,X karyotype, 279, 336, 339, 357
Xanthelasmas, in hyperlipidemia, 207,
208, 211
Xanthomas, in hyperlipidemia, 207, 208,
213, 214, 217
XX female infant, virilization of,
343–345
46,XX males, 338

XXY male (Klinefelter syndrome), 256,
330, 336, 358
46,XY females, 338
XY male infant, undervirilization of,
345–347

Y chromosome
in females, 283
in genetic sex determination,
336–338, 342f
pseudoautosomal region of, 337, 337f
sex-determining region of (SRY), 337,
337f, 339, 342f

Zoledronic acid, in hypercalcemia
treatment, 141–142